Dental Care of the
Medically Complex Patient

Commissioning Editor: Michael Parkinson
Project Development Manager: Hannah Kenner
Project Manager: Nancy Arnott
Designer: George Ajayi
Illustrator: Anne Olsen and Hardlines

Dental Care of the Medically Complex Patient

Fifth Edition

Edited by
Peter B. Lockhart, DDS, FDS RCSEd, FDS RCPS
Chairman, Department of Oral Medicine, Carolinas Medical Center, Charlotte, NC, USA

Consulting Editors
John G. Meechan, BSc, BDS, PhD, FDS RCPS
Senior Lecturer in Oral Surgery, School of Dental Sciences, University of Newcastle upon Tyne, UK

June Nunn, PhD, DDPH RCS, FDS RCS, BDS
Professor of Special Care Dentistry, Dental School and Hospital, Trinity College, Dublin, Ireland

wright

Edinburgh London New York Oxford Philadelphia St Louis Sydney Toronto 2004

WRIGHT
An imprint of Elsevier Science Limited

First edition 1985 *A Practical Guide to Hospital Dental Practice* published by
Medical Area Service Corporation (MASCO)
Second edition 1989 published by Corporate Visions Inc.
Third edition 1991 published by JBK Publishing Inc.
Fourth edition 1997 *Oral Medicine and Hospital Practice* published by the
Federation of Special Care Organizations in Dentistry
Fifth edition 2004 *Dental Care of the Medically Complex Patient* published by
Elsevier Science Limited

ISBN 0 7236 1090 8

British Library Cataloguing in Publication Data
A catalogue record for this book is available from the British Library

Library of Congress Cataloging in Publication Data
A catalog record for this book is available from the Library of Congress

Notice
Medical knowledge is constantly changing. Standard safety precautions must be
followed, but as new research and clinical experience broaden our knowledge,
changes in treatment and drug therapy may become necessary or appropriate.
Readers are advised to check the most current product information provided by
the manufacturer of each drug to be administered to verify the recommended dose,
the method and duration of administration, and contraindications. It is the
responsibility of the practitioner, relying on experience and knowledge of the
patient, to determine dosages and the best treatment for each individual patient.
Neither the Publisher nor the editors assume any liability for any injury and/or
damage to persons or property arising from this publication.
The Publisher

Printed in China

Contents

Preface

There is longstanding concern about the availability and quality of dental care for people with complicated medical and physical conditions, and those with non-surgical problems of the region of the oral cavity. Beyond the issue of funding as a barrier to care, there is a shortage of dental practitioners who are willing and trained to manage these patients. Dental students have minimal exposure to medically compromised patients and those with oral medical problems, and there is a need for more medical center-based training programs in general dentistry for both dental students and house officers. In addition to the demand for such training on the part of dental students in the US, there is increasing awareness on the part of the leadership of our profession that this is essential training for all dentists.

This book first appeared in 1985 as *A Practical Guide to Hospital Dental Practice*, and was intended to help dental house officers in 1-year training programs to manage a medically complicated patient population in a non-dental school environment; communicate with and work alongside healthcare administrators and other healthcare providers; and understand better the role of dentistry in the healthcare system. The title of the book has been changed to reflect a broadening of the subject matter from previous editions. It now better serves the needs of an increasing number of dental students, house officers and practitioners engaged in the care of both ambulatory and non-ambulatory patients.

This fifth edition represents a broad-based effort by twelve contributors to provide a portable text that spans the scope of oral medicine and special needs/hospital-based dentistry. Each chapter is designed to contain the important information that dental practitioners need at short notice concerning the medical history, laboratory values, risk assessment and management of a broad scope of clinical problems and patient populations. The contributors represent the fields of hospital dental practice, oral medicine, pediatric dentistry, oral and maxillofacial surgery, geriatric dentistry, community practice, maxillofacial prosthodontics, special needs and internal medicine. Contributions have been made to each chapter by at least four, and in some cases all of these individuals, thus ensuring uniformity and quality of content. This edition has also been reviewed and modified by consulting editors from the United Kingdom, Ireland, and Australia to ensure that the terminology is appropriate for non-North American practitioners. It should be noted that UK equivalents to drug names, words and expressions are given in square [brackets].

In addition to the present and past contributors to this book, I am indebted to my family and to my colleagues at Carolinas Medical Center, who maintain an environment conducive to this effort.

Peter B. Lockhart
2004

Acknowledgments

I wish to acknowledge the significant contributions made to prior editions of this book by doctors Susan Connolly Fiorillo, Kent Sargent, and Sandra Craig. I would also like to thank Louise Kent for her proofing and research skills, Anne Olsen for her talent as a medical artist, Katharine Cornell for her help with pharmaceutical tables, Tainika Bryant and Linda Burke for their proofing and word processing skills, my colleague Dr Philip Fox for his wisdom and helpful comments, and our house officers over the years, who have challenged and inspired us.

Contributors

Editor
Peter B. Lockhart, DDS, FDS RCSEd, FDS RCPS
Chairman, Department of Oral Medicine, Carolinas Medical Center,
Charlotte, NC, USA

Consulting editors
John G. Meechan, BSc, BDS, PhD, FDS RCPS
Senior Lecturer in Oral Surgery, School of Dental Sciences, University
of Newcastle upon Tyne, UK

June Nunn, PhD, DDPH RCS, FDS RCS, BDS
Professor of Special Care Dentistry, Dental School and Hospital,
Trinity College, Dublin, Ireland

Contributors
Lawrence E. Brecht, DDS
Director of Craniofacial Prosthetics, The Institute of Reconstructive
Plastic Surgery, New York University Medical Center, New York, NY,
USA

Michael T. Brennan, DDS, MHS, M SND RCSEd, M OM RCSEd
Oral Medicine Residency Director, Carolinas Medical Center, Charlotte,
NC, USA

Paul S. Casamassimo, DDS, MS
Chief of Dentistry, Children's Hospital, Columbus, OH, USA

Agnes Lau, DMD
Director, MGH Dental Group, Massachusetts General Hospital, Boston,
MA, USA

Lauren L. Patton, DDS, FDS RCSEd
Associate Professor and Director, General Practice Residency Program,
UNC Hospitals and University of North Carolina School of Dentistry,
Chapel Hill, NC, USA

Stanley R. Pillemer, MD
Senior Staff Physician, Gene Therapy and Therapeutics Branch,
National Institute of Dental and Craniofacial Research, Bethesda, MD,
USA

Mark Schifter, BDS, MDSc, M SND RCSEd, M OM RCSEd
Staff Specialist and Clinical Lecturer, Oral Medicine/Oral Pathology,
Westmead Hospital, Sydney, Australia

Kenneth Shay, DDS, MS, FDS RCSEd
Director, Network 11 Geriatrics & Extended Care, US Department of
Veterans Affairs; and University of Michigan, Ann Arbor, MI, USA

David Wray, MD, FDS, F Med Sci
Dean and Consultant in Oral Medicine, Glasgow Dental Hospital and
School, Glasgow, UK

Introduction

Special needs dentistry in the United States, often referred to as hospital dentistry, is practiced by a relatively small but dedicated group of dentists, most of whom have postdoctoral training in medical center-based residencies. Special needs patients make up a broad range of individuals with medical, physical and emotional problems, many of whom require dental care in non-traditional settings. Some of these patient populations are better cared for than others, as they have better access to clinical services and settings, more efficient funding sources, or stronger advocacy groups.

The existence of space and equipment to treat special needs patients is often the deciding factor in access to dental services. Frequently, larger hospitals will have an organized dental department that provides care to in-hospital patients, as well as to those who reside in the surrounding community and seek care on an ambulatory basis. Other facilities, such as those that care for people with intellectual and physical impairments or elderly people, may not have dental equipment on site, and thus patients have more limited access to general dental care. Such facilities will rarely have an on-site dentist. Rather, they rely on one or more practitioners in the community to provide dental services for a fee or on a voluntary basis. Mobile dentistry is gaining prominence in the delivery of care to some of those without access.

Formal, postdoctoral, hospital-based training programs for recent dental school graduates began in the United States in the late 1930s with the 1-year, elective 'rotating dental internship'. Over the following decades, these programs gained popularity among students, became more uniformly structured and, in the late 1960s, became known as general practice residencies (GPRs). Two-year programs had evolved by the mid-1970s, by which time the profession had developed formal accreditation guidelines that set minimal requirements and a uniform structure to the clinical and didactic components of those programs that are accredited by the American Dental Association (ADA).

In the 2000–1 academic year, there were 219 ADA-accredited, 1- and 2-year GPRs in the US, with over 1000 house officers, 86% of whom are based in general medical–surgical hospitals. In the late 1970s federal and private foundation funding became available in the form of grants for both the creation of new programs and the expansion of existing, accredited postdoctoral programs in general dentistry. This funding resulted in a new type of postdoctoral training, the Advanced Education in General Dentistry (AEGD) programs, which also have a focus on people with special care needs. There are currently over 600 graduate students in 94 such programs, primarily sponsored by, and based in, dental schools or military facilities.

Postdoctoral general dentistry programs have grown in popularity in the past 25 years and they help to compensate for the minimal exposure that American dental students have to such patients in the 4-year doctoral curriculum. The demands on current curricula in many dental schools in the US have meant that exposure to medically compromised patients has been sacrificed to other subject areas. Pressure on deans from a variety of professional and patient advocacy groups has done little to alter this. At the postgraduate level there are continuing education courses run by a number of organizations, as well as under-graduate programs, mostly devoted to preclinical teaching.

In the US, the goals for these formal training programs in special needs dentistry vary depending on the host institution (e.g. hospital, dental school, military), the institution's patient population and the clinical interests on the part of the dental faculty (staff). GPRs require formal rotations in departments of medicine, anesthesia and emergency medicine. Beyond some commitment to didactic instruction, the bulk of the remaining time is spent delivering dental care to a medically compromised patient population very different from that of the dental school. Some programs are more heavily weighted toward the medical side of the training spectrum, the goal being to have dental house officers totally integrated into the medical center, where they enjoy parity with their medical and surgical colleagues. GPRs should concentrate on aspects of clinical and didactic training not available in dental school, such as the management of severe cases of infection, trauma, bleeding, pain and a wide spectrum of oral medical problems. Such complex patient services require knowledge of general medicine, physical and risk assessment, principles of anesthesia and a variety of other skills. Medically complex patients also require the integration of dental with medical care plans through interdisciplinary teamwork. In most cases, full-time and volunteer faculty members, representing the clinical dental specialties, supervise the house officers' care of a wide variety of hospitalized and ambulatory outpatients who gain access to these services because of their significant degree of medical or physical compromise.

Graduates of GPR programs receive a Certificate of Training. Some seek positions in general medical hospitals or go on to specialty training, but the majority enter community-based, general dental practice. They are far more competent clinicians as a result of their hospital-based residency training, especially with regard to special needs patients. However, it must be said that these programs are heavily oriented toward medically compromised patients as distinct from people with only physical or intellectual impairments.

The only professional group formed specifically to support dentists with a commitment to these patient populations is Special Care Dentistry (originally known as the American Association of Hospital Dentists). This Chicago-based group has been in existence for over 30 years and has recently become a federation, with two additional groups representing people with disabilities and geriatric populations. Annual spring meetings are held in Chicago and include lectures, seminars, medical updates, organizational business and other activities where dentists with an interest and commitment to medically, intellectually and physically compromised patients can meet with colleagues who share common interests.

In Canada, there is more variation across and within the individual provinces. For example, in Ontario there is provincial funding for special care patients to receive up to five visits to a dental office each year for scaling and polishing, although other treatment items are not covered as comprehensively. In Alberta, there is funding for special care patients, and hospital dentistry and sub-specialties like gerodontology are recognized. Connections with the American and Canadian Dental Associations foster these developments.

In Brazil, Special Care Dentistry is recognized as a specialty. There are undergraduate programs in dentistry for people with disabilities, as well as postgraduate and continuing dental education courses, but there is no government support for treatment services outside of the universities.

The model of care in the United Kingdom is based on the National Health Service, with dental care theoretically available to everyone. A fee is payable as a proportion of the cost of treatment, the remainder being reimbursed by the government. Some patients are exempt from charges and many people with disabilities are eligible for free care. There is, however, an increasing reliance on the private sector for dental care. Many disabled people obtain dental care through general dentists in their community practices, but many also receive comprehensive care in the public dental service. More specialist services are offered, also free, from hospitals. Undergraduate training in the specialty is not well developed in most universities but the national society, The British Society for Disability and Oral Health (www.BSDH.org.uk) is working towards a set of guidelines for undergraduate training. Three universities in the UK offer masters or modular courses and a number of the dental hospitals run certificate courses in Special Care Dentistry for dental nurses. The Royal Colleges of Surgeons in London and Edinburgh both offer postgraduate qualifications, one of which is run as a distance learning program.

In mainland Europe the situation is variable. The Scandinavian countries are the most advanced and, indeed, have centers dedicated to the multiprofessional care of people with rare disorders – two in Sweden, one in Norway and a new center opening in Copenhagen, Denmark. Favorable funding has been secured for oral and dental care for people with disabilities in many of the Scandinavian countries; in Sweden, dental care is free up to 20 years of age, in Norway until 18 years. In Sweden, of the 7700 dentists and 3500 dental hygienists, 50% are in the public dental service, from which 95% of children and 50% of adults receive their care. Specifically, the groups covered within this are:

- people in residential or nursing home care
- people with intellectual impairments
- housebound people in receipt of social and other services at home
- people with severe psychiatric disease.

Additionally, there are schemes in place for free annual screening visits by dental hygienists to homes for people in residential or nursing home care. The people identified above are also eligible for necessary dental care at reduced cost, which includes care that is essential to ensure adequate nutrition or, at the very least, to reduce pain and discomfort. There is also the facility to provide dental care deemed necessary as part of medical treatment, for example, eradication of oral infection prior to surgery or transplantation and correction of dentofacial anomalies; the costs of which are paid in part by the patient.

However, educational input at either the undergraduate or post-graduate level is not generally available. In Norway, the Center for Rare Disorders in Oslo has a postgraduate program that incorporates telemedicine facilities for outreach teaching. Most of the Scandinavian countries engage jointly in continuing dental education courses for dentists with an interest in Special Care Dentistry, either with meetings on specific topics (e.g. ectodermal dysplasias or oromotor function) or meetings of special interest societies in the individual countries. They also publish their own journal on Special Care Dentistry.

Further south, in the Netherlands, community provision for people with disabilities is very comprehensive. People with disabilities are offered dental care from 23 centers throughout the Netherlands and there are plans to double the number in Rotterdam, because of pressure from mounting waiting lists. In addition, the universities offer undergraduate programs in Special Care Dentistry and there is outreach clinical care, including sedation facilities. Flanders has four centers in three provinces offering dental care for people with disabilities; some of these institutions also offer sessional care to the residents.

In Germany, most dental care for disabled people is offered from private dental offices. There is a budget for the funding of treatment for disabled patients but with an upper limit, above which the patient has to pay. More advanced dental needs are provided from one privately run university at which facilities for treatment of people with disabilities under general anesthesia are offered.

Similarly, in Turkey, all care for disabled children, delivered under general anesthesia, is provided only in universities. In 2003, a center for oral and dental care for people with disabilities will be constructed in Turkey.

Services in southern Europe are less well developed and tend to focus mainly on medically compromised people, especially in countries like Spain and Portugal. In Spain, however, the deans of the dental schools have given a commitment to undergraduate education with teaching of special care patients as part of the curricula. In Valencia there is a 3-year master's program based in the hospital. Within hospitals, dental care for these patients is free. In Greece, disabled people are entitled to free dental care up to 18 years of age (as it is for the rest of the population) but general dentists have no specific training in the care of disabled people. As in many countries, the origin of care for such groups rests in the specialty of pediatric dentistry. Once these patients grow older there is frequently no-one to provide for their continuing dental needs. People who are in residential care facilities are looked after by volunteer staff, working from a mobile unit that visits these centers and provides dental care on site. Undergraduate students have some exposure to this facility but most of the education is concentrated on the postgraduate students in pediatric dentistry, who have some exposure to disabled people in residential care in long-stay institutions. In Italy, similar arrangements exist for delivering care to people with disabilities with, in one area of the north, a mobile unit providing domiciliary, out-of-office care to disabled people.

The situation is similar in Israel where only pediatric dentists treat disabled patients, even though the subject area in the final year is dental curriculum. The national health service in Israel does not include general dental care, although dental treatment under general anesthesia has been included since 2000 and preventive care with a dental hygienist is offered once a year.

Australia has made significant provision for people with disabilities. The Royal Australian College of Dental Surgeons has developed a fellowship examination in Special Needs and the first diet of the examination was run in Adelaide in 2002. Several Australian and New Zealand postgraduate degrees in Special Needs Dentistry have been established and are further evolving. In both countries, representation has been made to the appropriate dental authorities and there is now the prospect of establishing the specialty of Special Needs Dentistry in the near future. In Australia, 1 in 4 people (including up to 80% of older adults aged 65+ years) are eligible for government benefits and public dental care, so that prioritizing those who receive this care is a constant challenge. Most states require public dental patients to make a co-payment, with Special Needs patients often exempted from these payments or giving a reduced co-payment. However, several key public Special Needs Dentistry centers operate in Sydney, Melbourne and Adelaide, providing a wide range of fixed clinic and domiciliary dental care for special needs dental patients who are hospital inpatients and outpatients, community-living and institutionalized. Recent government support has targeted geriatric dental service provision in several states, such as Western Australia, South Australia and Victoria. Also, an inaugural Professor of Special Needs Dentistry is currently being appointed at the University of Melbourne, and the funding base for research in Special Needs Dentistry is increasing.

The services in New Zealand are similar to those in the United States, in that the care is based in general medical hospital-based dental clinics.

The New Zealand Hospital Dental Surgeons' Association was formed in 1948 in recognition of the need to provide special oral health care to patients with special needs in the hospital setting. This association has recently expanded and renamed the New Zealand Society of Hospital and Community Dentists (NZSHCD) in recognition of the growing role of Special Needs Dentistry in the community. The NZSHCD has an annual conference that focuses on Hospital and Special Needs Dentistry and publishes the conference proceedings to attending delegates.

In Japan, there are many centers for such treatment, both in community-based clinics and in the university hospitals. The different organizations hold many postgraduate and special interest meetings each year and it is likely that the Japanese Society for Special Care Dentistry will introduce a program of continuing dental education in 2003.

Clearly, the number of people with special needs who lack access to comprehensive dental care is growing and significant barriers exist. Financial considerations, physical access to community dental practices and the limited number of dentists trained and willing to see such patients all require that the dental profession in all countries continue to identify and solve these problems. All the European countries have active societies that represent dentists who provide oral and dental care to special needs patients, some offering hands-on courses. In addition, over 3000 people belong to the International Association for Disability and Oral Health (www.IADH.org), which acts as a focus for national organizations and has the very specific aims of improving communication and acting as a forum for exchange of information, principally through the biennial congresses, the textbook and the news pages of the website. The Organization also serves to act as an advocate for people with disabilities and to work with governments and legislators as well as voluntary organizations. Increasingly, it is becoming involved in under- and postgraduate education in its links with the FDI.

International cooperation in the form of meetings and programs, common fellowship credentialing and evidence-based clinical research will translate into better care for these patient populations.

Chapter 1

In-hospital care of the dental patient

DENTAL ADMISSIONS

Introduction

The medical health and dental needs of patients must be considered when deciding on hospital admission. Admission to hospital should be considered whenever the required treatment could threaten the patient's well being, or indeed life, or when the patient's medical problems will seriously compromise the treatment.

Reasons for admission

Fractures of the mandible/maxillofacial structures

Admission is necessary if fracture of the mandible/maxillofacial structures necessitates fixation (wiring or plating) under general anesthetic or in-patient nursing after fixation (e.g. in children or patients with special needs).

Infection

Admission is necessary if the patient has an infection that:

- impairs oral intake (especially fluid intake, e.g. severe herpetic stomatitis in very young children, which might require hospitalization because of dehydration)
- compromises the airway (e.g. Ludwig's angina)
- involves the soft tissue planes that drain or traverse potential areas of particular hazard and so are a danger to the patient (e.g. periorbital or infratemporal swelling).

Oral surgical/dental procedures

Patients should be admitted if the oral procedure is inappropriate in the outpatient setting.

Compromised patients

Medically, mentally or physically compromised patients who are insufficiently cooperative to be treated in an outpatient setting should be admitted to hospital for their procedure. This category includes patients who might require 'chemical intervention' by means of general anesthesia or IV sedation and/or appropriate cardio-respiratory monitoring by an anesthesiologist during treatment.

Children

Young children who require treatment under general anesthesia because of the combination of poor cooperation and the need for a large number of dental procedures as a result of extensive caries and/or consequent infection.

Underlying medical problems

Patients suffering from the following medical problems should be admitted to hospital for treatment:

- unstable cardiac disease
- labile or uncontrolled hypertension, angina or ECG findings needing cardiac or electrolyte monitoring before, during and after surgery
- controlled seizure disorders or movement disorders (e.g. Parkinson's disease, Huntington's chorea)
- poorly controlled diabetes or hyper-/hypothyroidism
- coagulation disorders (that cannot be managed as an outpatient)
- hematologic malignancies or other immunologic problems that require parenteral therapy (platelets, coagulation factors (namely VII, VIII, and IX, FFP or cyroprecipitate) and/or antibiotics).

Patients who require heavy sedation or general anesthesia should also be admitted for treatment.

Medical consultations

Objectives

The objectives of medical consultations are to:

- determine and reduce peri- and postoperative medical risk to the patient from the planned oral surgical/dental procedures
- determine, and so lessen or indeed prevent, the effects of the proposed surgery/procedures on any medical illness

- ensure that the patient's underlying medical condition is being treated as optimally as possible and to ensure follow-up of the patient so as to manage postoperative care and limit any possible complications.

THE PATIENT'S MEDICAL HISTORY

Introduction

There is an art to eliciting the correct, pertinent and relevant information regarding a patient's current medical and physical status – taking an accurate, relevant and concise medical history requires repeated practice and experience. The goal is to obtain sufficient information from the patient to facilitate the physical examination and, in conjunction with the examination, to arrive at a working diagnosis(es) of the problem.

Old hospital records, if they exist, can be immeasurably helpful in providing information about past hospitalizations, operations (including complications) and medications, particularly if the reliability of the patient or guardian as an informant is in question.

Key points for taking a medical history
- Record the patient's positive and negative responses.
- Remember that the patient might not understand the need for, and value of, an accurate medical history in the dental setting.
- Be persistent and patient.
- Double-check the veracity of the information by asking the same questions but in a slightly different way (e.g. ask patients to list their current medical problems; a bit later ask for a list of their current medications; follow this up by asking the patient to detail what each specific drug/medication is used for).
- If you need to use an interpreter, try as much as possible to use a professional healthcare interpreter and not members of the patient's family.
- If you need to gain consent for minors and intellectually impaired adults or elders, make sure that the person whose consent you gain (patient's parent/guardian/carer) has the legal authority to provide consent.

Elements of the history

The following discussion of the components of the medical history is directed at providing a full and complete history. Often, a shorter form of the medical history will be sufficient for a healthy patient admitted for routine care (e.g. extraction of teeth).

Patient identification

A one-line note detailing the age, gender and general condition of the patient. For example '36-year-old man in no acute distress'. In note form, this would be written: 36 yom in NAD.

Informant and reliability

Note the name of the person or material used to obtain the pertinent information (e.g. patient, parent, relative, medical/nursing record).

Also note whether the informant was reliable – were your questions understood, was the informant coherent and knowledgeable and how well did he/she know the patient?

Chief complaint (CC)

Record what patients perceive to be the problem that brought them to hospital. The patient's own words should be used if possible.

History of present illness [complaint] (HPI)

Make a chronologic description of the development of the chief complaint. Record:
- when the problem started
- the course since onset – the duration and progression
- whether the problem is constant or episodic (if it is episodic, note the nature and duration of any periods of remission and exacerbation)
- the symptoms: character (e.g. sharp, dull, burning, aching) and severity (e.g. impact on daily living)
- any systemic signs and/or symptoms (e.g. weight gain or loss, chills, fever)
- previous diagnoses and the results of previous trials (success, partial resolution or unsuccessful) with treatment and/or medication related to the chief complaint.

Past dental history

You now need to gather as full a past dental history as possible. Ask the patient about:

- previous oral surgery, orthodontics (age, duration), periodontics, endodontics (tooth, date, reason), prosthetics, other appliances, oral mucosal problems (e.g. herpes, candida, aphthae), dental trauma
- frequency of dental visits (regular or emergency only)
- frequency of dental cleanings (when were the patient's teeth last cleaned?)
- experience with local anesthesia/sedation (if possible, find out what type was used) and general anesthesia (e.g. allergy, syncope)
- experience with extractions – was there post operative bleeding or infection? How well did they heal?
- history of pain, swelling, bleeding, abscess, toothaches, herpes, or other mouth sores/ulcers
- temporomandibular joint – history of pain, clicking, subluxation, trismus, crepitus
- habits – nail-biting, thumb-sucking, clenching, bruxing, mouth-breathing
- fluoride exposure – was this systemic or topical?
- home care – brushing method and frequency, instruction, floss or other aids; carer assistance required?
- food habits/diet. Ask about sucrose exposure (including liquid oral medicines). For children, the history and frequency of bottle and breastfeeding should also be included. Find out about nutritional supplements (form and consistency), liquid diets, tube feedings
- problems with saliva (hyper-/hypo-salivation) chewing, speech
- negative dental experiences.

Past medical history (PMH)

Direct questioning is probably the best way to elicit the patient's past medical history.

Ask the patient 'Are your being treated for anything by your doctor at the moment?' If the answer is 'Yes', ascertain how severe the condition is (the extent to which it interferes in daily living activities) and how stable it is. A severe condition (e.g. angina) might prove not to be a significant hindrance to planned dental treatment as long as it is well managed and stable. However, a patient with unstable angina should not be treated until the angina is stabilized or, if this is not practical, treatment should be planned while the patient is monitored, and possibly lightly sedated, to minimize stress and anxiety.

Ask the patient 'Have you been treated in the past, or currently being treated for ...

... rheumatic fever, heart murmurs, infective endocarditis, angina, heart attack, or an irregular heart beat?'

... asthma, emphysema, hay fever, or allergic rhinitis or sinusitis?'

... epilepsy, stroke, nervous or psychiatric conditions?'

... diabetes or thyroid conditions?'

... peptic or gastric ulcer disease, liver disease (e.g. hepatitis or cirrhosis)?'

... kidney problems – obstruction, stones or infection?'

... urinary problems – obstruction or infection?'

... gynecologic or women's problems?'

... rheumatoid or osteoarthritis, osteoporosis, back or spinal problems?'

... skin cancer or rashes?'

If the patient is currently receiving treatment for cancer, find out the mode of treatment (surgery, chemotherapy or radiotherapy). Finally, ask if the patient has ever required a blood transfusion or other blood products (platelets, plasma, or clotting factors).

Review of systems

As part of the past medical history, you will need to question the patient systematically about all the body systems. It is often possible to obtain significant additional symptoms or information not elicited in the discussion of the patient past and present illness(es). A positive ('Yes') response should be probed in depth and significant negatives ('No') must also be noted.

General Weight loss or gain, anorexia, general health throughout life, strength and energy, fever, chills, night sweats.

Cardiovascular Palpitations, chest pain and radiation, history of myocardial infarction, orthopnea (number of pillows), hypertension, cyanosis, edema, varicosities, phlebitis, congenital cardiac abnormalities, murmur, exercise tolerance, cardiac valve prosthesis, history of rheumatic fever/RHD/endocarditis.

Respiratory Cough (type), sputum production (taste, color, consistency, odor, amount/24 hours) hemoptysis, dyspnea, wheezing, cyanosis, fainting, pain with deep inspiration, history of pleurisy, pneumonia or asthma, seasonal allergies, bronchitis, emphysema.

Neurologic   Loss of smell, taste or vision, muscle weakness or wasting, muscle stiffness, paresthesia, anesthesias, lack of coordination, tremors, seizures, syncope, fatigue, aphasias, memory changes, paralysis.

Psychiatric/emotional   General mood, problems with 'nerves', bruxism/clenching, habits or tics, insomnia, hallucinations, delusions, medications. Ask children about sleeping patterns, night terrors/nightmares.

Endocrine   Goiter, hot/cold intolerance, voice changes, changes in body contours, changes in hair patterns, polydypsia, polyuria, polyphagia.

Gastrointestinal   Appetite, food intolerance, belching, indigestion and relief, hiccups, abdominal pains, radiation of pain, nausea and vomiting, hematemesis, cramping, stool color, odor, flatulence, steatorrhea, diarrhea, constipation, mucus in stools, hemorrhoids, hepatitis, jaundice, spleen or liver problems, alcohol abuse, ascites, ulcers.

Genitourinary   Urinary frequency (day and night), changes in stream, difficulty starting or stopping stream, dysuria, hematuria, pyuria, urinary tract infections, impotence, libido alterations, venereal disease, genital sores, incontinence, sterility.

Gynecologic   Gravida/para (pregnancies/live births) and complications, abortions or miscarriages, menstrual history, premenstrual tension, painful or difficult menstruation (dysmenorrhea), bleeding between periods, clots of blood, excessive menses (menorrhagia), frequency, regularity, date of last period, menopause (date, symptoms, treatment), postmenopausal bleeding.

Breasts   Development, lumps, pain, discharge, family history of breast cancer.

Musculoskeletal   Trauma, fractures, lacerations, dislocations with decreased function, arthritis, inflamed joints, arthralgias, bursitis, myalgias, muscle weakness, limitation of motion, claudication, gait, joint prosthesis.

Dermatologic   Hair or nail changes, scaling, dryness or sweating, pigmentation changes, jaundice, lesions, pruritus, biopsies, piercing, tattoos.

Head, eyes, ears, nose, throat (HEENT)

- Head: headache, fainting, nausea or vomiting, vertigo, dizziness, pains in head or face, trauma.
- Eyes: vision, glasses, trauma, diplopia, scotomata, blind spots, tunnel vision, blurring, pain, swelling, redness, tearing, dryness, burning, photophobia.
- Ears: decreased hearing or deafness, pain, bleeding or discharge, ruptured ear drum, clogging, ringing.
- Nose: epistaxis, discharge (amount, color, consistency), stuffiness, hay fever, colds, change in sense of smell or taste, polyps.
- Mouth and throat: pain, sore throat, dental pain, dental hygiene history, bleeding or painful gums, sore tongue, lesions, bad taste in mouth, loose teeth, halitosis, dysphagia, temporomandibular joint dysfunction, trismus, hiccups, voice changes, neck stiffness, nodes or lumps, trauma.

Hematologic.   Increased bruising, bleeding problems, nodes or lumps, anemia.

Family history

Find out what illnesses grandparents, parents, siblings and children have/had. If any of these relatives are dead, at what age did they die and from what? Ask about family history of tuberculosis, diabetes, heart disease, hypertension, allergies, bleeding problems, jaundice, gout, epilepsy, birth defects, breast cancer and psychiatric problems.

Social history

Ask about the patient's home life: education, occupational history (including military, if applicable), family closeness, normal daily activities, financial pressures, smoking and alcohol history. A good question to ask is 'What will you do when you get better?' For children, find out about the home environment (e.g. are there smokers present?) and parental arrangements and custody.

History for pediatric patients

Generally, history taking is the same for a pediatric patient as for an adult patient. However, special emphasis should be placed on:

Prenatal and perinatal history

Was the child full term or premature? Were there any complications during pregnancy? What was the perinatal course:

- hospitalizations: reasons and dates
- operations: procedures and dates, including anesthetic used and any complications
- allergies: medications, foods, tapes, soaps, latex. Include a note on the type of reaction. Be careful to differentiate between true hypersensitivity/allergy reactions and adverse side-effects
- medications past and present: dose and frequency, prescription and over-the-counter (including topical agents)
- potential exposure to dangerous or easily transmissible infections: tuberculosis, venereal disease, hepatitis, flu, HIV, and prion disease (UK)
- maternal immunizations: tetanus, rubella, hepatitis
- transfusions
- trauma
- diet while pregnant
- maternal habits: alcohol intake, tobacco, recreational drugs
- any psychiatric treatment.

Postnatal history

It is also important to look into:

- immunization status: is the child up-to-date or behind with immunizations?
- infection: recent exposure to childhood infections (e.g. cold, flu, chickenpox, rubella, or mumps) can be sufficient cause to post-pone elective surgery
- diet: was the child bottle- or breastfed. At what age was the child weaned? Does the child have any food allergies? Is there any history with fluoride?
- personal or family history of complications from general anesthesia
- developmental delays
- febrile symptoms
- cerebral palsy
- school status
- acute otitis history
- health of siblings: ages, are they living at home?

PHYSICAL EXAMINATION

Introduction

Depending on training and dental practice laws, dentists might be responsible for completing a full physical examination when admitting a patient; the admitting dentist will certainly be responsible for the detailed examination of the oral cavity and must be able to interpret the results of the history, physical examination and laboratory tests. Whenever possible, the physical examination should be completed in a systematic manner, so that nothing is omitted, although physical limitations of the patient might preclude this.

Elements of the physical examination

Start the physical examination by giving a statement of the setting in which the examination was performed and a gauge of the reliability of the examination (i.e. whether you were able to perform a full exam).

General inspection

Note the patient's apparent age, race, sex, build, posture, body movement, voice, speech disorders, nutritional/hydration status, facial or skeletal deformities.

Vital signs

- Pulse: if irregular, measure the apical pulse and note its beat as 'regularly irregular' or 'irregularly irregular'. Do this on the right and left sides.
- Blood pressure: take in both arms with the patient sitting, supine and standing.
- Temperature: note the site at which this was recorded.
- Respiratory rate.
- Height, weight (for a child record the percentile height/weight).
- Global pain score on a scale of 1 to 10 (1 = no pain and 10 = worst possible pain).

Skin

Note the color/pigmentation, texture, state of hydration (turgor), temperature, vascular changes, lesions, scars, hair type and distribution, nail changes, tattoos, piercing.

Head, eyes, ears, nose, throat (HEENT)

- Head: note the size (normally noted as normocephalic) and palpate for swelling, tenderness, injuries, symmetry. Take an actual measurement of the circumference in children.
- Eyes:
  - visual acuity: if corrected, the degree should be estimated
  - periorbital tissues: edema, discoloration, ptosis
  - exophthalmos/enophthalmos
  - conjunctiva and sclera: pigmentation, dryness, abnormal tearing, lesions, edema, hyperemia
  - oculomotor: PERRLA (pupils equal, round, react to light and accommodation), EOMI (extraocular movements intact) or gaze restricted, nystagmus, strabismus
  - fundoscopy: optic disc (size, shape, color, depression, margins, vessels), macula, periphery, light reflexes, exudates, edema.
- Ears: hearing (watch tick, hair manipulation, whisper, Rinne and Weber tests when indicated), external auditory canal, tympanic membranes, mastoids, wax, discharge.
- Nose: septum (position, lesions), discharge, polyps, obstruction, turbinates, sinus tenderness to palpation (if necessary, transilluminate).
- Mouth and throat:
  - lips: color, lesions
  - teeth: hygiene, decayed, missing or filled teeth, mobility, prostheses, occlusion. Record the developmental status in children (primary, mixed) and whether this is appropriate for the chronological age
  - gingiva: color, texture, size, bleeding, lesions, recession
  - buccal mucosa: color, lesions, salivary flow from parotid glands, Stensen's ducts
  - floor of mouth: color, lesions, salivary flow from submandibular/sublingual glands, Wharton's ducts
  - tongue: color, lesions, papillary distribution or changes, movement, taste (if indicated)
  - hard and soft palate: color, lesions, deformities, petechiae, movement of soft palate
  - oropharynx: tonsillar pillars, color, lesions, gag reflex
  - temporomandibular joint (TMJ): click, pop, crepitus, tenderness, trismus from a variety of problems (e.g. infection, micrognathia, scleroderma, arthritis)
  - muscles of mastication: tenderness, spasm.

Neck
- Lymph nodes: deep cervical, posterior cervical, occipital, supra-clavicular, preauricular, posterior auricular, tonsillar, submaxillary, sublingual, submental.
- Trachea: position, movement with swallowing.
- Thyroid: size, consistency, tenderness, mobility, masses, bruits.
- Throat/neck: dysphagia, carotid bruits, JVD, hoarseness.
- Cervical spine: mobility, posture, pain, muscle spasm.

Chest
- Observation: symmetry, size, scars, shape, anteroposterior dimension, respiratory excursions.
- Percussion: resonance or dullness and where located, tactile fremitus.
- Auscultation: breath sounds, stridor, wheezing, rales, rubs, rhonchi.

Breasts (see Box 1.1)
- Size.
- Symmetry.
- Lesions.
- Stippling.
- Discharge.
- Masses.
- Tenderness.
- Tanner stage (in children and adolescents)
- Gynecomastia (in males).

Box 1.1 Sensible precautions when examining a patient

Make sure that a chaperone is present during examination of the breasts, genitals or anus.

Cardiovascular
- Point of maximal impulse (PMI): inspect and palpate for PMI noting location and character, thrills, heaves.
- Auscultate: rate and rhythm, murmurs, friction rubs, gallops, other abnormal sounds. When indicated, changes in heart sounds with exercise or change of position should be noted.
- Edema: location, degree, extent, tenderness, temperature.

- Arteries: the aorta should be auscultated. The carotid, superficial temporal (facial), brachial, radial, femoral, ulnar, popliteal, posterior tibial and dorsalis pedis pulses should be palpated for strength, character and equality.
- Veins: pressure, varicosities, cyanosis, rubor, tenderness.

Abdomen
- Appearance: size, shape, symmetry, pigmentation, scars.
- Percussion: note borders of organs and fluid, areas of tympany, hyperresonance, dullness or flatness, shifting dullness, and tenderness.
- Palpation: size of the abdominal aorta and pulsations, liver, spleen, kidneys, masses, fluid wave, tenderness, guarding, rebound tenderness, hernia, inguinal adenopathy.
- Auscultation: bowel sounds, peristaltic rushes, bruits.

Genitalia

Male

Development, penile scars or lesions, urethral discharge, testes descended, hernia, tenderness, masses, circumcision.

Female
- External examination: hair, skin, labia, clitoris, Bartholin's and Skene's glands, urethral discharge, vaginal discharge, lesions.
- Internal examination: cervix, uterus, fallopian tubes, ovaries (masses, tenderness, lesions), indication of pregnancy.

Anorectal
Record hemorrhoids, skin tags, fissures, rectal sphincter tone, masses, strictures, character of stool, guaiac stool. In males, prostate size, consistency, nodularity and tenderness should also be noted.

Extremities
Proportions (to each other and to entire body), amputations, deformities, finger clubbing, cyanosis, koilonychia, edema, erythema, enlargement, tenderness, range of motion of joints, cords, muscle atrophy, strength, swelling, spasm, tenderness.

Spine

Alignment and curvature, range of motion, tenderness to palpation and percussion, muscle tone.

Neurologic

- Appropriateness, alertness, orientation to person, place, time, situation, recall for past and present. For adults aged 55 and older whose responses to questions seem inconsistent, the Mini Mental State Exam (MMSE) can be used to check the possibility of dementing illness or other insidious, progressive cognitive impairment that might call into question the patient's ability to provide informed consent and a thorough history. If there is evidence of injury or cortical disease, further tests are indicated.
- Impaired sensorium: degree and kind.
- Meningeal signs (if indicated): stiff neck, Kernig and Brudzinski signs.
- Cranial nerves (CN; Box 1.2).

Box 1.2 The cranial nerves	
I	Smell: test by asking the patient to identify common odors (e.g. coffee, peppermint, wintergreen) with the eyes closed and one nostril occluded (this is not usually done on gross examination).
II	Vision: the patient's vision can be compared at distance with examiner's visual fields.
III	Test that the pupils are equal, round and reactive to light and accommodation (PERRLA).
IV and VI	Test by asking the patient to move the eyes up, down and laterally.
V	Sensory: superficial touch (light/soft, sharp and two-point discrimination) at the forehead, malar and mandibular areas, corneal reflex. The motor function of V can be determined by symmetry and the tension of the masseter muscles when the patient clenches the teeth.
V and VII	Strength and mobility in the upper and lower face can be tested by the patient wrinkling the forehead, closing the eyes tightly and smiling.
VIII	Ears: auditory acuity can be tested using a watch tick for stimulus. Compare air and bone conduction (Rinne test). The presence or absence of rapid lateral movement of eyes on lateral gaze (nystagmus) should be noted.

IX and X	Test the 'gag reflex'. The sensory arm is conveyed by the IXth cranial nerve and the motor response by the Xth. Determine the mobility of the soft palate by asking the patient to say 'Aahhh'. Hoarseness and difficulty swallowing should be noted.
XI	The sternocleidomastoid and trapezius muscles should be observed and palpated for weakness or atrophy. Shoulder shrug.
XII	Tongue: bilateral muscle strength and coordination, symmetry of muscle mass, range of motion (ROM) and hypertonia of the tongue should be observed. The tongue, when protruded, should not deviate from midline.

Musculoskeletal

Check for tenderness, swelling or deformities of the joints. Look especially for limited mobility of the neck.

CONCLUDING THE ADMISSION WORKUP

- Assessment (problem list): list the patient's differential diagnosis derived from the history, physical examination and old records.
- Plan: include further tests, procedures, medical therapies or surgeries.

ADMISSION NOTES AND REQUEST (INSTRUCTIONS)

Introduction

These are generally the first orders written on a patient following admission. As such, they must include all aspects of the patient's care and comfort, taking into account both the environmental factors and the proposed therapeutic procedures. Orders are a major link between dental and nursing staff in providing patient care. Many needless phone calls can be avoided if the orders are precise, intelligible and legible. Like any other entry in the chart, they become part of the permanent medical record and, if necessary, legal record. They should be signed and dated, and the time should be noted.

Box 1.3 Elements of the admission notes and request

Disposition: admit to (floor, service and attending dentist).

Diagnosis (reason for admission): actual or provisional, other medical problems.

Condition: good, fair, poor and critical are adequately descriptive.

Allergies: allergies of any sort – food or drug – should be included, but specifically you should enquire as to penicillin and other antibiotics, aspirin, codeine, iodide preparations, latex and surgical tape. Also note any medications to be avoided secondary to concomitant disease(s) or medications (e.g. aspirin, warfarin/peptic ulcers; atropine/glaucoma).

Patient monitoring: vital signs should be monitored every 2, 4, 6 hours per shift, or per routine. Specific requests for varying monitoring will depend on the patient's condition (e.g. check for stridor, call house officer if temperature is > 101°F (38.5°C).

Activity: should be consistent with patient's condition (e.g. out of bed ad lib, bathroom privileges, up with assistance, chair, bedrest). For children: detail the required supervision, restraints (e.g. bed [cot] rails, consent for restraints).

Diet: should be normal [usual], soft, mechanical soft, full liquids, clear liquids, nil by mouth (NPO; indicate time). Diet can be modified if this is made necessary by concomitant disease state(s) such as diabetes, renal failure, hypertension (e.g. American Diabetes Association 1500 calories, no added salt (NAS), fluid restrictions, force fluids).

Diagnostic tests: hospitals have different requirements for admission testing [routing investigations]. Examples include:

– routine: complete [full] blood cell count, differential, electrolytes, prothrombin time with international normalized ratio (INR), partial thromboplastin time, type [group] and hold, or type [group] and crossmatch; sickle screen when indicated

– electrocardiogram, chest X-ray, urinalysis

– when indicated: blood gases, cultures, cytology, endocrine studies, liver enzymes, hepatitis and HIV studies, pulmonary function tests

– additional X-rays as indicated.

Pediatric patients: complete [full] blood cell count with differential and urinalysis. Sickle screen when indicated. Additional tests should be requested as indicated by medical history and physical examination. Same-day surgery admissions in many hospitals permit a fingerstick hematocrit for well children before elective surgery.

IV fluids: both composition of fluid and rate of infusion should be specified, taking into account existing and potential deficiencies.

Medications: routine medications taken by patient – the regimen might need to be adjusted according to present physical status and procedure planned. Also note the medications to be started on admission – dosage and administration schedule.

Input: amount and composition of fluid intake, both PO and IV.

Output: fluid lost from all sources (urine, vomitus, nasogastric tube, fistula, wound drainage). *Note*: Weight is often followed to monitor fluid balance.

Consults: service or individual to whom consult is directed, a brief description of the patient's current medical problem(s), planned procedures and specific information sought.

Special procedures:
  – monitors – electrocardiogram
  – Foley catheterization
  – ice packs/heat packs – location, time on/off
  – wound care – dressing changes, irrigation and precautions
  – specific preparations for additional tests
  – position of bed (e.g. head of bed elevated 30°C)
  – suction/lavage
  – cultures

Precautions: side rails, seizures, bleeding, respiratory, neutropenia, scissors or wirecutters at bedside, etc.

OVERVIEW OF PATIENT ADMISSION PROCEDURES

Admission arrangements

The admissions office will want to know the patient's name, address, telephone number, mother's or father's name (if the patient is under the age of consent), preoperative diagnosis, procedure to be performed and whether blood will be needed. Requests for admission, radiographs and any necessary laboratory work should also be made at this time.

Patient contact

Patients should be contacted and told of the admission and surgery dates and the scheduled time for surgery. Patients should be advised to continue taking all medications consistent with the anesthesia department's policies and not to stop taking appropriate medications before admission simply because they are 'going to the hospital'. Once in hospital, notes will be written to ensure that the appropriate medications are continued.

Hospital contact with patient

If your hospital has a preadmission questionnaire, patients should be asked to complete this and return it to the hospital.

A complete history and physical examination should be performed either on the day a patient is admitted to the hospital or before admission. The requested laboratory procedures will be completed and the results placed in the record while the patient is in hospital awaiting surgery. The surgical [and anesthetic] consent form should be completed, explained to the patient and signed according to hospital policy, if not already done prior to admission. If the patient is judged not to have the capacity to give consent because of intellectual impairment, then notwithstanding the legal guidelines, the agreement of parents or guardians [carers] must be sought.

PREOPERATIVE CONSIDERATIONS

Prophylactic antibiotics

Preoperative antibiotics are routinely given immediately before major surgical procedures are performed on some medically compromised patients. The appropriate national regimen for endocarditis prophylaxis (see Chapter 8) should be followed for patients at risk of developing this life-threatening problem – in America the American Heart Association (AHA) has developed guidelines; the UK follows the British Society of Antimicrobial Chemotherapy (BSAC) guidelines. Because an IV line is typically in place for OR [theatre] procedures, and the patient required to fast before surgery, the IV route is preferred.

Selecting the anesthetic technique

Local/regional anesthetic

Local/regional anesthetic should be used for minor procedures and as an adjunct to IV sedation or general anesthesia.

Nitrous oxide/oxygen

Consider whether the patient is suitable for conscious sedation using nitrous oxide and oxygen.

IV sedation

IV sedation should be considered for:
- anxious patients needing a procedure of any magnitude
- patients who are unresponsive and not cooperative
- patients in whom the risks of general anesthesia are too great – usually patients with severe cardiac disease or airway concern
- medically compromised patients needing stress reduction.

General anesthesia

General anesthesia should be administered for:
- extensive or very painful procedures
- patients with a profound gag reflex
- when protection of airway with endotracheal tube is desirable
- when hypotensive anesthesia is necessary

Risk assessment

Patient-related

This is the most critical type of risk. A thorough history and physical examination is necessary to ascertain the extent of patient-related risk. Cardiac and respiratory diseases are the greatest causes of increased perioperative morbidity and mortality. Be aware of the increasing use of medications, including complementary (e.g. St John's wort), which might interfere with blood coagulation or produce other drug reactions. Appropriate laboratory studies should be obtained to adequately evaluate clinical findings preoperatively.

The American Society of Anesthesiologists' (ASA) classification of physical status (Box 1.4) is the most common form of pre-anesthetic risk assessment.

Box 1.4 The ASA classfication of physical status

Class I	Healthy patient.
Class II	Patient with mild systemic disease (e.g. well-controlled diabetic, asymptomatic tobacco smoker, asymptomatic aortic stenosis, asthma).
Class III	Patient with severe but not incapacitating or stable systemic disease (e.g. patient with severe type 2 adult-onset diabetes but requiring insulin for glycemic control, patient with significantly limited exercise tolerance due to cardiac or pulmonary disease).
Class IV	Patient with incapacitating systemic disease that is a constant threat to life (e.g. immediately following myocardial infarction).
Class V	Moribund patient, not expected to survive beyond 24 h.
Class VI	Organ donor.

Procedure-related

Dental and oral/maxillofacial surgical procedures are typically associated with minimal morbidity or mortality. The treatment of severe infections with airway compromise and the management of maxillofacial trauma carry the highest risk.

Anesthesia-related

Recent advances in anesthetic monitoring equipment and techniques have reduced anesthetic-related morbidity and mortality. The most common risks include aspiration and other airway disturbances, hypo-/hypervolemia, and human error. Rare, but important, risks also include malignant hyperthermia, dysrhythmias, seizures, myocardial infarction and hepatitis.

Provider-related

Complications tend to decrease with practitioner experience and institutional experience. Outcomes assessment [audit] is necessary to ensure that the highest quality of care is given.

Laboratory studies

As a requirement for admission to many hospitals the patient will need to undergo:

- a hematocrit: to check for anemia
- a pregnancy test for females of childbearing age. Urine human chorionic gonadotrophin (hCG) is the most commonly used test. It is less expensive than others, but also less sensitive. Serum quantitative hCG is more accurate but more expensive
- urinalysis.

Other commonly requested tests based upon history and physical evaluation are shown in Box 1.5.

Box 1.5 Common tests for hospital admission

Most hospitals have established criteria for preoperative laboratory screening, which must be followed. Common tests include:

- Complete [full] blood count: hemoglobin, hematocrit (not always necessary for healthy children), leukocyte count, platelet count. Anemia, infection, immune status, platelet deficiency.
- Coagulation studies (prothrombin time/INR, partial thromboplastin time, bleeding time): bleeding disorders, anticipated extensive oral surgery.
- Serum electrolytes (Na, Cl, K, CO_2, blood urea nitrogen, creatinine, glucose): metabolic disturbance (e.g. kidney failure, diabetes).
- Toxicology screen: drug use, levels of seizure medication.
- Blood for typing: if there might be a need for transfusion.
- Urinalysis: urinary tract infections, hydration, kidney function.
- Liver function tests: ALT (alanine aminotransferase), AST (aspartate aminotransferase), LDH (lactic dehydrogenase), GGT (gamma-glutamyl transferase), bilirubin, alkaline phosphatase, acid phosphatase.
- PA and lateral chest radiographs: cardiorespiratory anomalies (e.g. pneumonia, hypertrophic cardiomyopathy).
- ECG: dysrhythmia, conduction abnormalities.

Prevention of aspiration

Patients undergoing IV sedation or general anesthesia should not consume anything by mouth ('nil by mouth'; NPO) within a specific number of hours prior to anesthetic induction, depending on institutional policy and the age of the patient. You must ensure that these instructions have been strictly followed by questioning the patient before going to the operating room (OR). An empty stomach decreases the gastric volume and hence the risk of aspiration.

Preoperative medication – an H_2 antagonist or proton pump inhibitor – can be given preoperatively to decrease the gastric pH; in the event of aspiration of gastric contents, the decreased acidity might improve the outcome. Ranitidine has also been shown to increase gastric emptying, thereby reducing stomach volume.

Pulmonary embolism prophylaxis

Pregnant, elderly and debilitated patients are at risk for development of deep vein thrombosis (DVT) and subsequent pulmonary embolism with significant morbidity and possibly mortality. The following prophylactic measures should be taken to decrease the occurrence of blood clots in the lower extremities due to venous stasis during surgery:

- Heparin: 5000 units SC 2 h prior to surgery and then every 8–12 h during the immediate postoperative time period can prevent 50% of pulmonary emboli. This small dose has not been shown to increase bleeding.
- Pneumatic stockings: placed after induction of anesthesia, these stockings alternately inflate and deflate to decrease venous stasis.
- Elastic stockings: can also be used to decrease pooling of blood in the lower extremities.

Prevention of homologous blood transfusion

Transfusion of homologous blood (i.e. blood from another person) for elective maxillofacial procedures in healthy patients can be avoided by having the patient make a predeposit of autologous blood. This is usually done 4–30 days before surgery. Ferrous sulfate and multivitamin therapy is given after donation of the autologous blood to aid in the production of new hemoglobin.

Prevention of adrenal crisis

Patients who have been or are currently on systemic steroids are potentially at risk for an adrenal (Addisonian) crisis during or after a stressful event like a surgical procedure or general anesthetic. The issue of prophylactic steroids prior to dental procedures is controversial, and the risk of an adrenal crisis in the dental setting is unknown. Keep in mind that topical and other non-parenteral sources of steroids can suppress adrenal function if prolonged and/or of high-enough dosage. Also, the likelihood of clinically significant adrenal suppression varies with the individual and no reliable 'cook book' formula (e.g. rule of 2s) exists to help the clinician. Adrenal crisis in the dental setting is extremely rare and steroid supplementation is often given because it is easy, inexpensive and non-threatening to the patient, in comparison with the potential outcome from an adrenal crisis.

PREOPERATIVE NOTE

Introduction

The preoperative note is a summary of the patient's general status and laboratory results. It is entered in the progress notes the night before surgery. Abnormal laboratory values should be assessed and orders and notes revised accordingly. Some hospitals combine the preoperative and admission notes in day-surgery cases.

Box 1.6 Elements of the preoperative summary

General statement: e.g. healthy, 16 yo intellectually impaired male admitted to (give the location) for (name the procedure or reason for admission).

Diagnosis: list all current medical problems.

Physical examination: indicate whether this was within normal limits or if there were abnormalities.

Vital signs.

Allergies.

Box continues

Box 1.6 continued

Chest X-ray: pertinent findings should be noted. If the film is clear, no active disease should be indicated.

Electrocardiogram: rate, rhythm, any abnormalities.

Chemistries: results should be shown, with any abnormalities noted.

Complete [full] blood cell count: any abnormalities should be listed.

Sickle screen: results should be noted and, if positive, electrophoresis requested to determine the percentage hemoglobin S.

Prothrombin time/INR and partial thromboplastin time: results, any abnormalities.

Urinalysis: results, any abnormalities.

Operative consent: signed and in chart.

Blood: if blood replacement is anticipated, the number of units requisitioned should be indicated and whether for type and hold or type and cross.

Plan: e.g. to OR [theatre] in am for full-mouth rehabilitation.

PREOPERATIVE NOTES AND ORDERS [REQUESTS]

Definition

These notes are written the night before surgery to prepare the patient for surgery.

Elements

Different institutions have different policies. Check your own – it might be different to the guidelines in Box 1.7.

> **Box 1.7 Elements of preoperative notes and orders (requests)**
>
> NPO after midnight: in children under 6 months, only clear fluids after midnight, NPO 4 h preoperatively; children aged 6 months to 5 years, only clear fluids after midnight, NPO 6 h preoperatively; children older than 5 years, NPO after midnight or 4 h preoperatively depending on hospital policy.
> Radiographs to be taken if not already done.
> Steroids/antibiotics on call to operating room.
> Void on call to operating room.
> Blood sample to blood bank: type and hold or type and crossmatch, number of units, if need for blood products is anticipated.
> Medication:
> - sleeping pill, if necessary
> - analgesics, if necessary
> - premedication: depending on the hospital, the house officer might write these or they might be per the anesthesiologist.

INTRAOPERATIVE CONSIDERATIONS

Positioning the patient

1. The patient should be placed in the reverse Trendelenburg position with the head elevated 10 to 20 degrees to prevent pooling of blood in the face.
2. Eye protection should be provided by the placement of ophthalmic ointment, taping the eyelids closed or using ocular occluders, and placement of gauze eye pads.
3. The endotracheal tube is secured using tape so that the head can be turned from side to side without extubation. A simple technique, if the patient is nasally intubated, involves taping the tube to the skin of the bridge of the nose and forehead with silk or cloth tape (benzoin application can improve adherence) and placing a folded pillowcase 'turban' around the head and securing the tube over the top of the head. Nasal intubation is generally preferred for most intraoral procedures and is mandatory if the patient needs to have bite-wing X-rays taken, the occlusion

checked or if maxillomandibular fixation is required during the procedure. Nasal intubation is contraindicated if the patient has epidermolysis bullosa, severe coagulopathy, nasopharyngeal carcinoma or nasal obstruction.

4. The height of the operating table is adjusted so that the operating field is at elbow level. A count is made of sponges [swabs, mops], etc.

5. The patient's arms should be tucked along his or her side so that they do not dangle over the side of the table. Foam padding should be placed under the arms and feet to prevent pressure injury. A 'donut' or headring can be placed under the head to prevent movement.

Prepping and draping

Surgical preparatory scrub solutions
- Iodine-containing compounds (Betadine), check for allergy first.
- Chlorhexidine (Hibiclens) [Hibiscrub].
- Alcohol.

Technique of mucosal and skin preparation
1. Suction the oropharynx.
2. Place a moistened throat pack (with radiopaque marker) into the oropharynx by layering.
3. Some clinicians brush the teeth and bathe the oral tissues with iodine or other antibacterial compound (this is optional, depending on the procedure).
4. Cleanse the face by applying prep solution in an expanding circular, non-overlapping fashion at least three times, each time with a different sponge. When applying the scrub solution, take care not to pass the same sponge over the area more than once. Be careful when applying surgical prep solutions around the eyes – only dilute iodine compounds are tolerated by the ocular tissues.

Draping for orofacial procedures
Place sterile towels or paper drapes around the operating field. Then use a larger sterile drape to cover the entire patient except for the operative field. A thyroid drape is usually ideal for intraoral procedures or procedures involving a segment of the face. Other styles of sterile drapes can be useful depending on the amount of surface area needed in the operating field.

Use of local anesthetic

Consider discussion in situations when there might be a contra-indication (e.g. epinephrine and severe aortic stenosis).

Type

To provide the most profound anesthesia and minimize the amount of endogenous catecholamine released, use a regional block when possible, using a long-duration local anesthetic with vasoconstrictor. When proper aspiration is performed, there are few contraindications to local anesthetics containing a vasoconstrictor. In the past, epinephrine-free solutions have been recommended for use when treating 'cardiac' patients. However, without epinephrine, the level of anesthesia is inadequate. The resultant pain response stimulates endogenous secretion of norepinephrine, which could have the same cardiac effects as a local anesthetic with vasoconstrictor. Therefore, short-acting local anesthetic agents without vasoconstrictor should be avoided except in cases where there is a clear contra-indication, such as left ventricular outflow obstruction (e.g. hyper-trophic subaortic stenosis, aortic valve stenosis). If using local anesthetic for pain control, with or without IV sedation, choose a local anesthetic agent that will provide profound anesthesia well into the postoperative period.

Profound local anesthesia will reduce the amount of general anesthetic agent needed. Consider giving additional regional blocks prior to emergence from general anesthesia to decrease post-operative discomfort.

Local anesthetic with vasoconstrictor is frequently infiltrated in the surgical site, principally to control bleeding. Exercise caution in very young or intellectually impaired patients, who might in-advertently self-mutilate soft tissues during the recovery period.

Quantity

The maximum dose of lidocaine to limit systemic toxicity is 4.4 mg/kg, but is elevated to 7 mg/kg if epinephrine is used. The dysrhythmic threshold for submucosal epinephrine is different depending on which inhalational agent is being used: 2 mcg/kg for Halothane, 6 mcg/kg for Desflurane, Isoflurane, and Sevoflurane, and 18 mcg/kg for Ethrane. Halothane and Ethrane are now rarely utilized due to the introduction of these newer agents. Always aspirate prior to injection to avoid a large intravascular dose of local anesthetic and/or vasoconstrictor. Notify the anesthesiologist of the dose and the percentage epinephrine prior to injection.

Block versus infiltration

If vasoconstrictor is used, the area of the surgical procedure could be infiltrated to decrease bleeding. If the local anesthetic is given for analgesia, a regional block might be more desirable.

Sequence of surgical procedures

The sequence in which procedures are performed will depend on the particular case. With the advent of antibiotic usage, rigid internal fixation and other technical improvements, many of the old sequencing rules no longer apply. However, it is important that the presurgical preparation includes not only the types of procedures to be performed, but also an order in which they will be done. Every case must be treated individually.

Hemostasis (Box 1.8)

Box 1.8 Procedures to ensure hemostasis

Vasoconstrictors: infiltration of vasoconstrictor (generally with local anesthetic) will decrease bleeding from small vessels.

Position: tilting the head upward will decrease accumulation of blood in the face.

Modified hypotensive anesthesia: controlled reduction of blood pressure can reduce blood loss, create a better operating field and reduce operating time. Indicated for procedures that might result in large amounts of blood loss, when the surgical field might be obscured by hemorrhage and/or there is a high risk of postoperative hematoma. The blood pressure is carefully lowered to a systolic pressure of 85–90 mmHg with inhalation agents, IV medications or a combination of these. Urine output should be measured intraoperatively, via a Foley catheter, to ensure adequate renal perfusion.

Electrocautery: electrical current can be used to seal small blood vessels. Advise the anesthesiologist first. The electrocautery unit can be used to incise and coagulate at the same time as well as to coagulate individual vessels. Contraindicated in patients with cardiac pacemakers.

Direct ligation: suture material might be necessary for bleeding from larger vessels. The vessel should be clamped with two hemostats with tips pointing toward one another, the vessel divided and the ends ligated.

Chemical cautery: limited nasal or oral mucosal bleeding can often be satisfactorily treated by application of chemical agents such as silver nitrate.

Direct pressure: until other, more definitive, measures can be taken, pressure applied directly over a bleeding vessel will usually stop the hemorrhage. In some instances, when the vessel cannot be controlled, gauze packing can be placed.

Occlusion: bleeding from alveolar bone can be controlled by crushing nutrient canals or applying bone wax.

Hemostatic agents: oxidized cellulose (Surgicel®) or topical tranexamic acid (5%) mouthwash, applied using gauze.

OPERATIVE NOTES

Introduction

Operative notes are a detailed summary of the surgery, preferably dictated or written immediately postoperatively before leaving the OR [theatre] suite.

Box 1.9 Elements of operative notes

Patient data: doctor (first and last names) dictating an operative report on (patient's name, hospital number). Patient's hospital location, service performing the surgery, and date of operation should be included.

Preoperative diagnosis.

Postoperative diagnosis.

Operation performed.

Box continues

Box 1.9 continued

Surgeon(s) and assistant(s).

Anesthesia: e.g. halothane inhalation with nasotracheal intubation.

Indications for operation: a succinct history of present illness. For the healthy child, give behavior history.

Description of procedure:
- introduction of anesthesia: smooth, stormy, tube in place
- prepping and draping of surgical site
- type of incision, steps in incision
- tissue removed: description of tissue
- pathology report (if any): disposition of any tissue removed (e.g. 'teeth sent to pathology for gross only' or 'tissue sent for preparation and histologic examination')
- irrigation solutions
- closure: steps and specific material used
- packs, drains, tubes, dressing placed (including throat pack)
- IV fluids
- intraoperative medications, other than those used by the anesthesiologist (e.g. antibiotics, steroids)
- surgery: when the procedure is done include operative dentistry, a description of procedures should include condition of the teeth and oral cavity. All procedures should be noted (e.g. examination, scaling, four periapical radiographs). Restorations should be described by tooth restored and material used (e.g. teeth #3, 12 and 18 were restored using occlusal amalgams over $CaOH_2$ liner). Some hospitals permit the use of universal numbering systems in medical records whereas others require use of the full name of the tooth (e.g. 'tooth #3' versus 'maxillary right permanent first molar').

Blood: estimated blood loss (EBL), and hematosis at completion of surgery.

Fluid replacement.

Complications.

Status on arrival in the recovery room: state of consciousness, with or without respiratory assistance, intubated or extubated in operating room, etc.

BRIEF OPERATIVE NOTE

Definition

This is a short note written in the medical records immediately following surgery.

Box 1.10 Elements of a brief operative note

Preoperative diagnosis
Postoperative diagnosis
Operation performed
Surgeon
Anesthesia
Estimated blood loss
Fluid replacement
Complications
Condition

POSTOPERATIVE ORDERS/REQUESTS

Definition

Following surgery, all previous orders are considered cancelled. Hence, postoperative orders, like admitting orders, must consider all aspects of patient care and comfort.

Elements

These are essentially the same format as for admission orders (Box 1.11).

Box 1.11 Elements of postoperative orders/requests

Disposition: admit to (location) via recovery room.

Diagnosis.

Procedure.

Condition.

Allergies.

Patient monitoring: indicated frequency of checking of the vital signs by the attendant nursing staff. The usual routine is every 15 min for the first postoperative hour, then every half hour until fully awake from anesthesia, followed by every hour for 4 h and then per routine, if the patient's condition is stable.

Diet: postoperative – clear liquids to full liquids as tolerated.

Activity: ambulation as soon as possible following surgery is helpful in clearing secretions from the bronchial tree. It also helps to prevent thrombophlebitis. Toward this latter end, the use of elastic stockings is a routine postoperative procedure in some hospitals. The level of supervision should be specified, especially for children and patients who are intellectually impaired.

Physiotherapy: until the patient is ambulatory, turning, deep breathing and coughing (unless contraindicated) are helpful in clearing the bronchial tree of secretions.

Respiratory assistance: consider in the immediate postoperative period when respiratory efforts are still depressed secondary to anesthesia and for pain. If an inhalation anesthetic was employed, and the patient is still blowing this off, supplemental oxygen is probably necessary and can be requested as 40% O_2 via facemask or tracheal collar (if trached × 8 h) to prevent hypoxia. Depending upon the patient's respiratory status, an incentive spirometer can be requested.

Daily weights.

Input and output.

Voiding: the patient with adequate fluid intake, either PO or IV, and adequate renal function can be expected to void within 6–8 h postoperatively. If a catheter was placed, a flow of 30–60 mL/h is adequate. The house officer should request notification if the patient fails to void or if rate is significantly decreased.

Tubes, catheters, drains, packs: type, location, number and care should be specified.
Bedside equipment: ice, Vaseline®, suction, wire cutters or tracheostomy set.
Monitors.
IV fluids: e.g. 'Continue type of solution at 75 mL/h until patient is taking fluids PO, then DC'.
Medications: preoperative medications are resumed when appropriate. Adequate analgesia is important in the postoperative period; too little can result in hyperventilation secondary to splinting, and too much can depress respiration at the central nervous system level. Antibiotics, antiemetics and antipyretics can be added. Avoid the tendency to undermedicate children, who tend to be more pain sensitive than adults.
Unusual conditions: notify the house officer (e.g. blood pressure > 150/100 mmHg or < 90/60 mmHg; temperature > 101°F (38.5°C); pulse < 60 or > 120 bpm; oral bleeding; protracted nausea and vomiting).

POSTOPERATIVE ORDERS/REQUESTS

Antibiotics

Infected wounds

Surgical principles for the removal of the etiologic agent and adequate drainage are of foremost importance. All infected wounds should be cultured for aerobes and anaerobes, antibiotic sensitivities should be determined and a Gram stain should be performed. However, the culture and sensitivity results will usually take days and these infections must be treated empirically until precise information is available from the microbiology laboratory.

Penicillin

The drugs of choice for most infected wounds in the oral cavity is penicillin VK 500 mg PO every 6 h or penicillin G 1 million units IV every 4 to 6 h, which covers Gram-positive aerobes and anaerobes. Bacterial resistance due to production of beta-lactamase is increasing. Modify dosage for a child (g/k body weight).

Metronidazole

This drug can be added to the therapeutic regimen to provide more anaerobic coverage. It is usually prescribed as 500 mg every 6 h IV or PO. Caution the patient against consuming ethanol when taking this medication because this can cause severe nausea and vomiting and profound hypotension.

Cephalexin

This is frequently used when staphylococci are shown or thought to predominate. Although it provides better activity against beta-lactamase-producing staphylococci, its spectrum of activity is otherwise similar to penicillin, except for poorer coverage of anaerobes. It is given as 500 mg every 6 h PO. There is a 5 to 10% chance that a patient who has a known penicillin allergy will have an allergic reaction to this cephalexin. Cefazolin, with a similar spectrum to cephalexin, can be given (1 g every 8 h IV) instead.

Erythromycin

This can be used in penicillin-allergic patients. It provides similar coverage to penicillin and is administered as 500 mg every 4–6 h IV. It should be continued for approximately 1 week at 250–500 mg PO QID. When given IV, erythromycin can cause burning at the IV site and phlebitis.

Clindamycin

This broad-spectrum antibiotic can be used in penicillin-allergic patients. It is also useful for infections containing penicillin-resistant organisms. It is administered as 600–900 mg every 6 h IV or 900 mg every 8 h, and continued as 300 mg PO QID for 1 week postoperatively. Although clindamycin has been implicated in the development of pseudomembranous colitis, alternative antibiotics have also been shown to cause this problem. If pseudomembranous colitis should develop, it will be caused by *Clostridium difficile* and characterized by gastric distress and blood in the stool. It has traditionally been treated by administration of PO vancomycin but alternative antibiotic regimens exist, including metronidazole.

Non-infected wounds

Prophylactic antibiotic coverage should be continued intraoperatively and postoperatively until the IV line is discontinued. Additional antibiotic therapy might be indicated via the PO route if the patient has a grossly contaminated wound, an unusually extensive operation, placement of a bone graft or a compromised immune status. PO antibiotics are administered to endocarditis susceptible patients according to the AHA [or BSAC] guidelines (see Chapter 8).

Fluid management

The management of fluids is outlined in Boxes 1.12 to 1.14 below.

Box 1.12 Calculation of postoperative fluid deficit

Estimated fluid requirement (EFR) per hour:
First 10 kg: 4 cc/kg (100 cc/kg per day)
Second 10 kg: 2 cc/kg (50 cc/g per day)
Above 20 kg: 1 cc/kg (25 cc/kg per day)

Example: EFR for a 70 kg patient $= (10 \times 4) + (10 \times 2) + (50 \times 1)$
$= 40 + 20 + 50$
$= 110$ cc/h

Estimated fluid deficit (EFD) = EFR times the number of hours since last oral intake:
Example: EFD for 70 kg patient NPO (nothing by mouth) for 8 h
EFR $\times$ 8 = 110 cc/h $\times$ 8 h = 880 cc

Replacement of blood losses:
Crystalloid fluid: 3 times estimated blood loss (EBL)
Colloid or blood: 1 times EBL
Example: For EBL of 400 cc, crystalloid fluid replacement should be $3 \times 400 = 1200$ cc

Total postsurgical fluid deficit (TPFD):
EFD + (blood losses $\times$ 3) – fluid replaced by anesthesia during surgery.
Example: A 70 kg patient is NPO for 8 hrs, has 400 cc of surgical blood loss, and receives 1500 cc of crystalloid during surgery.
TPFD = 880 cc + 1200 cc – 1500 cc = 580 cc
Insensible losses are generally negligible in most orofacial procedures.

Box 1.13 Physical assessment of fluid balance

Mental status: confusion, dementia.
Vital signs: temperature, pulse, respiratory rate, blood pressure (sitting, lying).
Cardiovascular: jugular venous distention, heart sounds.
Lungs: clear or congested.
Skin: turgor.

Box 1.14 Laboratory tests

Electrolytes.
Hemoglobin/hematocrit.
Urinalysis: specific gravity.

Types of intravenous fluid (Table 1.1)

The different types of intravenous fluid are outlined in Table 1.1.

Potassium

Abnormal levels of serum potassium can have an adverse effect on cardiac muscle function.

Table 1.1 **Types of intravenous fluid (milliequivalents/L)**

IV solution	NA	K	Cl	Bicarbonate	Calories
Ringer's lactate	130	4	109	28	0
Ringer's solution	147	4	155	0	0
Normal saline (0.9%)	154	0	154	0	0
Lactated Ringer's with dextrose	130	4	109	28	170
Dextrose 2.5% in NaCl 0.45%	77	0	77	0	85
Dextrose 5% in Ringer's lactate	148	4	156	0	170
Dextrose 5% in 2% NaCl	34	0	34	0	170
Dextrose 5% in 0.33% NaCl	56	0	56	0	170
Dextrose 5% in 0.45% NaCl	77	0	77	0	170
Dextrose 5% in 0.9% NaCl	154	0	154	0	170
Dextrose 10% in 0.9% NaCl	154	0	154	0	340
Dextrose 5% in water	0	0	0	0	200
Dextrose 10% in water	0	0	0	0	400

Hyperkalemia

Hyperkalemia is far more dangerous than hypokalemia. Clinical signs include confusion, weakness and hyperreflexia. ECG changes include peaked T waves, decreased R waves and a prolonged QRS complex. It should be treated by sodium bicarbonate 1 mEq/kg IV, followed by 25 g dextrose 50% in water IV, and 5–10 units regular insulin and by sodium polystyrene sulfonate (oral or enema). Calcium chloride 1 g IV stat should be given if the patient has cardiac rhythm abnormalities.

Hypokalemia

Hypokalemia is more commonly encountered than hyperkalemia. Clinical signs include weakness, anorexia and nausea. If it is decided to one to replace potassium, this should generally be performed slowly by administration of 20 mEq/L.

Acid–base balance

Conditions that affect the acid–base balance are discussed in Boxes 1.15 to 1.18.

Box 1.15 Metabolic acidosis

Causes: severe diarrhea, renal failure, or excessive production of acids.
Compensatory mechanism: hyperventilation.
Diagnostic tests: low arterial pH and low serum bicarbonate.
Treatment: treat the cause of acidosis; administer bicarbonate if the acidosis is severe.

Box 1.16 Respiratory acidosis

Causes: decreased ventilation.
Complications: these are the same as for metabolic acidosis.
Compensatory mechanisms: retension of bicarbonate, excretion of metabolic acids, increased ammonia formation.
Diagnostic tests: low anterial pH, elevated arterial pCO_2.
Treatment: treat the cause of acidosis, improve ventilation.

Box 1.17 Metabolic alkalosis

Causes: vomiting, gastric suctioning, diuretics, severe
hypokalemia, Cushing's syndrome.
Compensatory mechanisms: excretion of bicarbonate,
hypoventilation.
Diagnostic tests: elevated arterial pH, elevated serum bicarbonate.
Treatment: treat the cause of alkalosis; administer NaCl or KCl,
depending on etiology.

Box 1.18 Respiratory alkalosis

Cause: hyperventilation.
Compensatory mechanism: excretion of bicarbonate.
Diagnostic tests: elevated arterial pH, low arterial $p\mathrm{CO_2}$.
Treatment: treat the cause of alkalosis, CO_2 rebreathing, sedation,
IV calcium gluconate if tetany develops, careful administration
of KCl.

Water intoxication

This disorder is usually of iatrogenic origin as a result of fluid
overloading in the perioperative period. Clinical signs include
polyuria, soft tissue edema, pulmonary edema, confusion and
seizures. It is treated by water restriction with or without diuretic
administration. Hypertonic saline solutions should generally not be
given because rapid administration can lead to central pontine
demyelination.

Inappropriate antidiuretic hormone production

In this condition, usually following head trauma, excess water is
retained. The clinical signs are similar to those of water intoxication.
This problem is treated by water restriction and administration of
normal saline. If hyponatremia persists without volume excess,
hypertonic saline can be administered slowly and carefully.

Diet

Patients and their families should be made aware of dietary alterations that might be experienced as a result of the surgical pro-

cedure. The importance of maintaining adequate dietary intake for normal recovery should be stressed. Minimum daily requirements during convalescence include 160 g of protein and 3000 non-protein calories. The patient should also be encouraged to drink 3 L of fluid per day. Dietary supplements are often helpful in providing adequate nutrition during the immediate postoperative period.

Although maxillomandibular fixation is rarely necessary since the advent of rigid internal fixation, some patients undergoing orthognathic surgery or treatment of facial fractures will have their teeth wired together. These patients are at particular risk for nutritional disturbance. Blenderizing [liquidizing] in a blender will allow for ingestion of a broader variety of foods.

Pain management

Postoperative pain management can begin before leaving the operating room by giving small amounts of IV morphine, giving 30 mg ketorolac tromethamine IV, and by administering regional/local anesthetic nerve blocks with bupivacaine. Additional intravenous morphine in 2 aliquots can be given in the recovery room or after return to the hospital room [ward]. Meperidine [pethidine] 50 mg IM is commonly used for moderate to severe postoperative pain. Additional 15–30-mg doses of ketorolac can be given IV or IM every 6 h for a maximum of 5 days. Patients should be encouraged to abandon IV or IM medications for PO pain management as soon as possible. In small children, intra- or postoperative morphine can delay discharge.

Control of edema

Non-pharmacologic techniques:
- elevation of the head
- head dressings
- ice packs (for a maximum of 12 h).

Pharmacologic methods rely on the corticosteroid dexamethasone: 10 mg PO (at least 1 h prior to surgery) or 4–12 mg IV before the procedure. However, corticosteroids should not be used in patients with chronic infections, peptic ulcer disease, renal insufficiency, gastritis, severe cardiovascular disease or diabetes.

Management of perioperative complications

Nausea and vomiting

Anesthetic agents and swallowing blood can precipitate nausea. Nasogastric suction immediately before the patient emerges from general anesthesia can be beneficial if considerable ingestion of blood is suspected. Antiemetic medications such as prochlorperazine (Compazine) 10 mg IM [Stemetil 12.5 mg IM] every 4 h PRN nausea or promethazine [Phenergan] 12.5–25 mg IM or PR [ondansetron 4 mg IV or IM] can also be used.

Fever

If the temperature is < 100°F (38.5°C), the patient can be treated empirically with acetaminophen (Tylenol) [paracetamol] 1 g PO or PR and encourage fluid intake, deep breathing, and ambulation.

If the temperature is > 100°F (38.5°C), treat as above and consider using chest physical therapy (PT) and incentive spirometry if atelectasis is a possible cause.

Workup

1. Inspect wounds, IV sites and skin for inflammation or rash.
2. Pulmonary auscultation for diminished lung sounds or rales.
3. Chest radiograph to rule-out atelectasis, pneumonitis or pulmonary edema.
4. Urinalysis and urine culture.
5. Blood cultures for recurrent severe temperature elevation or persistent high-grade fever.

Table 1.2 **Treatment of infection (by type of infection)**

Cause of fever	Treatment
Surgical trauma	None
Transient bacteremia	Usually none
Dehydration	Encourage PO intake and/or increase flow rate of IV fluids
Atelectasis	Encourage ambulation, coughing and deep breathing, chest PT, incentive spirometry
Aspiration pneumonitis	Supplemental oxygen, antibiotics, bronchodilators
Urinary tract infection	Antibiotic therapy
Phlebitis	Remove IV catheter, change to another site, elevate the affected extremity

Treatments for the different types of infection are discussed in Table 1.2.

Hypertension
The causes and treatment of hypertension are discussed in Table 1.3.

Hypotension
The causes and treatment of hypotension are discussed in Table 1.4.

Airway compromise/decreased oxygenation
Upper airway obstruction should be treated with a nasal decongestant, for example xylometazoline (Afrin). If severe, obstruction of the nasopharyngeal airway might require reintubation or tracheostomy (if unable to reintubate). Pulmonary obstruction can be caused by:

- Atelectasis: the clinical diagnosis is rales, tachypnea, fever and tachycardia; treatment is by ambulation, coughing and deep breathing, chest PT, incentive spirometry.
- Aspiration pneumonitis: the clinical diagnosis is segmental lung hypoventilation, dyspnea, wheezing, rales, rhonchi, cough, fever;

Table 1.3 **Causes and treatment of hypertension**

Cause	Treatment
Pain	Increase analgesics
Hypervolemia	Fluid restriction consider diuretic
Urinary retention	Catheterization
Pre-existing hypertension	Consider a temporary increase in patient's medication or small doses of IV antihypertensive drugs

Table 1.4 **Causes and treatment of hypotension**

Cause	Treatment
Hypovolemia	Trendelenburg position
Drugs (narcotic analgesics, anesthetics)	Increase IV fluids (if no cardiac dysfunction)
Decreased cardiac output	Ephedrine 10 mg IV acutely; if hypotension is persistent, obtain cardiology consult and institute vasopressor drip (e.g. phenylephrine)*

*Exclude hypovolemia (actual or relative) before using pressors.
If a cardiac cause is suspected, obtain immediate cardiology consultation.

treatment is by supplemental oxygen, bronchodilators, sputum culture, antibiotics, IV steroids.

Pulmonary obstruction can also be a result of pulmonary edema, pulmonary embolism, pneumothorax and asthma or bronchospasm.

Urinary retention

Assistance should be given to any patient who has been unable to void within 12 h of surgery. This usually occurs as a result of anesthetic agents, opioid analgesics or a supine position. However, volume depletion, urinary tract infection and renal failure are also potential causes. The diagnosis is suprapubic fullness and the urge to urinate. Treatment is by:

- assisted ambulation
- heat packs to suprapubic region
- straight catheterization
- urinalysis to rule-out hypovolemia, urinary tract infection and renal failure.

THE POSTOPERATIVE NOTE

Definition

This is a short note discussing the status of the patient the evening of surgery. It is usually in a 'SOAP' format: subjective, objective, assessment and plan.

Box 1.19 Elements of postoperatve notes

Subjective: patient report of status.
Objective:
    – vital signs.
    – neurologic status: awake, alert
    – wound condition: draining, oozing, dry
    – respiratory status: auscultation results
    – input/output: e.g. diet, vomiting, voiding.
Assessment.
Plans.

FOLLOW-UP NOTES

Definition

Follow-up notes are brief comments concerning patient status and plans for treatment.

Box 1.20 Elements of follow-up notes

Subjective: information from the patient concerning nutrition, pain, swelling, limited movement, drainage, bleeding, etc.
Objective: information concerning vital signs, laboratory data, examination of wound/surgery site, healing.
Plan/Suggestions: for continuation or change in treatment (e.g. diet, rinses, medications, exercises, etc.).

DISCHARGE NOTES AND REQUESTS (BOX 1.21)

Box 1.21 Discharge notes and requests

Discharge diagnosis: all diagnoses should be noted.
Operation or procedure.
Condition.
Medications: prescriptions for antibiotics, analgesics should be included.
Discharge time.
Home care instructions.
Follow-up appointment: time, place, telephone number.

DISCHARGE SUMMARY

Introduction

As well as writing an order [notes] in the chart [records] that the patient is to be discharged, a discharge summary must be dictated. If this is a 'day surgery' case there is no need for a discharge summary.

Box 1.22 Elements of a discharge summary

Patient data:
- name
- medical record number
- service
- date of admission
- date of discharge
- attending physician/dentist.

History:
- patient's age
- number of admissions to this hospital
- symptoms and past treatment, if any
- pertinent past medical history
- pertinent review of systems
- pertinent family history
- allergies.

Past medical history: anything that has not already been covered.

Physical examination: positive findings only.

Laboratory data: positive findings only.

Hospital course: positive findings only.

Discharge diagnosis.

Operations or procedures performed.

Complications.

Medications on discharge: dosage should be included.

Condition on discharge.

Disposition: follow-up care should be noted.

Estimated disability.

Clinical course [treatment summary]

There might be a clinical course resume to be completed and placed in the chart prior to discharge. This is a fill-in-the-blank, very abbreviated discharge summary that, among other items, lists the person responsible for dictating the more detailed discharge summary.

EXAMPLES OF HOSPITAL CHARTS

The hospital charts in Appendix 1 (at the end of the book) show how to record the history and physical examination; orders [notes];

consult requests; and progress, operative and discharge notes. The correct required paperwork, forms, elements of the medical record and orders will vary from one hospital to another. Short-stay or same-day admissions (day surgery) are increasing, especially for elective surgery, and hospitals often abbreviate chart entries to allow for the short duration of the stay. Admission and preoperative notes are sometimes combined, as are admission and preoperative orders [records]. A discharge note might suffice instead of a discharge summary for a short hospitalization, recounting the entire hospitalization.

EXAMPLES OF EMERGENCY ROOM ADMISSIONS

Appendix 2 gives examples of emergency room admissions.

Chapter 2

Outpatient management of the medically compromised patient

Perhaps the most challenging responsibility for a dentist is to provide care for medically compromised outpatients. A thorough history is necessary to establish the existence and nature of any medical problems to decrease the likelihood of medical emergencies and to ensure appropriate dental management.

This chapter starts with a brief risk assessment for bacteremia and the need for prophylactic antibiotics and then goes on to consider specific medical problems that are of concern to dentists. Brief consideration is given to the significant, essential elements in the history, and medical and dental management.

RISK ASSESSMENT FOR BACTEREMIA AND THE NEED FOR PROPHYLACTIC ANTIBIOTICS

Past medical history

Many of the dental management issues with medically compromised patients revolve around the use of antibiotics, either as prophylaxis or treatment. With regard to prophylactic antibiotics, the medical history is essential because the indications are rarely evidence based. When taking the history from the patient, it is helpful to ask specific questions that cover critical issues in the identification of patients at risk for distant-site infection (e.g. infective endocarditis). These questions should elicit information about previous hospitalizations, surgery, allergies, medications and physician visits in recent years. Standard health questionnaires (Box 2.1) will often bring out significant positives in the history but cannot be relied upon as the sole source of information, due either to inaccuracies in filling out such questionnaires or to omissions. They should therefore be used as a starting point for a more thorough verbal history.

Box 2.1 An example of a standard questionnaire for taking a patient's past medical history

Hospitalizations: dates, reason(s) for admission, and findings.

Operations: surgery involving the brain (e.g. shunts), liver (e.g. transplant), joints, bone marrow, kidney, heart or other vascular structures might indicate a need for antibiotic coverage for invasive dental procedures.

Allergies: allergy to one or more antibiotics should prompt a search for the next best drug with consideration for the oral flora and risks involved.

Medications: drugs of particular concern.
- oral contraceptives: reported decreased contraceptive effectiveness with antibiotics and/or antifungals
- immunosuppressive drugs: steroids, cancer chemotherapy, organ anti-rejection drugs
- antibiotics, antifungals, antivirals: need to consider the effect on the oral flora and the risk of superinfection
- non-steroidal anti-inflammatory drugs (NSAIDs): including aspirin, because of their effect on platelet function, although there is no clear evidence that this is clinically significant.

Management guidelines for antibiotic prophylaxis

All patients must be considered individually and their host resistance factors assessed (e.g. immunity, drugs, disease, debilitation). If a patient is at risk, determine which antibiotic to use and the dose, route and duration based on the oral organisms most likely to cause infection. Oral antibiotics can be indicated for some procedures (e.g. prosthetic cardiac valves) but data are not sufficient to recommend routine prophylaxis for all of the conditions that are reported to put patients at risk.

ALLERGY

Significance of the problem

Fifteen per cent of the population have one or more significant allergies. Life-threatening reaction (anaphylaxis) can occur within seconds of exposure.

Significant elements in the history

- Sensitivity: to any medications, drugs, foods or materials such as latex, which can cause itching, rash, swelling or breathing difficulties. Details of prior experience with specific drugs that might be used in the course of dental treatment (e.g. antibiotics, codeine, aspirin-containing compounds) should be elicited from the patient.
- History of asthma or hay fever.
- Family history of atopy: if positive, there is a greater likelihood that the patient will also have allergies.

Evaluating for allergy

First, determine the nature of the allergy:

- Drug and dosage given: exclude overdose or adverse side-effects.
- Other medication(s) taken at the same time: exclude drug interaction.
- Time sequence: how soon after injection/ingestion exposure did the response occur?
- Reaction: syncope, tachycardia, peripheral vasodilitation, loss of consciousness, breathing difficulty or rash.
- Therapy: drugs administered and the response to them.

You also need to record the name(s) of the clinician(s) involved.

Second, when you have determined the nature of the allergy, differentiate it from other drug-related side-effects, such as syncope, GI upset and overdose.

You then need to give specific consideration to the following facts:

- Allergy to local anesthetics must be qualified:
  - procaine: allergic reaction is more likely than to other anesthetics but procaine is rarely used in contemporary dental practice
  - lidocaine: although it is extremely rare, allergy to lidocaine can occur. More commonly, however, a preservative is usually the cause of allergic reactions.
- First exposure to a drug will rarely cause allergic response.
- Anaphylaxis is as likely with oral as with parenteral administration and can last longer if the allergen is administered orally.
- Although many reactions to drugs and foods are not true allergies, do not challenge a patient with a substance that patient has identified as a possible allergen in a non-hospitalized, uncontrolled setting without access to appropriate resuscitation drugs and equipment.

- In cases of documented or suspected allergy, patients should be referred to an appropriate clinician (clinical immunologist or allergist) for testing and/or desensitization before exposure to the drug in the dental office [surgery].

Evaluating a suspected allergic reaction

- Take both supine and sitting blood pressure. If a postural fall in blood pressure is present, early circulatory collapse could be imminent.
- Use a stethoscope to auscultate the trachea for stridor and the lungs for bronchospasm (wheezes).
- Look for urticaria (hives or rash).
- Common drugs with significant allergic potential, and alternative medication(s) are shown in Table 2.1.

Table 2.1 **Common drugs with significant allergic potential and alternative medication(s)**

Medication	Substitute medication(s)
Antibiotics	
Penicillins	Roxithromycin
Ampicillin	Clindamycin
	Metronidazole
Analgesics	
Aspirin	Acetaminophen [paracetamol]
Narcotics	Non-steroidals can be substituted but allergy can occur
Antianxiety agents	
Barbiturates	Diazepam [flurazepam], chloral hydrate, hydroxyzine
Local anesthetics	
Esters	
Procaine	Lidocaine
Benzocaine	Diphenhydramine
Tetracaine	
Methylparaben preservative	Alternative preservative or anesthetic without preservative

BLEEDING DISORDERS

Etiology

Take a family history to determine whether the bleeding disorder is the result of an inherited or an acquired problem. Also ask the patient about:

- Prolonged bleeding after previous surgery (especially tooth extraction, tonsillectomy and adenoidectomy). Differentiate between local factors and systemic problems.
- Spontaneous bleeding (e.g. nosebleeds, heavy menstrual bleeding, hematuria).
- Easy bruising, petechiae or hematoma formation, or bleeding into joints.
- Anticoagulant medications (warfarin, heparin, aspirin) and interaction with other drugs.
- Liver, renal or bone marrow disease, or underlying malignancy.
- Significant exposure to radiation, benzene, cytotoxic chemotherapy, insecticides or other relevant chemicals.
- Malabsorption syndrome.

Laboratory screening

- Prothrombin time (PT)/international normalized ratio (INR): extrinsic pathway factors (I, II, V, VII, IX, X).
- Activated partial thromboplastin time (APTT): intrinsic pathway factors (all except III, VII, XIII). This could be within normal limits, unless the factors are less than 30% of normal.
- Platelet count: usually under 40 000 per microliter if bleeding is secondary to thrombocytopenia.
- Bleeding time: although often recommended, this test has little (if any) value in dental practice.

Specific coagulopathies

Hemophilia A (factor VIII deficiency)

The amount of factor VIII the patient needs depends on the procedure. In severe hemophilia A (factor VIII level < 1%), a single infusion of factor VIII concentrate should be considered (1 unit/kg will raise the plasma level of the patient by 2%):

- Invasive procedures: the goal is to raise the level to 25–50% transiently (the half-life of factor VIII is about 12 h). Surgical procedures, including extractions, might require raising the factor VIII level to 100% with a presurgical bolus injection. This can be followed by 4–6 g epsilon aminocaproic acid (EACA) four times daily for 6–8 days, beginning 6 h after the procedure.
- Less invasive procedures: in procedures requiring infiltration or block anesthesia (e.g. operative, prosthetic, deep periodontal scaling and root planing) the goal is to raise plasma level to 15–20% transiently.

Moderate (1–5%) and mild (5–25% factor VIII) hemophiliacs can often be managed with desmopressin to transiently increase plasma levels of factor VIII and epsilon aminocaproic acid (EACA) to prevent rebleeding, thus avoiding factor replacement. The decision should be made by discussion with the patient's physician.

Factor VIII antibodies (inhibitors) exist in 20% of patients who have received factor VIII in the past.

Hemophilia B (factor IX deficiency)

Treat either with factor IX concentrate or with fresh frozen plasma. Factor IX concentrates can contain activated coagulation factors and trigger thrombosis and embolism.

Hemophilia C (factor XI deficiency)

Treated with fresh frozen plasma. The patient's physician should be consulted.

von Willebrand's disease

This autosomal dominant disorder of platelet function and factor VIII activity is characterized by prolonged bleeding time and/or decreased platelet adhesiveness to glass beads. Replacement therapy, if indicated, as per patient's hematologist. Options include desmopressin cryoprecipitate or factor VIII concentrate. Desmopressin can be useful in patients with the most prevalent 'classic' form of this disease.

Thrombocytopenia

This is defined as a platelet count under 100 000 per microliter. It can be congenital, acquired or idiopathic, and adverse drug reactions are a common cause. It is characterized by prolonged bleeding following surgery and usually occurs with platelet counts below

50 000 per microliter. Spontaneous bleeding can occur with counts below 20 000 per microliter.

Avoid elective procedures, which can produce bleeding, because many thrombocytopenias are reversible. Irreversible disease or non-elective surgery might require platelet transfusion, as per the hematologist.

Medications that predispose to bleeding

Aspirin. This is commonly taken for its anti-inflammatory properties or prevention of coronary ischemic events. Some clinicians feel that aspirin should be discontinued at least 5 days prior to elective surgical procedures but there are no data to support this practice for routine dental care (including single tooth extraction).

Warfarin (Coumadin) [coumarin]. This is generally used for atrial fibrillation, atherosclerotic vascular disease, postmyocardial infarction (MI), postcerebrovascular accident (CVA) or prosthetic heart valves or grafts. It is usually taken orally for long-term anticoagulation therapy; prolongation of PT/INR persists for 3–4 days after the last dose.

Heparin. This is generally used in hospitalized patients as short-term treatment (e.g. pulmonary embolus or deep venous thrombosis) and immediate anticoagulation therapy. It is not fibrinolytic and remains active 5–6 h after the last IV dose, or 24 h after last subcutaneous dose.

Thrombolytics. Thrombolytics, for example streptokinase and tissue plasminogen activator (tPA), are fibrinolytic agents generally used for the short-term treatment of hospitalized patients (e.g. acute MI) when an immediate thrombolytic effect is desired.

Clopidogrel (Plavix) This antiplatelet agent is used to prevent athero-sclerotic events in patients with a history of MI, CVA or PVD. Normalization of platelet aggregation occurs 5–7 days after discontinuation.

Drug interactions. Broad-spectrum antibiotics interfere with the intestinal flora and mucosal absorption. Corticosteroids, some anti-fungals, oral hypoglycemics and cimetidine can all predispose towards bleeding.

Other bleeding disorders

Many less common bleeding disorders exist. The severity of the disease should be determined from the history and it is important to consult with the patient's physician or hematologist prior to scheduling a surgical procedure.

Management considerations

- Consultation: consult with patient's physician because replacement therapy might be required for block anesthesia, scaling, use of rubber dam clamps, and all surgical procedures.
- Infiltration anesthesia: this is the preferred technique because blocks (e.g. inferior alveolar) could potentially cause bleeding in the pharyngeal space; consider intrapulpal anesthesia for endodontic or intraligamental anesthesia for extraction procedures, especially in the mandible.
- Hemostatic measures: primary closure, tranexamic acid or EACA rinse, and absorbable gelatin packing, might be desirable. Use full liquid or soft diet following multiple dental extractions. With good surgical technique and the use of local measures, simple oral surgery, scaling and restorative procedures can usually be performed with an INR < 4, but individual cases must be evaluated to determine whether the risk of a thromboembolic event with discontinuation of anticoagulant therapy is greater than the risk of oral bleeding. INR level recommendations are controversial. Many authorities now feel that moderately invasive surgery (e.g. single tooth extractions) are safe up to an INR of 4. In general, the risk to the patient of altering the warfarin dosage (e.g. in stroke patients) far exceeds the potential problem of bleeding following a dental procedure. However, until more is known, the use of regional blocks should be undertaken cautiously.
- Aspirin: the number of people taking aspirin has increased greatly in recent years because of its use as a long-term anticoagulant. Take a careful history because patients might not list aspirin as a medication. Avoid aspirin and NSAIDs in patients with pre-existing bleeding disorders.
- Transfusions: multiple transfusions with blood products place patients at risk of hepatitis B and C.
- Desmopressin (DDAVP): can raise factor VIII levels sufficiently to treat patients with mild to moderate hemophilia and classic von Willebrand's disease. The patient's hematologist will conduct trials prior to any planned use to determine the individual patient's response to desmopressin. It shows a declining effect with repeti-

tive, frequent uses. Use care with any soft tissue manipulation (e.g. matrix bands, wedges).

- Loss of primary teeth: this is generally not a concern, as any oozing is usually controlled by pressure, or topical thrombin [Dirombin] if necessary.
- Oral disease: prevention of oral disease (e.g. frequent dental evaluation, fluoride use, strict oral hygiene, and diet control) should be stressed to minimize later need for invasive dental care.

CANCER

Of major concern is the patient's overall medical status and type(s) of cancer therapy. As dental disease worsens, perhaps giving rise to additional complications when ideal dental therapy becomes inadvisable because of the patient's medical status, emphasis should be placed on dental prevention. Problems that do arise are generally from two modes of medical therapy: radiation and chemotherapy.

Radiation therapy

Although radiation therapy (RT) for most cancers has no discernible effect on the oral cavity or the provision of dental care, RT for the management of head and neck cancer has a high incidence of oral sequelae. Review the patient's medical chart and discuss it with the radiotherapist/medical oncologist.

Significant elements in the history
- Date of diagnosis.
- Location and histology of the malignancy.
- TNM classification for staging head and neck tumors (Table 2.2).
- Previous therapy (e.g. RT, chemotherapy, surgery or combination, or the use of radio-sensitizers). Can be supplemented with the patient's medical chart.
- Field(s) (i.e. the area(s) receiving the direct beam), dose and fractionation (e.g. twice/day) of radiation. External beam radiation versus interstitial implant (brachytherapy). Note: 6000 rads = 6000 cGy (centigray) = 60 Gy, where Gy is a unit of radiation called a gray, the standard unit of absorbed ionizing radiation dose, and represents 1 joule per kilogram.
- Problems with xerostomia, ability to eat, taste, swallow (solids versus liquids), oral pain.

Table 2.2 **TNM staging for tumors of the lip and oral cavity**

Primary tumor (T)

TX	Primary tumor cannot be assessed
TO	No evidence of primary tumor
Tis	Carcinoma in situ
T1	Tumor 2 cm or less in greatest dimension
T2	Tumor more than 2 cm but not more than 4 cm in greatest dimension
T3	Tumor more than 4 cm in greatest dimension
T4	Tumor invades adjacent structures (e.g. through cortical bone, inferior alveolar nerve, floor of mouth, skin of face)
T4a	(Oral Cavity) Tumor invades through cortical bone, into deep [extrinsic] muscle of tongue (genioglossus, hyglossus, palatoglossus, and styloglossus), maxillary sinus, or skin of face
T4b	Tumor involves masticator space, pterygoid plates, or skull base and/or encases internal carotid artery

Regional lymp nodes (N)

NX	Regional lymph nodes cannot be assessed
NO	No regional lymph node metastasis
N1	Metastasis in a single ipsilateral lymph node, 3 cm or less in greatest dimension
N2	Metastasis in a single ipsilateral lymph node, more than 3 cm but not more than 6 cm in greatest dimension; or in multiple ipsilateral lymph nodes, none more than 6 cm in greatest dimension; or in bilateral or contralateral lymph nodes, none more than 6 cm in greatest dimension
N2a	Metastasis in single ipsilateral lymph node more than 3 cm but not more than 6 cm in greatest dimension
N2b	Metastasis in multiple ipsilateral lymph nodes, none more than 6 cm in greatest dimension
N2c	Metastasis in bilateral or contralateral lymph nodes, none more than 6 cm in greatest dimension
N3	Metastasis in a lymph node more than 6 cm in greatest dimension

Distant metastasis (M)

MX	Distant metastasis cannot be assessed
M0	No distant metastasis
M1	Distant metastasis

Biopsy of metastatic site performed ☐ Yes ☐ No

Source of pathologic metastatic specimen _____

Stage grouping

Stage 0	Tis	N0	M0
Stage I	T1	N0	M0
Stage II	T2	N0	M0

Table 2.2   continued

Stage III	T3	N0	M0
	T1	N1	M0
	T2	N1	M0
	T3	N1	M0
Stage IVA	T4a	N0	M0
	T4a	N1	M0
	T1	N2	M0
	T2	N2	M0
	T3	N2	M0
	T4a	N2	M0
Stage IVB	Any T	N3	M0
	Tb4	Any N	M0
Stage IVC	Any T	Any N	M1

Histologic grade (G)

GX	Grade cannot be assessed
G1	Well differentiated
G2	Moderately differentiated
G3	Poorly differentiated

Residual tumor (R)

RX	Presence of residual tumor cannot be assessed
R0	No residual tumor
R1	Microscopic residual tumor
R2	Macroscopic residual tumor

Lymphatic vessel invasion (L)

LX	Lymphatic vessel invasion cannot be assessed
L0	No lymphatic vessel invasion
L1	Lymphatic vessel invasion

Venous invasion (V)

VX	Venous invasion cannot be assessed
V0	No venous invasion
V1	Microscopic venous invasion
V2	Macroscopic venous invasion

Additional descriptors

T, indicates the size of the tumor and differs slightly according to tumor location (e.g. lip and oral cavity versus pharynx versus larynx).

N, classification for lymph node metastasis.

M, metastatic disease distant to the head and neck; most commonly to the lungs in the case of squamous cell carcinomas of the head and neck.

For identification of special cases of TNM or pTNM classifications, the 'm' suffix and 'y', 'r' and 'a' prefixes are used. Although they do not affect the stage grouping, they indicate cases needing separate analysis.

m suffix, indicates the presence of multiple primary tumors in a single site and is recorded in parentheses: pT(m)NM.

Table 2.2 **Additional descriptors continued**

y prefix, indicates those cases in which classification is performed during or following initial multimodality therapy. The cTNM or pTNM category is identified by a 'y' prefix. The ycTNM or ypTNM categorizes the extent of tumor actually present at the time of the examination. The 'y' categorization is not an estimate of tumor prior to multimodality therapy.

r prefix indicates a recurrent tumor when staged after a disease-free interval, and is identified by the 'r' prefix: rTNM.

a prefix designates the stage determined at autopsy: a TNM.

Notes:

Lip and oral cavity: superficial erosion alone of bone/tooth socket by gingival primary is not sufficient to classify as T4.

Major salivary glands (parotid, submandibular, sublingual): extraparenchymal extension is clinical or macroscopic evidence of invasion of soft tissues. Microscopic evidence alone does not constitute extraparenchymal extension for classification purposes.

Clinical and radiographic examination

- Location and size of tumor, if visible.
- Status of soft tissue: careful examination for xerostomia, mucositis, mucosal breakdown, exposed bone, evidence of bacterial (e.g. periodontal, caries) or fungal infection.
- Teeth: number, mobility, bone support, state of repair, caries (especially cervical areas), periapical or periodontal infection, impactions with or without potential for communication with the oral flora.
- Trismus or limited jaw mobility.

Dental treatment planning and management considerations

Indications for and methods of medical therapy depend on multiple factors, all of which must be considered before beginning any invasive treatment, including basic restorative procedures. Factors to consider include the following:

- Overall tumor staging (e.g. T1–T4) and patient's overall prognosis.
- Portals of radiation, the cGy dose to be given, the start date, plans for radiation stents.
- Plans for cancer chemotherapy prior to, during or after RT.
- Risk/benefit of maintaining each tooth (mandibular teeth, especially molars, present a greater risk for osteoradionecrosis if extracted immediately before, during or at any time after RT). Teeth with > 4 mm pockets should be considered for extraction preoperatively, especially mandibular teeth if the mandible is in the RT portal.
- Status of major salivary glands following radiotherapy.
- Location, degree and potential for odontogenic infection (i.e. periodontal, pericoronitis, caries).

- Carious teeth: if shallow (i.e. no pulpal involvement), these can be restored before or following RT. Use fluoride toothpaste or gel to help arrest lesions. If of moderate depth, ensure pulp vitality and restore before RT, or at least use an intermediate restorative material until more definitive care can be given.

Major oral complications of radiation

Mucositis

Caused by thinning of mucosa from direct killing of cells by radiation. Mucostitis is usually a short-term, but potentially serious problem that can limit the RT dose and interrupt the schedule of radiation. If it is mild to moderate, try topical rinse anesthetics or systemic opioids. For example:

- 1:1 mixture of kaolin/pectin combination and elixir of Benadryl®; or Maalox® and Benadryl®; or 2% viscous lidocaine; or 20% benzocaine spray; or dyclonine; or a lidocaine/Benadryl combination. If available, benzydamine [Difflam] might be helpful.
- Benzocaine/tetracaine combination spray: as tetracaine is toxic systemically and absorbed rapidly through the mucosa, caution must be used to avoid spraying the vocal area and hypopharynx.
- If topical anesthetics fail, use systemic analgesics/opioids. These might be necessary when the topical anesthetic activity is short (5–20 min), they might cause stinging sensation and the taste might not be well tolerated. They can be used in conjunction with above agents. NSAIDs or synthetic opioids should be tried first, with escalation to stronger oral opioids as necessary.

Xerostomia and secondary infection

This often accompanies mucositis. It can be palliated by the use of saliva substitute or water (ice-chips). Alternatively, pilocarpine hydrochloride 5–10 mg 3–4 times/day can help to increase salivation. Begin at 5 mg and increase to 7.5 or 10 mg as needed for efficacy, but decrease the dose if systemic signs appear (excessive sweating, GI cramping, blood pressure changes). Cevimeline [Pilocarpine] 30 mg TID, which has been approved for Sjögren's disease, has been suggested and could have fewer side-effects. Caution should be exercised when using these muscarinic agonists in patients with asthma and cardiac problems.

Osteoradionecrosis (exposure of alveolar bone)

This is most likely to occur in patients receiving > 5000 cGy to the mandible, although the maxilla can also be involved. It is caused by permanent damage to bone and blood supply. The patient remains at indefinite risk of mucosal breakdown and exposure of bone and this can occur under dental prosthesis due to trauma to compromised mucosa, following oral surgery, from infection or spontaneously. Hyperbaric oxygen (HBO) can promote healing.

Invasive dental procedures are best done prior to RT, with at least 7 (ideally 14) days for healing. Teeth unlikely to become abscessed from caries or periodontitis can be maintained by aggressive preventive care. Following RT, compromised teeth should ideally be removed during the hyperemic stage (about 3 months after RT) as atraumatically as possible and with careful alveoloplasty, with primary closure of the mucosa, and antibiotic coverage against staphylococcal organisms. Preoperative HBO should be considered for patients who have received high-dose RT and who require mandibular extractions. Some authorities recommend no new removable prosthesis for 6–24 months after RT, but the literature suggests that the vascularity does not improve and that it might continue to deteriorate with time. Orthodontic appliances should be removed before RT that involves the dentition.

Radiation caries

This results from dry mouth rather than from direct damage to the teeth. Parotid gland tissue, if in the radiation field, will usually recover from < 3000 cGy but can remain non-functional from > 5000 cGy. Saliva production might drop to < 5% of normal within weeks. Protective immunoglobulin A and the buffering and remineralizing capacity of saliva are lost, with a resultant salivary pH of approximately 2.5. A neutral sodium fluoride rinse, brush-on gel or fluoride trays should be used every evening after careful tooth brushing and flossing. Some saliva substitute solutions have fluoride and/or calcium and phosphorus that can help to remineralize teeth. Patients need dietary counseling along with routine and careful follow-up until the dry mouth resolves, or indefinitely for patients who continue to have any degree of dry mouth or an increased incidence of caries.

Taste loss

This is a common problem when the tongue is in RT portals, but is usually transient except with high doses. The greatest resolution occurs within 3 months of treatment. Tongue hygiene and dietary considerations are important.

Infection

Bacterial. Gingival organisms might not survive during RT but inflammatory conditions can worsen as a result of direct RT on the mucosa, decreased oral hygiene, increased cariogenic diet and dry mouth.

Fungal. Candidal infections are common. Begin clotrimazole troches 4–5/day at the onset of infection and continue for the duration of RT. Dissolve clotrimazole troches in water if xerostomia prevents them dissolving in the mouth. Miconazole is an alternative. Nystatin troches contain sucrose and should therefore be avoided in dentate individuals. Fluconazole is an option for systemic therapy.

Tooth and bone development

Radiation has a major impact on the developing teeth and on active growth areas of the mandible.

Chemotherapy

The major concerns with dental management are related to the direct and/or indirect toxicity to the oral mucosa from cytotoxic chemotherapeutic agents. Mucositis, mucosal infection and bacteremia from ulcerative mucosa during myelosuppression are common problems.

When assessing a patient who is receiving cancer chemotherapy, you need to consider:

- Medical diagnosis: this determines prognosis and chemotherapy protocol employed.
- Overall status: nutrition, current blood counts, debilitation, ability to tolerate dental treatment.
- Timing of chemotherapy: if within the previous month, the oral mucosa and bone marrow might be significantly compromised.
- Blood counts: exercise caution if the patient has:
  - a total white blood cell count < 2000 and, more importantly, absolute polymorphonuclear leukocytes (PMN or polys) < 500

○ platelets < 40 000, if contemplating surgery prolonged mucosal/gingival bleeding unlikely with platelet count > 25 000.

- Risk of infection and/or bleeding from dental treatment: the dental treatment employed depends on the urgency. Sequelae from no treatment must also be considered. For uncomplicated healing to occur postsurgery or extractions, platelet counts must be durably maintained above 20 000, for anticipated clot turnover for the following week, and the absolute neutrophil count should be maintained at greater than 1000 for 7–10 days. Patients might have a coagulopathy from their disease (e.g. leukemia and poor platelet function) as well as from treatment (myelosuppression following chemotherapy).

Oral complications

Prevention of oral complications is imperative. Prior to chemotherapy, if the systemic condition allows and there is sufficient time before the severe myelosuppressive effects occur, the following measures should be taken:

- Patients should have a thorough oral examination, including a full-mouth series of radiographs.
- Extraction of hopeless periodontally or cariously involved teeth.
- Thorough oral prophylaxis and oral hygiene instruction. Patients should be educated as to the relationship between odontogenic disease and problems during chemotherapy.
- Orthodontic appliances are almost always removed when intensive chemotherapy is planned, given the potential for gingival inflammation and problems with oral hygiene.
- Oral antifungal prophylaxis (miconazole, or fluconazole) is used in secure settings when the white count or absolute poly count is significantly depressed, especially with prolonged periods of neutropenia.
- Fluoride: neutral rinse, if the patient can tolerate it, or fluoride gel. Discontinue if mucosal burning sensation occurs. Dose and timing is important with regard to other oral care, such as mouth care, topical anesthetics and antifungals, so as not to interfere with the benefit of each. For example, mouth care should be done first. Topical anesthetics and antifungals should not be followed by another oral medication/rinses until sufficient time for their efficacy has abated.

- Leave appliances out of the mouth during neutropenia or thrombocytopenia. Consider removing orthodontic appliances if chemotherapy will be prolonged or mucosal side-effects are anticipated.
- Brushing and flossing of teeth might need to be discontinued during a period of severe neutropenia or thrombocytopenia, as this can result in gingival bleeding. Give frequent (e.g. every 2 h) rinses with sterile saline, or bicarbonate or even plain water to debride the mouth and reduce bacteria levels. Commercial mouthwashes often contain alcohol and can sting ulcerated mucosa, and should therefore be avoided.
- Chlorhexidine mouth rinses have been suggested but they should be used only for short-term, atraumatic control of plaque if routine mouth care cannot be accomplished, due to the concern for selection and overgrowth of pathogenic bacterial organisms, and poor compliance and/or tolerance by patients.

Infection (periodontal abscess, dental abscess)

During severe neutropenia (absolute neutrophil count < 500 microliter), manage with broad-spectrum parenteral antibiotics. The patient needs cover for Gram-negatives and anaerobes (e.g. *Bacteroides* sp., *Escherichia coli*, *Serratia*, *Pseudomonas* and *Klebsiella* spp.) in addition to the usual Gram-positive oral flora. Elective dental treatment must wait until absolute neutrophil count rises to > 1000 and platelets to > 50 000.

Bleeding

This usually occurs from the gingival crevice with a very low platelet count (< 15 000–20 000). If pressure from a wet 2 cm × 2 cm sponge fails to stop the bleeding, a topical thrombin-soaked sponge should be applied to area and held in place for several minutes. Remove the sponge gently so as not to disturb the new clot. There is a degree of concern over the use of topical thrombin – because of sensitivity – and this should be discussed with the patient's physician. Avoid any gingival manipulation (e.g. brushing) within 48–72 h of oral bleeding or until the platelet count shows a steady increase.

Mucosal pain

Begin with one of several topical anesthetics (e.g. benzydamine, viscous Xylocaine®, dyclonine [ilyclonine] and/or a topical anti-inflammatory (e.g. Kaopectate/Benadryl [Benadryl pectate] 50:50). Change to systemic opioids if ineffective.

Nutrition

Weight loss can be a temporary side-effect of a sore or dry mouth/ throat, nausea/vomiting, poor appetite or diarrhea. Consult with a dietitian. For sore, dry or ulcerated mouth:

- Frequent rinses with a bland solution (e.g. baking soda and water).
- Soft and/or liquid diet: ice cream and watermelon are ideal. Avoid tart or acidic foods (e.g. citrus juices and fruits, seasoning and spices), alcohol, cigarettes and very hot or cold foods. Sugarless candy [sweets] or mints can stimulate saliva production, although sharp edges can injure the oral mucosa.

CARDIOVASCULAR DISORDERS

In general, consult the patient's primary care physician or cardiologist for details concerning the cardiac condition before dental treatment. The decision on management rests with the treating dentist, who takes ultimate responsibility for such issues as antibiotic coverage.

Considerations concerning bacteremia

The oral cavity, and the gingival crevice in particular, has a large and varied population of organisms and bacteremia containing oral microorganisms are common. However, there are only anecdotal data to suggest that invasive oral procedures are a more important cause of cardiac or prosthetic infections than the chronic low-grade routine bacteremia arising from other non-professional or naturally occurring sources (e.g. tooth-brushing, chewing food).

Other considerations

- Any manipulation of the gingiva can cause a bacteremia and a single dental extraction causes a bacteremia in virtually 100% of cases.
- Routine cleaning (scaling) of teeth is likely as 'invasive' as extraction(s) with respect to causing bacteremia.

- The extent of odontogenic disease (e.g. caries, periodontitis) might not be a factor in the risk of bacteremia but is thought to increase with the number of teeth extracted because of the more prolonged and invasive procedure.
- Polymicrobial bacteremias are common during extractions.
- The usual duration of a bacteremia is at least 10 min and might be as long as an hour, depending on host factors and the volume of organisms entering the circulation. Antibacterial mouth rinses have little if any effect on the incidence of bacteremia.
- Systemic antibiotics alter the nature and reduce the incidence and duration of a bacteremia, but it is not clear to what extent antibiotics reduce the risk of distant site infection (e.g. infective endocarditis).

Infective endocarditis (IE)

This is an infection of the myocardium of the heart by circulating organisms. The mitral valve is affected more often than the aortic valve. Together, these values account for over 90% of cases of IE. Mitral valve prolapse is a common predisposing lesion. A previous history of IE and prosthetic valves puts patients at higher risk. Children have a lower prevalence of IE than adults.

Rheumatic heart disease (RHD) and cardiac murmurs

Major concerns are the identification and management of patients at risk. Rheumatic heart disease and other conditions such as mitral valve prolapse (MVP) are of greatest concern in the presence of regurgitation, and echocardiography might be necessary to rule out the need for antibiotics. If unsure, consult the patient's physician to determine if the murmur is organic or functional — the patient's verbal history is often unreliable.

If there is an organic problem or an indeterminate history, and the patient must have an invasive procedure, current guidelines suggest coverage with appropriate antibiotic prophylaxis (see Chapter 8). However, it has been suggested that risk of anaphylaxis-induced death from antibiotics is greater than the risk of infective endocarditis from no coverage in patients with some types of murmurs (e.g. mild–moderate MVP without regurgitation).

Antibiotics might lessen the likelihood of IE, although there is no proof of this, but they do not eliminate the possibility. Some references suggest that presurgical antimicrobial rinses (e.g. chlorhexidine, Listerine) reduce the risk or severity of bacteremia but the data are controversial.

Fever, malaise or a change in the nature of murmur in the first 2 weeks after an invasive dental procedure should be reported to the patient's physician.

Congenital heart disease

Congenital cardiovascular malformations can be cyanotic (dominant right-to-left shunting), non-cyanotic (dominant left-to-right shunting) or no shunting.

Cyanotic defects include tetralogy of Fallot, transposition of the great vessels, anomalies of the tricuspid valve, pulmonary atresia, pulmonary stenosis, Eisenmenger's syndrome, Ebstein's disease and hypoplastic left heart syndrome (aortic atresia). Surgical correction of these defects is often accomplished in infancy and early childhood.

Non-cyanotic defects include ventricular septal defect (VSD), coarctation of the aorta, aortic valve stenosis and mitral valve prolapse.

Considerations in dental management

- Congenital cardiac defects are associated with many syndromes (including trisomy 21 or Down syndrome), inborn errors of metabolism (e.g. homocystinuria) and connective tissue disorders (e.g. Marfan syndrome, osteogenesis imperfecta, lupus erythematosus). A careful cardiac history should be taken in these patients. Review by a cardiologist and supplemented by an echocardiogram might be prudent prior to undertaking invasive dental procedures.
- Patients might be at higher risk of developing infective endocarditis from a bacteremia and require antibiotic prophylaxis (see Chapter 8) while a cardiac defect is present and for up to 6 months after surgical correction. Discuss with the patient's physician.
- Concern for the presence of congestive heart failure leading to arrhythmia and cardiac arrest.
- Consult the patient's physician when considering sedation or with questions concerning anticoagulation, exercise tolerance, or risk from invasive/stressful procedures.

Medication

- Respiratory depressants such as opioids, barbiturates and other sedatives can worsen the cardiovascular status.
- Atropine and similar agents produce tachycardia.
- Nitrous oxide/oxygen relative analgesia can be used safely in cardiac patients, but the oxygen content must not drop below 25%.
- Use of local anesthetics with vasoconstrictors is controversial with some cardiac defects. The benefits of vasoconstrictors (e.g. more profound and longer anesthetic effect) probably outweigh the risks in most cases but restricted outflow track defects (e.g. aortic stenosis, hypertrophic cardiomyopathy) are an exception. Avoid concentrations of epinephrine > 1:100 000 [1:80 000] and restrict the volume of local anesthetics. & C of EP(n) /aspiratin syring

Cardiac/vascular prostheses

Prosthetic heart valves, (as opposed to porcine-derived valves, most commonly require life-long anticoagulation therapy, most commonly with warfarin. Discuss the implications of this with the patient's cardiologist or thoracic surgeon before treatment.

Appropriate laboratory tests for patients with cardiac prostheses are INR and APTT. Occasionally, warfarin might need to be adjusted to bring the INR within the safe range – usually INR < 3.5–4.0. The risks of decreasing the INR (stroke, thrombosis) probably outweigh any risk of prolonged bleeding from extraction(s).

Patients who have received prosthetic valves used to be considered to be at higher risk for infective endocarditis, and parenteral antibiotic regimen were preferred for such patients. However, the latest AHA guidelines, plus extensive overseas experience, indicates that properly functioning prosthetic valves are at no higher risk of infection than natural damaged valves (i.e. such as mitral regurgitation). Therefore, oral rather than parental antibiotic prophylaxis might be preferred. However, the consequences of prosthetic valve infection tend to be more catastrophic for the patient so ensure good levels of oral hygiene, and removal of any possible active sources of oral sepsis.

Cardiac pacemaker

The increased risk of cardiac infection due to a pacemaker is very low or non-existent. Use of certain electronic dental devices, including ultrasonic scalers, electric pulp testers and electrosurgery units, should be avoided because of possible interference with pacemaker function. Cell phones compete with some monitoring devices. No data exist to demonstrate a benefit from using antibiotics to prevent bacteremia-induced infection of pacemaker leads.

Angina

The major concern is to reduce the possibility of an anginal attack. Question the patient as to precipitating factors (e.g. exercise, stairs, emotional stress), frequency, duration, timing, severity of attacks and response to medication.

Elective treatment

This is reasonable if, when it occurs, the angina is stable and well controlled by 1–2 nitroglycerin tablets, and if episodes are less frequent than one per week. Avoid elective treatment if these limits are exceeded because in these cases the angina is considered unstable (labile). Crescendo (increasing frequency) angina patients are at high risk for MI. Consult the patient's physician before treatment.

Assess the vital signs at each appointment. Consider cardiac monitoring during the elective procedure, if this option is available.

The patient's nitroglycerin tablets or spray should be readily available during the procedure. If attacks are more than one per week, or if the patient is fearful, and non-elective care is planned, consider nitroglycerin use at the start of the appointment.

Stress reduction protocol

Short appointments and consideration of nitrous oxide or Versed® [midazolam] for sedation. Do not oversedate because there is a risk of hypotension. Valium is not indicated for patients over age 65 – use lorazepam or alprazolam for this age group.

Epinephrine

The use of epinephrine is controversial but the benefit to the patient of prolonged and more profound anesthesia probably outweighs the risk of increased systemic epinephrine resulting from inadequate anesthesia. For restorative treatment on elderly patients, particularly in teeth with existing restorations, pulpal discomfort is likely to be minimal; this should be discussed with patient in advance. If local is used, avoid concentrations of epinephrine greater than 1:100 000 [1:80 000] units. Aspirate prior to injection.

Myocardial infarction (MI)

The major concern is prevention of additional infarction and heart muscle damage. Consult the patient's physician concerning coronary vessel and myocardial involvement, arrhythmias, medication, the presence of other vascular disease and whether or not the patient has a pacemaker or defibrillator.

- MI within 6 months: clinical dogma and textbooks suggest that elective procedures should be avoided during this period, but this is based on data that more MIs occur during general surgery and under general anesthesia in the 6 months after an MI. Data are not available concerning the risk of outpatient dental treatment.
- MI over 6 months ago: it is advisable to consult the patient's physician.
- Warfarin: the patient may be on warfarin (Coumadin) or aspirin therapy for anticoagulation. The INR should be < 3.5–4.0 for invasive (e.g. scaling, extraction) procedures.

Avoid long and/or stressful procedures; multiple short appointments are best. Use cardiac monitoring if this is available and be cautious if using epinephrine as a vasoconstrictor in local anesthetic. Consider nitrous oxide, diazepam [or midazolam] for sedation. Be aware that gingival hyperplasia can occur with calcium channel blockers.

Coronary artery bypass graft (CABG)

The major concern is myocardial infarction. Consult the patient's physician, asking the questions outlined in the MI section above. Some clinicians feel that the same time determinants apply as for patients with a history of MI, but cardiac circulation should be much improved following surgery and there is no documented need to wait longer than 6 weeks. There is no evidence of a risk of infection of grafted coronary vessels.

Heart transplantation

The major concerns are immunosuppression and current cardiac status. Patients will be on specific T-cell suppressants, such as cyclosporin [ciclosporin], and/or other immunosuppressant drugs (i.e. the more broad-acting corticosteroids), with a correspondingly altered immune response to infection.

Bacterial endocarditis is an issue, as valve damage might follow catheterization after heart muscle biopsy for evidence of rejection. Consider using antibiotics for invasive procedures and steroid supplementation for stressful appointments. Oral candidiasis can occur secondary to steroids, and xerostomia and cyclosporin-[ciclosporin]-induced gingival hyperplasia are also problems, although the use of the anti T-cell agents tacrolimus and serolimus can lessen the severity of gingival hyperplasia associated with these agents.

Patients might be anticoagulated and should be tested for INR with warfarin and evaluated as per patients following MI.

Patients might be best managed by having dental treatment either before or after cardiac transplantation, depending on their overall status and the nature of the dental treatment. A severely compromised patient in cardiac failure is likely at greater risk from dental treatment of any kind before transplantation, in spite of the concern for post-transplant immunosuppression. Avoid elective treatment during a rejection episode.

Congestive heart failure (CHF)

You need to understand the status of the CHF. The patient will have variable levels of compensation and might be on multiple medications and dietary measures to control and balance cardiac function.

If well compensated, patients can undergo elective dental treatment. If not, treatment should wait until the patient is stable. Signs of poor compensation and high risk for stressful dental procedures include:

- Paroxysmal nocturnal dyspnea (PND): patient awakens at night short of breath as a result of pulmonary congestion.
- Orthopnea: patient might have to sleep with two or more pillows to prevent pulmonary congestion.
- Shortness of breath (SOB) or dyspnea on exertion (DOE): ask how many steps or flights of stairs the patient can climb without having to stop and rest.
- Pedal edema: this results from right heart failure. Question the patient about swollen ankles and examine for a depression left after pressing a swollen ankle with a finger (pitting edema).

- Body weight: this can fluctuate by a pound or more per day. It is used as an indicator of therapeutic measures and reflects changes in body water.

Management considerations

- Patients with orthopnea will probably have a low tolerance for the supine position in the dental chair. Consider conducting dental treatment with the patient in the upright position. As patients can have orthostatic hypotension (as a result of their medication), raise them to a sitting position in several stages over several minutes. Ask them to sit with their feet on floor for 2 min before standing upright.
- Patients might have urinary urgency during morning appointments in response to a diuretic. Ask if they would like to use the bathroom before the procedure.

Cerebrovascular accident (CVA; stroke)

CVA can be caused by:

- Thrombus of a small or large vessel (e.g. carotid): usually in people with hypertension and diabetes. It comes on more slowly than an embolus. A transient ischemic attack (TIA) might be a warning of an impending CVA.
- Embolus: usually originates from the heart or neck (bifurcation of carotid). The patient might have atrial fibrillation. The deficit is sudden and improves only slowly.
- Hemorrhage: usually spontaneous, or secondary to hypertension or aneurysm; occasionally from coagulopathy. The onset of symptoms is sudden. Be concerned about hypertensive patients on anticoagulants.

CVA presents as paralysis or weakness, often involving the facial muscles. The patient might have headache, nausea and vomiting, and numbness or paralysis of one side of the body. Confusion and aphasia (inability to speak) are also common.

Patients with CVA might be on anticoagulant (e.g. warfarin, aspirin). An INR test, in the case of warfarin, is necessary to evaluate risk of bleeding from invasive dental procedures.

Arrhythmias

There is a wide range of arrhythmias, and also of degrees of concern for dental practice. Consult with the patient's physician. The patient might be anticoagulated (because of atrial fibrillation) with an increased risk for bleeding. Arrhythmias following MI are usually managed with medication. Epinephrine is not recommended and patients should be monitored carefully during dental procedures.

Hypertension

Hypertension is defined as resting blood pressure in excess of 140 mmHg systolic and/or 90 mmHg diastolic: it is found in up to 20% of adults on random screening. Hypertension is also a problem of childhood but routine blood pressure measurement in children has a low yield.

Classification of hypertension (Table 2.3)

Major concern is precipitating hypertensive crisis, stroke or MI. Patients often show poor compliance with blood pressure medications and diet. They need reinforcement concerning the importance of medications in preventing vascular problems.

Side-effects of blood pressure medications

Side-effects of antihypertensives include orthostatic hypotension, synergistic activity with narcotics and potassium depletion. Beta-blockers will decrease the response to medications (e.g. epinephrine) used to treat anaphylaxis.

Epinephrine

The use of epinephrine in dental practice is controversial. However, the benefit from prolonged and more profound anesthesia is thought to outweigh the risk of systemic effects. Do not use concentrations greater than 1:100 000 [1:80 000]. Aspirate the syringe prior to injection and avoid intravascular injection.

When to treat

Poorly controlled or uncontrolled patients should not be treated until their hypertension is under control. Elective treatment should be avoided if the blood pressure is significantly above the patient's baseline or if > 180 mmHg systolic or > 100 mmHg diastolic. Patients in pain might have some lowering of their pressures after local anesthesia. Monitor the blood pressure before, during and after treatment.

Table 2.3 Classification and management of blood pressure for adults*

BP Classfication	SBP* mmHg	DBP* mmHg	Lifestyle Modification	Initial drug therapy Without compelling indication	With compelling indications
Normal	< 120	and < 80	Encourage		
Pre-hypertension	120–139	or 80–89	Yes	No anti-hypertensive drug indicated.	Drug(s) for compelling indications[‡]
Stage 1 Hypertension	140–159	or 90–99	Yes	Thiazide-type diuretics for most. May consider ACEI, ARB, BB, CCB, or combination.	Drug(s) for the compelling indications.[‡] Other anti-hypersentive drugs (diuretics, ACEI, ARB, BB, CCB) as needed.
Stage 2 Hypertension	≥ 160	or ≥ 100	Yes	Two-drug combination for most[†] (usually thiazide-type diuretic and ACEI or ARB or BB or CCB).	

DBP, diastolic pressure; SBP, systolic blood pressure.
Drug abbreviations: ACEI, angiotensin converting enzyme imhibitor; ARB, angiotensin receptor blocker; BB, beta-blocker; CCB, calcium channel blocker.
* Treatment determined by highest BP category.
† Initial combined therapy should be used cautiously in those at risk for orthostatic hypotension.
‡ Treat patients with chronic kidney disease or diabetes to BP goal of < 130/80 mmHg.
From: National Heart, Lung, and Blood Institute (NHLBI), National Institutes of Health, and the US Department of Health and Human Services. Reproduced with permission.

DIABETES MELLITUS

Major concerns in dental management are preventing hypoglycemia and the poor response to dental and periodontal infections. Issues of increased risk of oral infection and impaired wound healing are controversial.

Classification

- Type 1 (formerly insulin-dependent or juvenile onset): patients produce little or no insulin. This type accounts for about 10% of all diabetics. There is a greater tendency to ketoacidosis than with type 2.
- Type 2 (formerly non-insulin-dependent or adult onset): non-ketosis-prone diabetes; the insulin receptors display diminished sensitivity to insulin.

Significant elements in history

- Age of onset.
- Compliance with therapy.
- Symptoms: excessive thirst, nocturia, malaise, decreased appetite leading to nausea, vomiting, hyperpnea, and coma (diabetic acidosis).
- Treatment: make a note of the patient's diet, insulin dosage, route, frequency and timing of injection. The type of insulin should also be noted, including newer forms of insulin, such as Humalog, which is taken with meals and Lantus, which produces even levels of insulin over a 24-h period (Table 2.4). Some patients might use an insulin pump to deliver steady doses of insulin.
- Admission: record any hospital admissions for uncontrolled state (e.g. insulin reactions, diabetic coma).
- Problems with infection: admission might be indicated for type 1 patients with severe oral infection.

Hyperglycemia

Hyperglycemia can result in diabetic coma, which can be severe, with the patient in a hyperosmolar state. The patient will show poly-

Table 2.4 **Types and durations of insulin therapy**

Type of subcutaneous insulin	Effect begins (hours)	Maximum action (hours)	Action effect (hours)
Regular (crystalline)	0.25	2–5	6–8
Semilente	0.5	4–6	10–12
NPH	3	8–12	18–24
Lente	3	8–12	18–24
Ultra Lente	3–4	16–20	30–36

dipsia, polyphagia and polyuria (the 'polys'); there might also be abdominal pain, nausea unconsciousness.

Signs include a flushed face, dry skin, dry mouth, weakness, dehydration, Kussmaul (very deep and rapid) respirations, elevated pulse, decreased blood pressure and lethargy.

Hyperglycemia can occur as a result of an infection (most common), weight gain, pregnancy, hyperthyroidism, steroids, fever, dehydration or non-compliance with medical care. It can lead to impaired granulocyte phagocytosis and chemotaxis. Data are unclear as to risks for postoperative infection following dental procedures.

Hyperglycemia can progress to ketoacidosis and coma over several hours or days in patients with type 1 diabetes mellitus.

Treatment
Early recognition and basic life support if indicated. Sugar solution by mouth if awake or IV glucose if unable to give by mouth (to distinguish from insulin shock). Get medical assistance.

Hypoglycemia – insulin shock

Loss of consciousness (LOC) occurs rapidly if the blood glucose falls to < 50 mg/100 cc. Common causes of hypoglycemia are omission or delay of meals, excessive exercise prior to meals, overdose of insulin or oral hypoglycemic agents, and stress. Hypoglycemia usually appears first as decreased cerebral function, mental confusion, headache, dizziness, changes in mood, hunger, nausea, increased epinephrine activity (sweating, tachycardia, piloerection, increased anxiety) as an endogenous reaction to raise blood glucose. The patient can appear intoxicated and might progress to unconsciousness, convulsions and coma.

Treatment
- Early recognition.
- Give the patient oral or parenteral simple carbohydrates.
- Basic life support.
- Get medical assistance.

Management considerations

In well controlled diabetes

- Patients should be scheduled for morning appointments and receive their normal insulin dose if they are able to eat after the procedure, otherwise reduce the insulin dose.
- Ensure that patient has eaten a normal breakfast, supplemented with orange or other sugar-containing juice.
- Have glucose available during the treatment.
- Antibiotic coverage is usually not indicated for surgical procedures. Although there is *in vivo* evidence to suggest an increased risk of infection (from decreased neutrophil function) this is not evident clinically. However, diabetics do not tolerate infection well and their management can be complicated by even asymptomatic oral infection (e.g. generalized periodontitis).
- Resume normal insulin and oral intake immediately after the procedure.

In poorly controlled diabetes

- Consult the patient's physician and consider hospitalization for extensive periodontal or oral surgical procedures.
- Avoid stressful procedures.
- Although antibiotic coverage is often recommended for surgical procedures, there are no data to support this practice. Anticipate slower healing.
- Insulin requirement might be affected by poor tolerance for oral infection or generalized periodontal disease: insulin dose might need to be adjusted after treatment.
- Be aware that type 1 diabetics might have significant atherosclerotic deposits at a younger age than non-diabetics and can therefore have asymptomatic, but significant, vascular disease at an earlier age. Diabetes is the major reason for kidney disease under the age of 25 and the main cause for dialysis at any age.
- Children with type I diabetes must be managed carefully in close coordination with their physician. Adolescents pose a risk of a 'honeymoon' period and then a denial phase.

DRUG ABUSE

The patient's history and medical chart are important for determining the nature of the drugs and the degree of abuse.

Treatment considerations

- Keep meticulous records. Prescription numbers should be written out to avoid forgeries (e.g. 'Disp: 10 (ten) tabs').
- There is an increased incidence of hepatitis and human immuno-deficiency virus (HIV) in parenteral abusers. Liver function and coagulation tests should be checked for decreased drug metabolism, coagulopathy and possible chronic hepatitis.
- There is an increased risk of cardiac problems: infective endo-carditis, arrhythmias, dyspnea, orthopnea and murmurs.
- The risk of interaction between prescribed and abused drug(s) should be discussed with the patient.
- Rampant caries can occur as a result of xerostomia, excess refined carbohydrates in diet, poor oral hygiene and overall neglect.
- It is possible that the patient will be suffering from accompanying psychiatric illness. Have assistance available if needed.
- Do not do elective procedures on patients who are under the influence of cocaine. Cocaine can potentiate cardiac arrhythmias in the presence of certain drugs (e.g. epinephrine).
- Tattoos and body piercing indicate increased likelihood of hematogenous viral disease.

ALCOHOLISM

Management considerations

- Morning appointments are best.
- A patient who is uncooperative or incoherent should not be treated because of the risk of injury, decreased gag reflex and problems of informed consent.
- Screens: bleeding potential (PT/INR to cover vitamin-K-dependent factors II, VII, IX, X), hepatitis screen, liver function tests; HIV (if indicated).
- A history of delirium tremens or gastrointestinal bleeding is important.
- There is a possible increased risk of oral cancer; this is greatly increased if there is concurrent tobacco use.
- Avoid using opioids.

FEVER OF UNKNOWN ORIGIN (FUO)

Evaluation for an oral source is important for a patient with true FUO, that is, a fever that is over 3 weeks duration and has no other identified source. Although asymptomatic oral infection is rarely a documented source of FUO in non-immunosuppressed patients, it is difficult to rule out an oral source. Evaluation should include:

- A thorough oral exam to include periodontal probing, evaluation of salivary ducts and percussion of teeth.
- Full mouth radiographs with apical imaging to help exclude odontogenic infection, caries and/or periodontitis.
- Correlation of the clinical findings with the oral symptoms, laboratory values (e.g. WBC and differential), systemic disease, other culture results and fever curve.

Remember that FUO in disabled children is rarely the result of dental infection and far more often the result of dehydration or aspiration pneumonia/respiratory infection.

HUMAN IMMUNODEFICIENCY VIRUS (HIV) INFECTION

HIV is a lymphotropic virus that infects the T4 (CD4) lymphocytes. Its routes of transmission include sexual contact, vertical transmission (from mother to fetus at birth), contaminated needles and transfusion of contaminated blood or blood products (usually pre-1985).

Without antiviral treatment, HIV leads to acquired immunodeficiency syndrome (AIDS), with widespread and severe defects in cell-mediated immunity, and consequent opportunistic infections:

- Viral infections: herpes simplex, varicella, Epstein–Barr, cytomegalovirus and Kaposi-associated virus (HHV-8).
- Fungal infections: candida and other less common species.
- Protozoal infections: *Pneumocystis carinii*, toxoplasmosis and cyptococcus.
- Mycobacterium infections: including atypical species (*Mycobacterium avium*).

In addition to the late-development endothelial cell (Kaposi's sarcoma; KS) and lymphoid malignancies, HIV-related encephalopathy and wasting syndrome can also occur. The time from infection to the development of AIDS, which is defined as an opportunistic infection or malignancy or T4 cell count less than 200/mm^3 can be greater than 10 years.

Antibody detected with ELISA and Western blot blood tests is usually present within 12 weeks of infection. The presence of the antibody does not mean the patient has AIDS.

Treatment

Since the introduction of protease inhibitors in the mid-1990s, optimum therapy has consisted of multiple antiretroviral agents, commonly referred to as highly affective antiretroviral therapy (HAART). At present, treatment is aimed at prevention (often by prophylaxis of opportunistic infections), slowing of viral spread and preventing the destruction of the main regulatory cells of the cell-mediated immune system – the CD4 cells – by using a combination of antiviral agents that inhibit the virus at crucial times in its synthesis and replication.

HAART

The combination of drugs used in HAART is made up of nucleoside retroviral inhibitors, non-nucleoside retroviral inhibitors and proteases. Although no effective vaccine is currently available, trials of a unique DNA vaccine that holds great promise are underway. Traditional nucleoside analogs such as: zidovudine (AZT; Retrovir®); didanosine (DDI; Videx®); dideoxycytidine (DDC; Zalcitabine®); stavudine (D4T; Zerit®) and abacavir (ABC; Ziagen®) are used in combination with non-nucleoside reverse transcriptase inhibitors: nevirapine (Viramune®); delavirdine (Rescriptor®), and efavirenz (Sustiva®) and/or protease inhibitors: indinavir (Crixivan®); nelfinavir (Viracept®); amprenavir (Agenerase®); ritonavir (Norvir®); saquinavir (Invirase®; Fortavase®) and lopinavir/ritonavir (Kaletra®) to suppress viral replication and thus maintain or improve immune system function (T4 count). Side-effects/toxicities are common and patient non-adherence is a problem. Non-adherence leads to drug-resistant mutations in HIV strains, thereby reducing antiretroviral drug effectiveness in some individuals. *Pneumocystis carinii* pneumonia (PCP) prophylaxis, which is common in patients with < 200

T4 cells, is accomplished with trimethoprim–sulfamethoxazole [sulfamethoxazole] or pentamidine.

Infection control precautions

These are as for hepatitis B and C. There is an increasing incidence of multidrug-resistant tuberculosis (MDR-TB) in patients and AIDS patients can be anergic and therefore do not respond to the TB (PPD) skin test.

Management considerations

- Oral hygiene: good oral hygiene is necessary to prevent periodontal infection. Aggressive management of HIV-associated periodontal diseases is debridement using Betadine® or chlorhexidine irrigation; consider metronidazole or amoxicillin therapy for 5–7 days after debridement.
- Antibiotic cover: consider brief antibiotic coverage for invasive procedures if neutrophil counts are < 500 cells/µL because there is an increased risk of fungal overgrowth with prolonged antibiotics. The literature suggests a low incidence of complication following extractions.
- Falling T4 count: watch for signs of a falling T4 count, (e.g. hairy leukoplakia, oral candida, Kaposi's sarcoma, lymphoma). Salivary gland enlargement, non-healing ulcerations, acute necrotizing periodontitis, and herpes simplex infection can occur.
- Low T4 count: a T4 count < 500 increases concern for secondary problems but oral manifestations do not usually occur above 300. The CD4 is a fair marker of patient's overall condition but neutrophil counts are better indicator of the ability to withstand invasive procedures. Quantitative HIV levels are a better predictor of viremia and viral disease progression. HIV viral load is quantified as number of HIV RNA copies/cc plasma using reverse transcriptase polymerase chain reaction (RT-PCR) technology. The goal of HAART is to achieve and maintain an undetectable (< 50 copies/cc) viral load.
- Fungal infections: require aggressive management for a longer than normal duration. Recurrence of infection is common. Consider miconazole or Mycelex® troche (1 tablet 5× a day) if the T4 count is high and not widespread throughout the mouth. Systemic medication (e.g. fluconazole, Diflucan®) might be necessary if

there is no response to Mycelex® within 24–48 h. Consult the patient's physician if the patient is refractory to oral antifungal agents.
- Children: children with HIV often have extensive oral health needs as a result of their lower socioeconomic status.

INTELLECTUAL DISABILITY

This includes a wide variety of conditions (such as Down, fragile X and other syndromes), pervasive developmental disorders (autism and schizophrenia), attention deficit hyperactivity disorder (ADHD) and microcephaly. In addition, physical impairments such as cerebral palsy and spina bifida can have an accompanying defect in intellectual functioning. A large number of people will have an intellectual impairment of unknown origin.

Down syndrome

This is one of the most commonly occurring syndromes with intellectual impairment as the characterizing feature. It is a chromosomal disorder with three distinct aberrations: trisomy, translocation and mosaicism. In trisomy 21 there are 47 chromosomes, with three in place of the usual two at chromosome 21. In translocation the additional 21 chromosome is translocated to chromosome 15; mosaicism is as a result of non-disjunction. It occurs at chromosome 21 and arises as a mistake rather than a meiotic event.

Down syndrome is characterized by:
- congenital cardiac anomalies
- impaired immune systems
- altered craniofacies
- and increased risk of celiac disease (3.6%) and acute lymphoid and non-lymphoid leukemia, as well as gastric and testicular cancer in males. Otherwise, the standardized mortality ratios for other tumor types are low, patients have fewer atherosclerotic risk factors (reduced insulin resistance syndrome) with lower fasting plasma glucose and systolic blood pressure.

Dental considerations
- Fifty per cent will have CHD (endocardial cushion defect, ventricular septal defect (VSD), tetralogy of Fallot) and, along with

gastrointestinal and other malformations and infections, account for a significantly increased rate of hospital admissions. Many of the patients with CHD will require antibiotic coverage for invasive procedures (see above).

- Most children with Down syndrome are functionally independent, apart from the need for support and supervision for communication, tasks relating to social skills and complex items of self-care.
- Young people are at risk for arthritis, diabetes, neck subluxation (as a result of congenital laxity of the transverse ligament between the atlas and odontoid processes of the vertebrae and the atlas and occipital condyles at the base of skull), and so are vulnerable during general anesthesia – exercise care when handling or fit a neck collar.
- Obesity is an issue in older patients and might preclude general anesthesia as an adjunct. Adults are also at higher than normal risk of dementia, at widely varying ages, because of factors influencing beta-amyloid. The risk of cardiac disease is increased in up to 71% of older Down syndrome patients, with mitral valve prolapse in 52%, associated tricuspid valve prolapse in 14% and aortic regurgitation in 12%. The prevalence of hepatitis B, especially in those people living in residential care, is also higher than normal.
- Seizures are commonplace and psychiatric and behavioral problems assume a greater significance than normal.

Oral and dental features

Orally and dentally, features observed are:
- Relative midface hypoplasia.
- A mongoloid slant to eyes.
- A tendency to squints. The epicanthic folds are prominent and there are brushfield spots on the iris.
- Tongue protrusion/open mouth posture: observe for angular cheilitis and lip fissuring (candidal infection).
- Intraorally the vault of the palate may be high. A relative class III malocclusion might be present.
- Retention of primary teeth is common, with delay in shedding lasting into the third decade (and sometimes longer) and delay in eruption or agenesis of successor teeth.
- Periodontal disease is relatively more common, resulting in tooth mobility and early loss due to impaired phagocytic function of

monocytes and neutrophils as well as enhanced PGE_2 production, increased activity of plasminogen activators and thus collagenase activity.
- The teeth might be diminutive, hypoplastic and worn – attrition and erosion – due to grinding and reflux/acidogenic diet, respectively.

Fragile X syndrome

Observe similar precautions as for Down syndrome with respect to risk of CHD (mitral valve prolapse). Affected males and heterozygous females can show signs of autistic behavior.

Autism

This is a range of childhood psychiatric, organically based neuro-developmental disorders with pre- or perinatal insults and chromosomal abnormalities as possible etiological factors. Autism is characterized by abnormal development before 3 years of age.

Features
- Impairment of social interaction, communication and repetitive and stereotyped patterns of behavior.
- Males affected (the male:female ratio is 4:1).
- Associated conditions include intellectual impairment (in 70–90% of cases), epilepsy (in 25–30%), fragile X syndrome (in 2–8%) and tuberous sclerosis (in 1–3%).
- Function in certain areas can be very high in the Asperger's syndrome variant.

Treatment
Cure is not possible but intensive behavioral therapy, instituted early in a child's life, might be beneficial. Drugs used in the treatment of autism include methylphenidate hydrochloride (a CNS stimulant that interacts with anticonvulsants), thioridazine (an anti-psychotic that enhances the antimuscarinic effects of other drugs), diphenhydramine hydrochloride (a sedative thought to be linked with narcolepsy, possibly to porphyria and perhaps even to sudden

infant death syndrome); and anticonvulsants, depending on the type of seizure control required.

Dental considerations

Any significant behavioral disturbances will need to be taken account of. There is a need for patience and routine, which might not be feasible in the emergency room. Elective approaches involve behavior shaping and drug therapy. Medication might interfere with drugs used in dental procedures (see above).

Attention deficit hyperactivity disorder (ADHD)

This developmental disorder affects 3–5% of school-aged children in the US. The male:female ratio is 3:1.2.

Features

There is an early onset (between 3 and 4 years). The children have normal IQ but poor sustained attention, impaired impulse control or delay of gratification. There is excessive task-irrelevant activity (flitting from one thing to another) and poor auditory memory – they cannot retain lengthy instructions.

Management

Behavior modification, educational and pharmacological measures:
- psychostimulants (methylphenidate hydrochloride if the child is over 6 years of age)
- dexamphetamine: side-effects are anorexia, sleep problems, irritability, abdominal pain and headaches
- clonidine (an antihypertensive)
- antidepressants (e.g. SSRIs, TCAs, MAOIs)
- neuroleptics.

LIVER AND SPLEEN

Hepatitis

Hepatitis A. Also known as infectious hepatitis, hepatitis A is spread primarily via a fecal–oral route. The incubation time is 2–6 weeks.

Some people display lifetime immunity. There is no known carrier state and hepatitis is rarely, if ever, fatal or parenterally transmitted.

Hepatitis B. Also known as serum hepatitis. Hepatitis B is transmitted primarily by parenteral inoculation, but it can also be spread by saliva, nasopharyngeal washings, semen, menstrual fluid, vaginal secretions, razors or toothbrushes; and also vertically (mother to fetus). Over half of dialysis patients are chronic carriers and have a persisting concentration of hepatitis B surface antigen. Unlike hepatitis A, the incubation period is 2–6 months. Five per cent of people infected develop chronic active hepatitis, 5–10% are carriers for 1–6 months and 2% are carriers for life. Factors that increase the risk of exposure include drug abuse, long-term residential or institutional care, transfusions of blood and blood products, newborns of women with hepatitis B, recent immigrants from south-east Asia.

Hepatitis C. Also known as transfusion-associated hepatitis, hepatitis C accounts for the majority of non-A, and non-B hepatitis. It is often transfusion associated and there is a high prevalence among injecting drug-users. Sexual partners and household contacts are at risk of infection. The incubation period is from 6–9 weeks to 6 months. There is an icteric period with anorexia, nausea, right upper quadrant pain for 6–8 weeks. Eighty per cent are chronic carriers and most improve in 2–3 years. However, 20% develop cirrhosis and in 1% of cases infection is fatal.

Hepatitis D (delta virus). The epidemiology, transmission and concern in dental practice are the same as for HBV and HCV. Transmission is parenteral, through blood–blood contact and via sexual intercourse. HBV vaccine also protects against HDV.

Clinical symptoms
- Gastrointestinal: nausea, vomiting, severe anorexia and a flu-like fever.
- Jaundice: can occur within a few days of the prodromal symptoms.
- Extrahepatic: possibly as a result of circulating immune complexes:
  - transient serum-sickness-like symptoms: urticaria, rash, poly-arthralgia or arthritis. These generally occur 1–6 weeks prior to the onset of clinical symptoms

- polyarteritis nodosa
- glomerulonephritis.

Differential diagnosis

Exclude biliary obstruction, primary biliary cirrhosis, Wilson's disease, alcoholic hepatitis, drug toxicity and drug hypersensitivity.

Laboratory tests

- Serum aspartate aminotransferase (AST or SGOT) and alanine aminotransferase (ALT or SGPT).
- Hepatitis B antigen test, hepatitis C test.
- Bilirubin.
- Blood tests:
  - total protein
  - WBC: often leukopenic; possible have lymphocytosis
  - serum albumin: decreased
  - serum globulin: increased
  - LDH
  - alkaline phosphatase.
- Liver biopsy.

Management considerations

- Hepatitis A and B: almost all hepatitis A (and over 85% of hepatitis B) patients resolve completely:
  - hepatitis B surface antigen persists in the remainder
  - cases are often mild or subclinical with only increased transaminase levels
  - carriers might be without a history of hepatitis and might have normal liver function tests
  - hepatitis B surface antigen is found in acute or chronic cases of hepatitis B, and also in healthy carriers
  - hepatitis B surface antigen concentration in patients with acute hepatitis B is usually transient. If it persists more than 4 months then a chronic disease state is possible.
- Hepatitis C (non-A, non-B hepatitis): can be transmitted by 0.0001 cc plasma. Infection rate is 1 in 27 parenteral exposures.
- Avoid elective treatment on active hepatitis patients.
- Evaluate liver function prior to prescribing certain medications (e.g. diazepam) because of poor drug metabolism. This also applies to some local anesthetics, analgesics, sedatives and antibiotics.

Liver-dependent factors involved in hemostasis should be checked prior to surgery; the PT/INR test is the most valuable.

Course of the disease

Hepatitis A. Peak virus levels are present in the stool 6–11 days before liver abnormalities are detectable. In the acute stage, there is a brief hepatitis A surface antigen viremia as well as increased levels in liver, stool and bile. The patient is most infective 2 weeks before jaundice appears until 2 weeks after jaundice disappears.

Hepatitis B. Generally lasts less than 10 weeks, although some patients remain carriers. There is a 5–20% likelihood of relapse. Hepatitis B surface antigen is detected with onset of clinical symptoms. Hepatitis B surface antibodies appear 3–6 weeks later.

Prevention

Hepatitis A
- Virus is stable at room temperature for 1 h, and for years when frozen.
- Hand-washing after bowel movements and before meals.
- 0.5% NaOCl (1:10 Clorox®), autoclaving at 100°C for 5 min, and ultraviolet light for 1 min at 1.1 W will inactivate hepatitis A virus.
- Immune serum globulin (ISG) offers 80–90% likelihood of passive protection if it is given within 1–2 weeks of exposure. However, it is useless 6 weeks after exposure.

Hepatitis B and C
- Methods of inactivating hepatitis B virus: 0.5% NaOC1 with low concentration of protein, 5.0% of NaOCl with whole sera for 3 min, autoclaving at 100°C for 10 min, ethylene oxide, 2% activated glutaraldehyde solutions yielding a pH of 2.4 for 6 h.
- Instruments must be washed well before sterilizing. Disposable syringes and needles should be used.
- Handpiece lines should be flushed with 1% sodium hypochlorite solution.
- Specific hepatitis B immune serum globulin, which contains high concentrations of hepatitis B surface antibodies, is useful if exposed to the virus. Immune serum globulin is of little value in hepatitis B surface antigen exposure.

The wearing of masks, gloves and protective eyewear is recommended with all patients, regardless of known medical status.

All cases of hepatitis, especially hepatitis B, should be reported to public health officials. If a hepatitis B surface antigen carrier is identified, he or she should be educated on the methods of transmission.

Liver failure and transplantation

Pretransplant considerations

- Poor drug metabolism: use caution with drugs metabolized in the liver.
- Bleeding disorders from decreased liver-dependent factors, and a low platelet count.
- Impaired wound healing.

Post-transplant considerations

- Immunosuppression: increased risk for infection even though T-cells are targeted. Bacteremia and sepsis should be avoided, particularly in the 6 months following transplant when immunosuppressive agents are given in high doses.
- Adrenal suppression secondary to the use of prednisone.

Asplenia

The functions of the spleen are filtration and immunologic destruction and processing; it removes unwanted red cells, intracellular debris and organisms. It is an important source of IgM antibodies and opsonins.

The lack of a spleen can be congenital, the result of infarcts or the result of surgical removal. Some splenectomized patients are predisposed to infection, although this is rare in patients who are otherwise healthy. About half of the infections are caused by *Streptococcus pneumonia* and the other half by *Staphylococcus aureus*, group A streptococci, *Haemophilus influenza* and *Neisseria meningitides*. Children can be at greater risk for the above infections.

No data exist to implicate dental treatment as a cause of systemic infection in splenectomized patients. However, antibiotic coverage is justified in splenectomized patients with primary disease such as Cooley's anemia, Wiskott–Aldrich syndrome, histiocytosis and lipidosis.

Glycogen storage diseases

Glycogen storage diseases are the result of a deficiency of enzyme system(s) involved in glycogen metabolism. They involve the liver and cause hepatomegaly, except types V and VII – muscle and/or RBCs. Ten different types have been identified. Patients have hypoglycemia, lactic acidosis, hyperlipidemia, hyperuricemia and a bleeding tendency (impaired platelet function and prolonged bleeding time).

Oral/dental considerations
- Severe periodontal disease and oral ulceration (defects in neutrophils and decreased chemotaxis).
- High/frequent NMES diet (complex carbohydrates and cornstarch dietary supplements) and caries risk.

Investigations
Blood chemistry and liver biopsy.

NEUROLOGIC DISORDERS

Neural tube defects – hydrocephalus

Neural tube defects result from the non-fusion of one or more posterior vertebral arches and/or protrusion of meninges. Accompanying hydrocephalus (caused by obstruction to the circulation of CSF) is present in 95% of cases. Patients with hydrocephalus, unless arrested, have a shunt fitted with a valve to control the flow of CSF from the ventricles.

Between 50 and 60% of cases are genetic, with the remainder being caused by environmental factors, teratogens, and so on. Neural tube defects are more common in females than in males. Epilepsy is present in 25% of people with neural tube defects and 30% have intellectual impairment.

Types
- Spina bifida occulta: (seen only on X-ray): apparent in 50% of unaffected children, and of no consequence.
- Spina bifida cystica: meningocele (meninges protrude through vertebrae in sac, this rarely produces a neurological defect but

20% might have hydrocephalus) and myelomeningocele (spinal cord protrudes into the sac, usually in the thorax–lumbar region, at motor level L3 and above).

Consequences

Flaccid paralysis, spinal deformity (severe kyphosis or scoliosis), loss of sensation, neurogenic bladder.

Dental considerations

- Prevention of dental disease is crucial. Patients might be taking antibiotics as prophylaxis for persistent UTIs.
- Antibiotic cover is required for ventriculoatrial shunts only, not for ventriculoperitoneal shunts.
- Be aware of the potential for latex allergy depending on the material used for the patient's shunt. There is an above average occurrence of latex allergy due to intermittent/continuous catheterization.
- Handling and moving skills need to be learned for safe transfer of patients from wheelchair to dental chair, preferably with a hoist or wheelchair adaptation of dental unit. Patients should be moved regularly, especially if there is a tendency to pressure sores.
- Scoliosis can produce problems of ventilation and are a consideration if general anesthesia is planned.

Parkinson's disease

Significance of the problem

This progressive degenerative disease affects approximately 1 million Americans, nearly all of whom are over the age of 50. It involves dopamine-producing nerve termini of the corpus striatum. Major effects on dental status include impaired oral hygiene and poor control of oral secretions. Symptoms that can affect dental care include uncontrollable tremor (worsened by anxiety), rigidity (compromising transfer, mouth opening, and chair and head positioning) and impaired control of the airway.

Management considerations

- Impaired self-care: involve caregiver (spouse, relative, nurse) in oral hygiene instructions and insertion/removal/care of prostheses. Fluoride rinses/gels and frequent recalls will aid preservation of the dentition.

- Tremor and rigidity: schedule dental appointments approximately 2 h after antiparkinsonian medications (e.g. levodopa, carbidopa, amantadine, bromocriptine). Employ mouth props and moldable cervical pillows.
- Swallowing dysfunction/airway control: keep patients as upright as possible. Use rubber dam whenever possible; employ high-volume suction. The patient might already have a fine-bore suction to help clear secretions from the airway.

Seizures and epilepsy

A sign or illness characterized by recurrent, unprovoked seizures; it affects 0.4% of the population. Distinguish from reflex anoxic seizures, vasovagal syncope, breath-holding attacks, migraine, cardiac arrhythmias, Munchausen's syndrome and 'pseudo' seizures, all of which are provoked. Epilepsy is caused by brain damage, CVA, brain tumors, alcohol intoxication or idiopathic (25% cases).

Etiology

There are many causes (including trauma, fever, tumor, stroke, epilepsy, diabetes, alcoholism and hyponatremia/kalemia). Children with a specific epilepsy syndrome will have a cause identified in 25–30% of cases only. There is a genetic predisposition: one parent affected results in a 4% chance; both parents affected to a 10–14% chance. Genetic conditions associated with increased prevalence include Sturge–Weber, Down and fragile X syndromes. Other conditions with seizures as a feature are cerebral palsy, tuberous sclerosis, von Recklinghausen's neurofibromatosis and IEM. Brain tumors are responsible for 1–2% of childhood epilepsy.

Types of seizure

Partial (focal) seizure

- Types: simple and complex.
- Signs: autonomic manifestations common. Face flushing, drooling, increased blood pressure and pulse, urination (differentiates from syncope).
- Has post-ictal phase after seizure. Patient is confused and with headache (this is not seen with syncope).

Generalized seizures

- Major motor seizures: the most common of which are tonic:clonic seizures (grand mal). Symptoms are loss of consciousness first

followed by apnea ('epileptic cry' as air is expressed), jaw muscle contraction, eyes move up, dilated pupils, high amplitude/frequency movement of all extremities for 3–7 min.
- Absence seizures: in children aged between 2 and 9 years. Duration 6–8 s. Can occur 30–80 times/day. Staring is the main symptom. They might be precipitated by hyperventilation. EEG has classic findings.

Significant elements in the history
- Type of seizure and frequency.
- Medication: type, dose, frequency and compliance.
- Precipitating factors: stress, pain, fever, anxiety, etc.
- Occur despite medications, or only when medications are not taken.
- 'Aura' before seizures: not a common phenomenon.
- Loss of consciousness.
- Facial trauma from falling.

Dental management considerations
- No contraindications to routine dental care. Consult the patient's physician.
- Condition active if seizures reported within the preceding 2 years.
- Awareness of staff of potential for seizure, which is usually self-limiting. Patients should be well controlled on medications for elective dental treatment. Check level of seizure control at each dental visit and potential for other drug interactions (e.g. aspirin, NSAIDs, antifungals and phenytoin; erythromycin with carbamazepine and valproate).
- Up to 70% of people can be managed on one drug alone. Consider obtaining blood levels of medications prior to involved surgical procedures.
- All anesthetic agents are cerebral irritants. Nitrous oxide sedation is safer.
- Seizures that are prolonged are considered status epilepticus, which is a medical emergency.
- Scrupulous oral hygiene necessary to help control gingival hyperplasia with certain antiepileptics.
- Be aware of the side-effects of seizure control drugs, such as oral ulceration with ethosuximide, benzodiazepines (e.g. clonazepam) and midazolam/flumazenil. Common problems with current drugs are sedation, pharmacokinetic interactions, teratogenesis and, in the longer term, weight gain, gingival hypertrophy and seizures despite combination therapy.

- Altered bone turnover/density: can be due to underlying seizure history or medication.
- Note platelet effects of valproate and bleeding potential after surgery. Preventive care is vital because of medication effects (xerostomia, sugar-based liquid oral medicines, gingival hypertrophy, potential for dental trauma).

Outlook

Between 70 and 80% of people progress to seizure-free episodes but 50% of these need maintenance drugs. Mortality rate is increased depending on the etiology and type of seizure. Death occurs due to status epilepticus, accidents during a seizure, drug effects, asphyxiation/bronchopneumonia due to aspiration and cardiac-related causes in 1:200–1200 epileptics annually.

Cerebral palsy (CP)

This is a significant cause of physical impairment acquired pre-, peri- or postnatally. There are six movement forms:
- spastic: hypertonic (70%)
- athetoid (16–20%)
- ataxic
- rigid
- hypotonia
- mixed.

These range in their effects depending on the extent of cerebral damage: one limb (monoplegic) or all limbs (quadriplegic).

The use of nitrous oxide sedation or oral benzodiazepines might reduce muscle hypertonicity, as will well-positioned supports. Some patients are prescribed intramuscular botulinum A injection to improve limb function. Conditions often associated with CP include epilepsy, intellectual impairment, sensory and emotional disorders, speech and communication defects and dysphagia (care in aspiration to avoid choking). Many patients with CP exhibit failure to thrive and supplemental feeding (high in NMES) and/or placement of a gastrostomy tube (PEG) is indicated. The latter might exacerbate gastroesophageal reflux disease (GERD) and cause dental erosion.

Dental considerations

- Periodontal disease (gastrostomy tube feeding increases prevalence of calculus if no oral intake occurs). Calculus should be removed because of a reported increase in aspiration pneumonia.

- Drug-induced gingival overgrowth.
- Untreated malocclusions.
- Enamel hypoplasia.
- Tooth wear (bruxism, GERD leading to erosion).
- Drooling/decreased parotid flow: CP patients with surgical correction (duct repositioning/ligation, salivary gland ablation) for drooling might have parotitis, rampant caries, especially of lower incisors and paradoxical hypersalivation.

Dementia

Significance of dementia

A progressive degenerative neurological syndrome characterized by loss of short- and long-term memory, impaired reasoning and personality change (including paranoid delusions and strong aversions to unfamiliar people, locations and situations).

Features of dementia

Patients eventually progress to total dependence, inability to communicate and, ultimately, coma and death. Dementia affects approximately 5% of those over age 65, and 20–45% of those over age 85. Approximately 50% of cases are termed Alzheimer's disease, in which degeneration in function is correlated with insoluble protein plaques and neuritic tangles in the cerebral cortex. The second most common cause involves multiple small infarcts ('multi-infarct dementia') (< 1 cm^3) in the cerebral cortex.

Alzheimer's disease (AD)

AD accounts for 50% of cases of dementia in older people (5% of people aged > 65 years and 20% > 85 years). Cases are sporadic but there might be an AD inheritance; genetic interest in the apolipoprotein E locus. Early brain trauma might be an etiological factor.

Presenting features

- Loss of short-term memory initially.
- Personality changes (frontal lobe involvement).
- Purposeful wandering secondary to memory loss.
- Confusion (due to delirium, dementia, depression).
- Deterioration of personal hygiene – may be dyspraxia related.

- Loss of language skills.
- Immobility.
- Incontinence.
- Generalized wasting of whole body.

AD should be distinguished from vascular dementia and dementia with Lewy bodies.

Investigations

- Clinical history.
- Mental state exam.
- Cognition tests: MMSE (Mini Mental State Examination) as a baseline for efficacy of treatments.
- Physical exam: exclude other causes of apparent dementia – thyroid dysfunction, benign cerebral tumors.
- Bloods and U+Es; thyroid, liver and renal function tests; vitamin B_{12} and folate deficiency.

Treatment

- Cholinesterase inhibitors monitored 3-monthly with MMSE tests.
- Other potential drug therapies: hormone replacement therapy (HRT), anti-inflammatory drugs, high-dose vitamin E. No clinical trials support alternative therapies as yet.

Dental management considerations

Impaired self care

Involve caregiver (spouse, relative, nurse, etc.) in oral hygiene instructions and insertion/removal/care of prostheses. Fluoride rinse/gels, salivary substitute if indicated. Frequent recalls.

Adverse behavior

Attempt non-pharmacological management strategies first. Schedule treatment at a time of day when the patient is known to display most cooperative behaviors. Have a familiar person (e.g. spouse, nurse) present, at least initially. Explain upcoming treatment steps in concrete, simple terms, one step at a time (e.g. 'I am going to put something cold into your mouth. Now I am going to pull on your cheek'). Minimize distractions such as conversation not involving patient, music, interruptions, etc. If this approach fails, consider oral, short half-life anxiolytic drugs such as alprazolam, lorazepam or oxazepam. In advanced or otherwise unmanageable cases, sedation or even general anesthesia might be necessary.

Progressive cognitive decline

Self-care and ability to cooperate in the dental environment will likely continue to degenerate along a time course of one to several years. Dental treatment planning must take this into account. Patients in the early stages of the disease (memory loss, anxiety) will have a greater likelihood for accommodating to new oral hygiene regimens and new prostheses. In later stages (disorientation, personality changes), more radical treatments might be necessary, such as extracting questionable teeth and limiting prosthetic care to immediate dentures, or reline or replacement of existing prostheses. In terminal stages (non-ambulatory, total care), treatment might be limited to removal of severely diseased and/or inaccessible teeth and management of symptomatic mucosal disease.

Consent for care

Many dementia patients will not have decision-making capacity but plans for care should be discussed with them out of respect for their right to self-determination and because their impairment might not have totally clouded their comprehension of the procedures. The patient might have the capacity to consent for certain things. Even if patient is still legally able to provide consent, decisions of care should also be discussed with the guardian or caregiver, with the patient's permission.

Degenerative neuromuscular disorders

Muscular dystrophies

The muscular dystrophies are genetic disorders involving voluntary muscle with progressive weakness and wasting. Muscle fibers are replaced by fatty and fibrous tissue. There are a number of types – Duchenne (which affects males only), Becker and those based on the affected muscle groups:

- Duchenne muscular dystrophy: an X-linked disorder caused by mutation of the dystrophin gene: two-thirds of mothers of isolated cases are carriers, 50% of female siblings will be carriers and 50% of sons will be affected.

- Becker muscular dystrophy: a less severe variant; survival is longer than with Duchenne.
- Facioscapulohumeral type: this affects the masticatory muscles more than the other facial muscles leading to weakness of the circumoral muscles and so-called 'transverse smile'.

Death is usually as a consequence of respiratory muscle involvement in the second decade of life. Scoliosis, muscle contractures, pseudohypertrophy of the calves evident in later stages, loss of walking (7–13 years) and reduced intelligence.

Dental considerations

- The swallowing reflex can be affected and oral clearance is poor, so efficient aspiration is essential during treatment.
- General anesthesia is contraindicated (require ICU admission, possibly for weeks, postoperatively).
- Reduce dosage of local anesthesia – tolerance poor.
- Malocclusions can arise as a consequence of altered soft tissue balance.
- Flaccid soft tissues, an open-mouth posture and muscle weakness mean oral hygiene might be poor.

Myasthenia gravis (MG)

An autoimmune disease (antibodies produce loss of acetylcholine receptors) in which muscles exhibit extreme painless, fatigability, provoked by infection or stress. Seen transiently in neonates (distinguish from congenital myasthenia) when antibodies cross the placenta but can produce arthrogryposis multiplex congenita (joint contractures and other deformities). MG can occur from 1 year of age, after childbirth and after muscle relaxants used in general anesthesia.

Symptoms

Ptosis or diplopia; bulbar (difficulty in swallowing, speaking or chewing), neck or limb weakness. Respiratory weakness can be life-threatening.

Treatment

- Symptomatic with anticholinesterase drugs: e.g. pyridostigmine (Mestinon®), prednisolone for ocular myasthenia.
- Thymectomy in generalized myasthenia.

- Immunosuppression (prednisolone/azathioprine) if the above measures fail. Patients might be on atropine to reduce the salivary secretions.
- Myasthenic crisis – life-threatening bulbar or respiratory weakness – immediate airway control, ventilatory support and nasogastric intubation. A rapid-onset anticholinesterase, edrophonium chloride (Tensilon®) may be of benefit. Plasma exchange (3–5 weeks of improved strength) or IV immunoglobulin for short-term control of symptoms, otherwise anticholinesterase drugs for previously untreated patients.
- Cholinergic crisis (overdosage of anticholinesterase drugs) – hypersalivation, lacrimation, increased sweating, vomiting and miosis.

Dental considerations

- Aspiration risk. Difficult airway control and therefore protection with use of rubber dam and efficient suction is essential.
- Be aware of the potential for drug interactions as detailed above, as well as for cholinergic crisis.
- Long-term atropine can produce the usual dry mouth sequelae of dental caries.
- Lipomatous atrophy of the tongue can result in a furrowed and flaccid clinical appearance. Attempts at smiling may result in a snarl. Lack of strength in the muscles of mastication can inhibit sustained chewing effort. Dysphagia may result in poor nutritional status, dehydration and hypokalemia.
- Drugs (including procaine, erythromycin, gentamicin, neomycin, polymixin B, bacitracin and clindamycin) may acutely potentiate myasthenic weakness. All local anesthetics should be used with caution.
- Oral infection and psychological stress should be minimized. Arrange short appointments in the morning (or appointments scheduled 1–2 h after ingestion of oral anticholinesterase medication) to minimize fatigue and take advantage of the typically greater muscle strength in the morning.
- Presurgical plasma exchange might be recommended for the myasthenic with severe exacerbations. If respiratory collapse occurs, an open airway and adequate respiratory exchange must be established. Poorly controlled myasthenics might need oral hygiene aids and/or might have difficulty managing complete dentures.

Motor neuron disease

A progressive condition of older people. Its origin is unknown and it involves degenerative changes in anterior horn cells, cranial nerve nuclei and pyramidal pathway. It is characterized by bulbar or pseudobulbar palsy – lower cranial nerve involvement, weakness of head and neck muscles, eating and swallowing difficulties.

Dental considerations

Are the same as for other conditions where airway impairment is profound eg myasthenia gravis and muscular dystrophy.

Multiple sclerosis (MS)

MS is a chronic, autoimmune, demyelinating disease of CNS that affects young adults (age 20–40 years), the majority of whom are female. In a Finnish cohort, there was 64% survival at 40 years.

MS is characterized by periods of remission and relapse. There are four types:

- Benign: mild attacks and complete recovery (with little/no disability after 15 years).
- Relapsing/remitting (25%): with increasing disability after each relapse.
- Secondary progressive (40%): relapsing/remission initially progressing after 15–20 years to no remission period.
- Primary progressive (15%): steadily worsening with little/no remission.

Symptoms

Symptoms depend on area of CNS affected and extent of demyelination:

- transitory weakness
- sensory disturbance affecting a limb
- cognitive effects – personality, mood (cerebrum)
- coordination – tremor (cerebellum)
- vision (optic neuritis or diplopia)
- dysphagia
- slurred speech and hearing defects (cranial nerve)
- breathing, bladder and bowel control (pyramidal tract)
- motor control (spinal cord)
- chronic pain.

Signs
- Trigeminal neuralgia (managed with carbamazepine or phenytoin or sodium valproate).
- Trigeminal sensory neuropathy and facial palsy.
- Lateral gaze defect.
- Abnormal perioral hypersensitivity or anesthesia.

Treatment
- Physiotherapy.
- Reduction of acute episodes with steroids/ACTH, beta-interferon (delaying disease progression/disability), immunomodulatory treatment (30% success rate).
- Oral baclofen, tizanidine, dantrolene, gabapentin and diazepam all reduce muscle spasticity to varying degrees.
- Drugs for bladder dysfunction can produce a dry mouth.
- Cannabis assists in spasticity and bladder control.
- Other drug effects: antidepressants, anticholinergics (incontinence), antihistamines (dizziness), antispasmodics, cytotoxics and beta-interferon oral ulceration and blood dyscrasias.
- Aggravating factors – infections, anesthetics/operations (and other stressful events).
- No causal link between mercury from amalgam fillings and MS established.

Dental considerations
- Trigeminal neuralgia may be presenting sign to a dentist, treat as above.
- Cannabis has significant oral side-effects – gingivitis, white patches, candidiasis (from steroids also), epithelial dysplasia/carcinoma and xerostomia, interference with LA and IV sedative agents.
- Side-effects from drugs – dry mouth, oral ulceration and blood dyscrasias. Glatiramer acetate (Copaxone®) mimics myelin basic protein but, paradoxically, appears beneficial in the treatment of MS.
- Significant physical disability can mean that patients use a wheelchair and allowances will need to be made for delivery of dental care, including manual handling skills for safe transfer from the wheelchair to the dental chair if necessary.

ORTHOPEDIC AND BONE DISORDERS

Arthritis

Significance of the problem

A reported history of arthritis should alert the clinician to the likelihood for chronic use of salicylates (aspirin) or other non-steroidal anti-inflammatory agents that might alter platelet function. Although poorly documented, either could contribute to prolonged oral bleeding as well as exaggerated ecchymosis following an invasive procedure. Long-term corticosteroid therapy results in the risk of adrenal insufficiency.

Children with juvenile rheumatoid arthritis (JRA) and related conditions can have considerable erosion of primary teeth from chewing salicylates. Severe JRA and related conditions can lead to temporomandibular joint disorders and impaired mandibular growth in children.

Severe rheumatoid arthritis is a relative contraindication to hyperextension of the neck, in ankylosing spondylitis the neck vertebrae may be fused, with resultant rigidity of the neck. Patients can have problems with oral hygiene secondary to impaired dexterity; they might also have difficulty rising from the dental chair without assistance. A patient in a wheelchair should always be transferred to the dental chair, for the patient's and the clinician's well-being.

Significant elements of the history

- History of rheumatic fever.
- Use of salicylates or other anti-inflammatory agents: record the drug name, dosage and duration of use.
- Prosthetic joint surgery.

Management considerations

- If the patient has a history of steroid use it might be necessary to adjust the dosage for stressful procedures. Discuss with patient's physician.
- If there is a prior history of rheumatic fever, question about cardiac involvement and evaluate for organic heart murmur. Assess for the need for premedication with antibiotics for endocarditis prophylaxis, and for steroid use.

- If possible, children with JRA should be taught to swallow rather than chew medication(s). Fluoride might slow the process of erosion. Eroded primary teeth might require full coverage restorations.

Prosthetic joint considerations

According to the US National Center for Health Statistics 117 000 hips and 160 000 knees were replaced in 1991, and currently this figure may be over 500 000/year.

Significance of the problem

The major concern is to prevent bacterial seeding of a prosthetic joint from the oral cavity. Any risk from dental procedures is extremely low but case reports (mostly poorly documented) do exist. The need for antibiotic prophylaxis for invasive oral procedures is controversial and the risk of anaphylaxis from an antibiotic likely outweighs the risk of sequelae from oral bacteremia, except perhaps in specific high-risk patients.

Significant elements in the history

Date of surgery. • Name of hospital and surgeon. • Type of joint for each operation. • Current or past use of steroids. • History of arthritis, diabetes, chemotherapy and immune deficiency.

Management considerations

- Aggressive treatment of overt dental infection with antibiotics, assisted by culture and sensitivity tests.
- Patient should contact orthopedic surgeon if experiencing pain in a prosthetic joint that was previously pain free.
- A joint panel of the American Academy of Orthopedic Surgeons, American Dental Association and specialists in infectious diseases recommends antibiotics prior to all invasive dental procedures for 2 years after replacement of a prosthetic hip joint. After 2 years, antibiotic coverage should be employed in patients who are immunocompromised, are insulin-dependent diabetics, are on a corticosteroid regimen, have a history of rheumatoid arthritis or have a history of previous joint infection.
- There are no data to suggest prophylactic antibiotics prior to dental treatment for patients with a joint prosthesis in any joint other than the hip. Hip prosthesis recommendations are based on

the relative risk from death due to anaphylactic reaction to antibiotics rather than an infected joint, and it is therefore reasonable to assume that the risk of death from infection of smaller joints will always be less than the risk of death from anaphylaxis.

- Patients taking steroids:
  - Might be at higher risk for infection.
  - The major consideration is suppression of adrenal capacity to respond to stressful situations, however the risk of this occurring during dental treatment is probably overstated and supplemental steroids are rarely indicated. Consult the patient's physician to determine the reason for and duration of steroid therapy, and regarding adjustment of steroid dose prior to stressful dental treatment if the patient's adrenal glands function poorly or not at all. The general goal for supplementation is to have 80–100 mg hydrocortisone available systemically for stressful (surgical or psychological) procedures. Patients on very low or high doses of steroids, or those undergoing non-surgical dental procedures probably do not require supplementation.
  - Consider dose adjustment for patients currently on steroids or who have been on steroids up to 6 months prior to dental treatment. General guideline is to increase to 2 times normal the day of treatment and 2 times normal the day after treatment (if still in pain). Consideration might be given to steroid supplementation 12 h after the procedure.
  - Patients off long-term high-dose steroids for over 6 months can have the drug instituted the day prior to treatment, at the discretion of the physician.
  - Keep in mind that a major precipitating factor in an adrenal crisis is hypovolemia. Therefore, ensure that the patient is well hydrated prior to the procedure.
- Dental evaluation and management of the patient with a prosthetic joint infection should include:
  - Joint culture results of bacteria specific to the oral cavity are necessary to suggest a dental source. Usually organism is staphylococcus from skin or wound infection, or a gastrointestinal organism.
  - Thorough oral exam, full mouth series of radiographs, and treatment to rule out or eliminate sources of possible hematogenous route of bacteremia from oral cavity.

Osteogenesis imperfecta

A group of inherited connective tissue conditions of type 1 collagen, characterized by increased bone fragility and lax joints. There are six types, based on clinical groups, severity and features, for example blue sclera (which is age dependent) and dentinogenesis imperfecta. Type II is fatal and there is increased mortality for type III and for younger children with types 1B, IVA and IVB.

Associated signs/symptoms
- Hearing loss.
- Mitral/aortic valve defects.
- Bruising.

Treatment
- Intramedullary fixation of long bones to prevent and treat fractures and subsequent deformities using expanding rods to allow bone growth is gold-standard treatment.
- Biphosphonates (inhibitors of osteoclast-mediated bone resorption), usually delivered by monthly IV infusion to increase bone density, mobility and wellbeing.

Dental considerations
- Possible cardiac defects needing antibiotic prophylaxis.
- Dentinogenesis imperfecta in 50% of cases with gray, discolored dentin; more marked discoloration in earlier erupting teeth and dentition.
- Pseudo class III malocclusion.
- Excessive wear and sensitivity necessitating full coronal coverage to maintain occlusal vertical dimension.
- Other, similar inherited dentin defects include Ehlers–Danlos syndrome, vitamin-D-resistant rickets, vitamin-D-dependent rickets and hypophosphatasia.

Osteitis deformans (Paget's disease)

This is a common disorder of older males (4% of population > 40 years). The maxilla and heavy long bones more often affected.

Etiology
Probably a slow virus disease – persisting measles or RSV. Osteoclasts

are morphologically abnormal, resorption is followed by increased osteoblastic activity.

Signs/symptoms
- Bony deformity (leg bowing, altered skull shape).
- Warmth over affected area (increased vascularity).
- Deafness (nerves trapped).
- Osteoarthritis.
- Osteogenic sarcoma.
- Serum Ca and PO_4 levels are normal but alkaline phosphatase is elevated (osteoblastic activity).

Dental considerations
- Oral: maxilla may expand, altering the fit of prostheses.
- Problems of root resorption: excessive bleeding after extractions (surgical removal indicated due to heavy cemental deposits on root surfaces).
- Ischemic bone in advanced disease can predispose to delayed healing and post-extraction infections.

Osteomalacia

This is a defect of bone mineralization (rickets in growing bone). It is mainly seen accompanying deficiency of vitamin-D or altered vitamin-D metabolism in inadequate dietary intake, renal disease or from anticonvulsant therapy. Treatment is by remedying the underlying cause and vitamin D/calcium.

Signs/symptoms
Bone fracture/deformity in children. The long bones are affected primarily in adults.

Dental considerations
Teeth eruption is affected only if the disease is severe.

Osteopetrosis

A rare condition, dominantly inherited (Albers-Schönberg disease) with autosomal recessive forms. It is the result of markedly decreased bone resorption, leading to bony deformities. The marrow spaces are occluded, resulting in anemia. BMT in the infantile form of the disease might allow some dental development. Prednisolone treatment in the malignant form in the infant might produce a cure.

Dental considerations

Osteomyelitis can complicate dental infections.

Osteoporosis

Arises as a consequence of physiological loss of bone, accelerated by aging, estrogen decline (in postmenopausal women) and immobility. Pathologically, it is seen as a consequence of lifestyle – smoking, excess alcohol ingestion, certain drugs (e.g. heparin) and some endocrine conditions. In older people, fractures and the associated morbidity impact on quality of life. Osteoporosis is a public health issue because of the aging population. Prevention is aimed at regular exercise, adequate diet, avoiding excess of alcohol and smoking cessation. Hormone replacement therapy, despite side-effects, might be advantageous in older (70+) postmenopausal women.

PREGNANCY

Oral manifestations

- 'Pregnancy gingivitis' secondary to hormone changes and inadequate oral hygiene.
- Pyogenic granuloma (pregnancy tumor): can be excised, preferably postpartum. If small, it might shrink without intervention after delivery.

Management considerations

Timing

Elective treatment should be avoided in the first trimester because of concern for susceptibility to teratogens and abortion. Dental prophylaxis and non-deferrable dental treatment are best provided in the second trimester. Elective procedures are not recommended in the third trimester because of the risk from anemia, hypertension, hypotension and nausea due to compromised venous return from fetal compression of inferior vena cava in the supine position.

Radiographs

Although risk is negligible, radiographs can usually be deferred until postpartum, unless needed for diagnosis of an acute problem. During the first trimester, radiographs should be taken only for emergency care, and a double lead apron should be used for psychological wellbeing.

Drugs

The FDA has a ranking of drugs based on the degree to which available information has ruled out risk to the fetus balanced against the potential benefits of the drugs to the patient (see Chapter 8 and Box 2.2).

Box 2.2 Drugs for use during pregnancy

Local anesthetics: safe in therapeutic doses but minimize the use of vasoconstrictors.

Antibiotics: penicillin, cephalosporin, vancomycin and erythromycin (except estolate form) are safe. Obstetrician should be consulted if other antibiotics are needed. Tetracyclines are absolutely contraindicated due to adverse effect on teeth and skeletal bone. Do not use sulfa drugs.

Analgesics: usually preferable to treat the cause of pain rather than to treat patient symptomatically with analgesics. Acetaminophen [paracetamol], hydrocodone, oxycodone and codeine are considered safe. Non-steroidal anti-inflammatory agents (including aspirin) and opioids (other than those mentioned above) should be avoided. Avoid Naprosyn®, ibuprofen, Darvocet® and aspirin. Obstetrician should be consulted if other analgesics are needed.

Sedatives: should be avoided. Obstetrician should be consulted if sedation needed. Diazepam and nitrous oxide (in early stages) are absolutely contraindicated.

Prolonged time periods in a dental chair can increase the risk of thromboembolic event.

PSYCHIATRIC DISORDERS

Do not assume that the patient has adequate decision-making capacity to provide valid informed consent (due to illness or drugs). Patients can be uncooperative or difficult to interview. However, it is important to discover what medications the patient is taking – record the types and dosages. Precautions exist for the use of sedatives, opioids, epinephrine and other drugs that could interact with the patient's medications.

Tardive dyskinesia is caused by phenothiazines, butyrophenones (used commonly for treatment of schizophrenia) and, less frequently, by metoclopramide and tricyclic antidepressants. These involuntary movements can compromise the success of complete dentures. All dental restorations placed in patients with uncontrollable movements should be designed to offer maximal resistance to shearing stresses. Balancing contacts should be avoided; working side contacts are only advisable if part of a group function. Alprazolam or buspirone may be effective in limiting movements during dental treatment. Xerostomia is a probable side-effect of neuroleptic and other behavior-managing medications.

The patient should be on a rigorous recall schedule and have dietary counseling, with particular attention to refined carbohydrate intake. Use fluoride supplementation with dentifrice, rinses, gels, or mouth trays. Involve the caregiver in all preventive and oral hygiene counseling. Use non-opioid analgesics if possible.

Depression

Medications used for depression can cause xerostomia, with resultant destruction of the dentition. Refractory depression remains an indication for electroconvulsive therapy (ECT).

ECT

The electrodes utilized for ECT are placed supra-auricularly, so that they directly stimulate the anterior temporal and masseter muscles, despite the patient's pretreatment with the alpha-paralytic agent. For this reason, reliable bilateral support of the mandible at or near the physiological dimension of occlusion is necessary.

Prior to ECT, complete dentures should be removed unless unusually retentive; partial dentures must be stable and retentive if they are to remain in place. Edentulous areas and unopposed dental segments can be stabilized with custom-fitted bite guards or rolled cushions of gauze. Such intraoral splints must be able to accommodate the obligatory airway tube that is needed to support respirations if the patient is paralyzed.

Schizophrenia

Avoid confrontation and ensure adequate medical management before treatment.

RENAL/ADRENAL DISORDERS

Hyperadrenocorticism (Cushing's syndrome)

This is hypersecretion of glucocorticoid as a result of various diseases affecting the hypothalamus, anterior pituitary or adrenal gland itself. Features include:

- Hypertension, muscle weakness, 'moon facies', truncal obesity, hirsutism.
- Diabetes, osteoporosis, bleeding diathesis – microcirculation does not respond appropriately. The result can be poor wound healing, easy bruising and increased risk of infection.

Hypoadrenocorticism (Addison's disease)

Hyposecretion of the glucocorticoid cortisol as a result of autoimmune destruction of adrenal cortex, exogenous steroid therapy, therapeutic bilateral adrenalectomy or damage to the pituitary gland. Features include:

- Hyperpigmentation: buccal and labial mucosa and gingivae.
- Weakness, fatigue, malaise, mental confusion, weight loss, fever, orthostatic hypotension, syncope (sodium depletion), depressed vasoconstrictor response.
- Poor response to stress. Could precipitate cardiovascular collapse.
- Nausea and vomiting, thirst, polyuria, hyperkalemia, arrhythmia, cardiac arrest.

Clinical considerations for adrenal insufficiency

Consultation with patient's physician to determine the present adrenal status. Increasing the steroid dose for surgical procedures is rarely necessary but it is difficult to predict who might have an adrenal crisis under stress, and the risk from increasing the steroid dose is minimal to non-existent. Patients who have had prolonged or significant dental infection will benefit most from supplemental corticosteroids, particularly if surgical extractions are anticipated.

The normal daily output of hydrocortisone is 20 mg. Patients taking low doses for short time periods do not likely need a supplemental dose. For patients on larger doses or for longer periods, consider either doubling the patient's daily dose the morning of surgery up to physiologic output of adrenal glands, or 100–200 mg of intramuscular or intravenous hydrocortisone 30 min prior to the planned procedure. Patients on high doses (> 40 mg/day) of prednisone would not normally require a supplemental dose, except perhaps for major surgery and/or general anesthesia.

The steroid dose for mild to moderately stressful procedures should be doubled on the day of surgery. For highly stressful procedures in patients at high risk, consider prednisone 60 mg or hydrocortisone 100 mg on the day of surgery, tapered rapidly over next 3 days back to the patient's usual replacement dose. Sedation should be considered to minimize stress.

Management considerations for renal patients

Renal dialysis
- Some authorities recommend antibiotic prophylaxis prior to invasive dental treatment for patients with arteriovenous shunts, but supportive data are lacking. Do not measure blood pressure in arm with a shunt.
- Potassium-containing penicillins are acceptable for short-term use (several days) but not for long-term use, due to high potassium levels. Erythromycin is an alternative. Aminoglycosides, tetracyclines and cephalosporins should be avoided due to nephrotoxicity.
- It is desirable to treat soon after dialysis, and to avoid the day before dialysis because of the problem of increasing uremia, and consequent failing platelet function. Concern about the heparin needed to prevent clotting of the vascular access shunt is overstated, since the volume is so small. Patients are usually tired after dialysis and might not tolerate dental appointments at that time. Renal failure and uremia predispose to bleeding secondary to poor platelet function. Consider use of desmopressin (DDAVP,

vasopressin); discuss with the patient's physician. The morning after dialysis is probably the best alternative.

- Patient might be chronically anticoagulated due to increased risk of thromboembolic disease. PT/INR should be obtained prior to surgical procedures if patient is on warfarin.
- There is a higher incidence of hepatitis B and C, and anemia.
- The serum calcium/phosphorus ratio is altered and there is an increased risk of the development of tertiary hyperparathyroidism, which can present with osteolytic 'Brown's tumors' of the jaws.
- Antibiotic prophylaxis: dialysis patients (and former dialysis patients, and therefore by definition, most renal transplant recipients) are at risk of uremia (chemical trauma) related heart valve damage and therefore antibiotic prophylaxis should be considered. Protection of the dialysis shunt or the transplanted kidney is not the main concern.

Renal transplant

- Patients are often on chronic prednisone and/or other immunosuppressive drugs. This might dictate the desirability for antibiotic and steroid prophylaxis. Watch for gingival overgrowth if the patient is taking cyclosporine. Oral infection should be treated aggressively and may require hospitalization.
- Cautious use of drugs requiring renal clearance (see Chapter 8).
- Laboratory tests: BUN and serum creatinine.

Drug therapy in renal failure

Renal patients are often on multiple drugs to manage both the renal disease and its complications. The dosage or frequency of administration of a given drug may have to be altered in order to obtain constant blood levels due to altered renal clearance and dialysis. Many drugs should be used with caution (see Chapter 8).

Drugs with major excretion route via kidneys

Antibiotics

- Penicillins: amoxicillin, ampicillin, carbenicillin, dicloxacillin, methicillin, oxacillin, penicillin, ticarcillin.
- Tetracyclines: tetracycline, doxycycline, vancomycin.

- Aminoglycosides: amikacin, gentamicin, streptomycin.
- Cephalosporins: cephalexin, cephalothin, cefamandole [cephapirin, cephradine].

Analgesics
- Non-opioid:
  - acetaminophen [paracetamol] (hepatic excretion): nephrotoxic with chronic use
  - aspirin: rarely nephrotoxic
  - non-steroidal anti-inflammatory drugs: most are nephrotoxic.
- Opioids: most have the liver as the major route; < 20% have the renal route.

RESPIRATORY DISEASE

Cystic fibrosis

In Europe, 1 in 25 people are carriers (normal) of this autosomal recessive disorder; it is the most common serious, inherited disease in Caucasians. Median survival is 30 years.

Etiology
Gene encoded on chromosome 7 (Cl channel), 400 mutations identified, four account for all mutations in northern Europeans.

Investigations
High concentration of chloride ions in the sweat (> 60 mmol/L, Na ≥ 70 mmol/L) identified via pilocarpine iontophoresis; 1:10 patients in the US are not diagnosed until adult life.

Symptoms/signs
- Respiratory: progressive bronchiectasis, hemoptysis, pneumothorax, nasal polyposis, chronic sinusitis, finger clubbing (adults).
- GI tract: neonatal meconium ileus (distal intestinal obstruction syndrome), rectal prolapse, pancreatic insufficiency (up to 15% of CF children are pancreatic sufficient), focal biliary cirrhosis/portal hypertension.
- Endocrine/reproductive: diabetes mellitus, male infertility.

Treatment
- Pancreatic supplements.
- Prophylaxis against *Pseudomonas aeuroginosa* (nebulized antibiotics delay colonization) with new third-generation cephalosporins.
- The beta-lactam, meropenem.
- Macrolides, for anti-inflammatory action, can help lung function.
- Nebulized Dornase alfa (recombinant human Dnase) for DNA-rich infected sputum decreases viscosity of sputum (decreases DNA strand) and causes a small increase in lung function.
- Transplant of cadaveric donor heart–lung or double-lung gives a current 1-year survival of 80%; 3-year survival = 50%.
- Living transplant: related lobe donation to overcome transplant shortage needs two donors, usually blood relations – lower lobectomy. Considerable ethical issues and some morbidity for donors.

Dental considerations

- Salivary gland enlargement.
- Enamel hypoplasia.
- Delayed eruption.
- Relative caries resistance due to high pH of saliva, tendency therefore to accumulate calculus deposits.
- Some older patients may have tetracycline-stained teeth.
- Water lines in dental offices should be scrupulously clean to avoid contamination with *P. aeuroginosa* for CF patients in particular.

Asthma

A syndrome of episodic and reversible acute or subacute narrowing of the airways, or bronchospasm. Decreased ciliary activity and increased secretions are early manifestations and an inflammatory reaction occurs later on. Constriction of smooth muscle with edema of bronchial mucosa and formation of tenacious mucous, predisposing to infection.

Significant elements in the history
- Age at which attacks began: onset before 10 years in 50% of cases.
- Frequency and severity of attacks: hospitalizations and/or frequency of emergency room visits.

- Precipitation of attacks: stress is an important factor in dentistry. Also cold air, pollutants, respiratory infection, exercise, aspirin, medical non-compliance.
- Medications used and response to medications: patients on steroids have severe asthma.
- Use of nebulized beta-agonists (isoproterenol, albuterol [salbutamol]) in acute episodes (Table 2.5).
- Patients might be taking drugs between attacks to avoid recurrence. If steroids are used, be alert for possibility of adrenocortical insufficiency and oral candidiasis. If patients are taking theophylline or aminophylline, use of erythromycin or clindamycin will increase the theophylline level and may result in theophylline toxicity.
- History of problems with aspirin or stress.
- 5% of asthma patients have multiple nasal polyps and aspirin sensitivity.

Table 2.5 **Medications used in asthma**

Medication	Use	Action	Caution
Methylxanthines Aminophylline Theophylline	Oral	Bronchodilation	Avoid epinephrine
Beta-2 receptor agonists Isoetharine [orciprenaline sulphate] Metaproterenol Isoproterenol Albuterol [ventolin]	Inhaled	Bronchodilation	Avoid epinephrine
Corticosteroids	Systemic inhalant	Decreased inflammation	Systemic: hyperglycemia Inhaled: not for acute attacks
Mast cell inhibitors Gastrocrom® (cromolyn) [cromoglycate] Tilade® (nedocromil)	Inhaled	Decreased mast cell mediator release	Not for acute attacks

Types

Extrinsic (allergic) asthma

- Usually children and young adults. Usually inherited predisposition.
- Attacks usually precipitated by specific allergens such as dust, feathers, animal dander, fungal spores, plant pollen, foods, and drugs such as aspirin/NSAIDs, penicillin, barbiturates. Attacks may disappear after adolescence.
- Airway obstruction usually develops within minutes of exposure to allergen.
- Immunoglobulin E antibodies produced: type I hypersensitivity reaction.

Intrinsic asthma

- Half of all asthmatics: usually develops in adults. Usually more severe than the extrinsic type.
- Usually precipitated by non-allergic factors such as infection, air pollutants, smoke, cold air, exercise, stress, emotional upset or physical exertion.

Clinical manifestations

Attack characterized by wheezing and, rarely, cyanosis. May have shortness of breath, cough, tachypnea, prolonged expiratory phase and apprehension.

Prevention of attack

Avoid treatment during respiratory infection. Avoid aspirin and NSAID-containing drugs and antihistamines. Ask the patient to bring medications to each appointment and keep the appointments short. Eliminate stress as much as possible. Sedation may minimize risk of attacks. Minimize the use of epinephrine. Consider prophylaxis with puff prior to treatment.

Management of attack (see Chapter 6)

1. Stop procedure and allow patient to sit upright.
2. Have patient use a beta-agonist inhaler – multiple puffs. Doses higher than prescribed are safe in acute episodes (4–8 puffs).
3. Monitor pulse if moderate-risk patient.
4. Consider supplementing oral steroids in a patient with history of steroid use.

5. Consider use of antibiotics if the patient is on steroids or if there is a risk of oral infection complicating medical management.
6. Consider hospitalization for dental care if the patient is moderate to high risk.

Bronchopulmonary dysplasia

Syndrome of increased resistance to airflow, reduction of elasticity of the lung and frequent lower respiratory tract infections. Usually occurs in young children with a history of premature birth and prolonged use of a respirator in infancy.

Management considerations
- Patients might be taking steroids; be alert for the possibility of adrenocortical insufficiency and oral candidiasis.
- Avoid sedatives, tranquilizers and other respiratory depressants.
- Emphasize prevention of dental problems: syrup-based medications might be harmful to teeth.

Chronic obstructive pulmonary disease (COPD)

Chronic bronchitis or emphysema.

Pathophysiology
Bronchospasm with increased resistance to airflow and destruction of alveolar units and with a decrease in elastic recoil, bronchial fibrosis, air trapping and alveolar distention. There are excessive secretions and mucosal swelling. COPD is usually the result of cigarette smoking.

Management considerations
- Patients may be taking steroids. Be alert for possibility of adrenocortical insufficiency and oropharyngeal candidiasis. Consider need for steroid supplementation for stressful procedures, and antibiotics for active oral infection.
- Patients are likely to be on theophylline or aminophylline; use of erythromycin should be avoided because it will result in increased theophylline levels and possible toxicity.
- Avoid sedatives, tranquilizers, hypnotics and opioids. Avoid high-flow oxygen because it could take away respiratory 'drive'.

Pulmonary tuberculosis (TB)

This is one of the least transmissible respiratory diseases. However, given the emergence of multidrug-resistant forms, masks must be worn as a preventive measure. Workplace modifications and use of HEPA filter respirators decrease risk of occupational transmission.

Refer the patient to a physician for chest film, cultures and purified protein derivative (PPD), if unsure of status. Avoid elective treatment in patients with active disease or positive sputum or who are still coughing. Most patients have negative sputum cultures after 3–4 weeks of therapy (streptomycin, isoniazid, rifampin [rifampicin], ethambutol, etc.) and are non-infective.

Multidrug-resistant (MDR) TB strains have evolved due to patient non-compliance with anti-TB drug therapy. MDR-TB is more prevalent in the HIV-infected population.

SICKLE-CELL ANEMIA

Significance of the problem

Eight per cent of African Americans have sickle-cell trait (heterozygosity for a hemoglobin S mutation of the beta hemoglobin chain); a smaller number have sickle-cell anemia (homozygosity for the hemoglobin S gene). A smaller number of individuals (usually of Mediterranean descent) are heterozygous or homozygous for beta thalassemia (a mutation of the beta hemoglobin chain):

- Sickle-cell trait: individuals are usually asymptomatic but severe hypoxia might trigger vaso-occlusive phenomena.
- Sickle-cell anemia: homozygous hemoglobin S:
  - Patients experience crises, which can be vaso-occlusive (sickled red blood cells block small blood vessels), sequestration (large amounts of blood accumulate in the liver or spleen) or aplastic due to failure of bone marrow production. Patients have chronic anemia. Vaso-occlusive crises are most common and can be triggered by local or systemic hypoxia and infection.
  - Mucosal pallor (from chronic anemia), jaundice (from hemolysis), hypoplastic enamel and delayed eruption of teeth can be observed.

- Enlargement of marrow spaces may result in abnormal alveolar trabeculation pattern on radiographs and a class II malocclusion (due to enlargement of the maxilla).
- Mental nerve neuropathy and non-specific dental pain can occur. Sickle-cell disease affects the small vessels of the dental pulp.
- Surgical removal of the spleen or autosplenectomy from multiple infarcts can result in reduced filtration of encapsulated organisms. Coverage with antibiotics suggested by some sources, but data are lacking.
- Thalassemia minor: heterozygous beta-thalassemia trait. Individuals may have mild anemia but are otherwise normal.
- Thalassemia major: homozygous beta-thalassemia. Significance is similar to sickle-cell anemia, but the shape of the red blood cells is different. Multiple transfusions are common and maxillary alveolar bone hyperplasia may be seen.

Significant elements of the history

- Frequency and type of crisis: number of hospitalizations and reason for each.
- History of transfusions.
- Laboratory values (hemoglobin electrophoresis, hemoglobin, hematocrit).

Management considerations

- Major concern is for acute oral infection that can precipitate a sickle-cell crisis.
- Emphasis should be on preventive dental care because of the serious sequelae of infection.
- Some patients require antibiotic prophylaxis prior to extensive procedures. The patient's physician or hematologist should be consulted.
- Dental pain may be due to a pulpal vascular crisis.
- Local anesthesia:
  - Agents associated with methemoglobinemia (e.g. prilocaine) should be avoided.
  - Use of vasoconstrictors is controversial. The benefits of vaso-constrictors probably outweigh the risk of local impairment of

circulation in most cases. Concentrations of epinephrine greater than 1:100 000 [1:80 000] should be avoided.

- General anesthesia, when necessary, may be preceded by blood transfusion by the patient's physician or hematologist.
- Sedation: nitrous oxide may be used, but oxygen must be 50% or greater. Avoid excessive barbiturates and narcotics that will suppress respiration.

DISORDERS OF THE THYROID GLAND

Hyperthyroidism (Graves' disease)

This usually affects women, who can present with exophthalmos. Thyroid storm (thyrotoxic crisis) can be precipitated by stress, trauma or acute infection if patient is not well managed. Use pharmacologic management of oral infection until under control (i.e. antibiotics/analgesics). Look for evidence of thyrotoxicosis – fever, altered mental status, tachycardia, hypertension and exophthalmos.

Use caution with stressful procedures. Prevention of infection is important to avoid crisis. Avoid epinephrine.

Hypothyroidism

Caused by a congenital defect, hypothalamus or a pituitary defect, Hashimoto's thyroiditis or radiogenic (e.g. radioactive iodine therapy).

The risk from inadequate management is poor response to stress, infection and trauma resulting in hypothyroid coma. Signs include hypotension, bradycardia, decreased temperature, and weight gain. Use caution with sedatives and opioids.

VISUAL IMPAIRMENT

Defined as visual acuity < 3/60 in better eye with optical correction (normal vision = 20/20). Blind = corrected field of vision < an angle of 20° or visual acuity of 20/70 in better eye with optical correction.

Etiology

- Genetic disease, cataracts, perinatal disease, non-congenital malformation (microphthalmos, congenital glaucoma), congenital infection (rubella), diabetic retinopathy.
- In developing countries, in addition: corneal scarring, vitamin A deficiency, measles, herpes simplex virus, malnutrition, trachoma and leprosy.
- Cataracts, macular degeneration and glaucoma account for 60% of blindness in older people.
- Associated conditions: severe disabilities (e.g. cerebral palsy, epilepsy, learning difficulties). Considerations must be made for 'seeing eye' [guide] dogs and decreasing noise in the operatory [surgery].

Chapter 3

Oral medicine: a problem-oriented approach

The wide variety of non-surgical problems of the oral cavity and maxillofacial region can be subdivided into those that are local versus those that represent oral manifestations and complications of systemic disease and medical therapy. The proper identification of such manifestations is important for several reasons. First, this might be the initial manifestation of a potentially serious or life-threatening systemic disease or condition. A classic example of this is leukemic infiltrate of the gingiva. Second, certain oral manifestations might represent a worsening systemic disease, such as the onset of oral hairy leukoplakia in a patient with advancing HIV disease. Early recognition of an oral manifestation of a systemic disease increases the likelihood for early diagnosis and a more favorable management of a number of medical conditions.

The starting point in oral medicine, as in all dental and medical disciplines, is the medical history. Developing the skill – indeed the art – of taking a medical history that is succinct, relevant but also comprehensive is essential. This is particularly important with regards to understanding a patient's medications (prescribed and otherwise), both from the standpoint of oral side-effects of drug therapy and also from consideration of the interaction of medications prescribed to patients by different clinicians. This chapter serves as a problem-oriented approach to the more common oral medical problems. It is not intended as a substitute for textbooks of oral medicine or oral pathology.

Patients with an oral medical problem that has systemic significance will most often present with one of the following subjective or objective indicators.

POSSIBLE ORAL/DENTAL INDICATORS OF SYSTEMIC DISEASE

Mucosal conditions or changes

- Lesions (localized or generalized):
  - ○ ulceration/erosion
  - ○ infection
  - ○ swelling
  - ○ pigmentation/color changes.
- Xerostomia.
- Halitosis/odor.
- Poor healing.

Pain and/or altered sensation or special senses

- Discomfort/pain.
- Anesthesia/paresthesia/dysesthesia/hyperesthesia/hypoesthesia.
- Altered taste/smell.

Radiographic changes

- Teeth.
- Bony changes.

NON-ODONTOGENIC PROBLEMS REFLECTED IN SIGNS AND SYMPTOMS OF THE ORAL CAVITY

White lesions

The nature of a white lesion is important, given the malignant potential of some of them (Fig. 3.1).

If the lesion rubs away easily with gauze
Consider an infectious etiology.

Infectious etiology
Most likely pseudomembranous candidosis. More rarely, secondary syphilis or diphtheria.

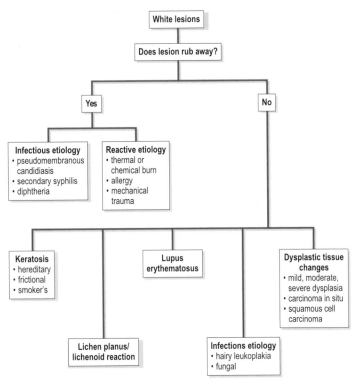

Fig. 3.1 **White lesions.**

- History: candidal infection, no matter what form or clinical presentation, is a marker of immunosuppression.
- Local causes: xerostomia, use of corticosteroid inhalants, altered local oral microflora secondary to the use of broad-spectrum antibiotics.
- Systemic causes: immunosuppressed secondary to cytotoxic agents, high-dose steroids, bone marrow impairment or HIV/AIDS.
- Signs: white plaque(s) on an erythematous mucosa base.
- Symptoms: generally asymptomatic.
- Tests: KOH smear, culture for candidosis, or VDRL to exclude secondary syphilis.

- Treatment: identify and correct contributing etiology. Local causes must be addressed and systemic causes screened for and identified (e.g. diabetes, HIV disease). Topical antifungals (e.g. clotrimazole troches) or systemic antifungal agents (e.g. Diflucan) (see Appendix 3).

Reactive etiology

- Differential diagnosis: includes trauma, which can be thermal, chemical or mechanical burn, or more rarely allergy (e.g. toothpaste, mouthwash, 'pizza burn').
- History: recent trauma or use of a new oral care product.
- Clinical signs: white sloughing tissue with or without erythema.
- Tests: after excluding traumatic causes, consider stopping or changing any product that might have a temporal association with the onset of the lesion(s).
- Treatment: re-evaluate in 2 weeks; consider biopsy if no etiologic agent identified.

If lesion does not rub away easily

- Differential diagnosis: includes keratosis (hereditary or reactive), autoimmune conditions such as lichen planus/lichenoid eruption, lupus erythematosus, infectious etiology or dysplastic or neoplastic tissue changes. If family history, consider hereditary keratosis (e.g. white sponge nevus).
- History: present since childhood, other family members affected.
- Clinical signs: localized or panoral.
- Tests: biopsy
- Treatment: none. Reassurance to the patient of the innocence of the condition.

If on an occlusal line

Consider a reactive traumatic frictional keratosis:

- History: cheek chewing (associated with anxiety?).
- Signs: affecting an area that can be traumatized.
- Symptoms: mild discomfort.
- Tests: biopsy, if etiology unclear.
- Treatment: reassurance. Consider splint therapy if significant damage to mucosa. Consider psychologic source and referral.

If patient is a smoker

Consider smoker's keratosis:

- History: smoker, bad taste, dryness.
- Signs: prominent minor salivary gland ducts on palate, associated tobacco malodor and tooth staining.
- Tests: biopsy, if suspicious for dysplasia/malignancy.
- Treatment: cease tobacco use.

If lesion is striated

Consider lichen planus:

- History: mucosal sensitivity and roughness.
- Clinical signs: usually bilateral; might be eroded; might be skin lesions and/or possibly symptomatic genital lesions as well.
- Tests: biopsy. Consider histology and direct immunofluorescence to differentiate from lupus.
- Treatment: topical and systemic steroids, for symptomatic ulcerative disease (see Appendix 4).

If lesion is unilateral or asymmetric

Consider lichenoid eruption:

- History: positive drug history. Temporal association with the start of the lesions and the commencement of a specific drug or medication. Medications implicated include non-steroidal anti-inflammatories, antihypertensives and diabetic medications.
- Lesions in direct contact with amalgam restorations (so called 'kissing lesions').
- Tests: biopsy, confirm diagnosis and exclude dysplastic feature and/or consider patch-test screening of possible causative dental restorative materials and planned replacement materials.
- Treatment: with lichenoid reaction, consider altering medication. Consider removing amalgams if lesions are in contact.

If lesion is striated but atypical

Consider systemic lupus erythematosus (SLE):

- History: long-standing with or without systemic disease.
- Clinical signs: erosions with annular striations, particularly on the palate.
- Tests: biopsy, for both histology and direct immunofluorescence; serology, especially screening for SLE (ds-DNA antibodies, and rheumatoid factor).
- Treatment: topical steroids (see Appendix 4).

If lesion on the lateral border of the tongue

Consider hairy leukoplakia:

- History: known HIV or high-risk activity.
- Signs: vertical corrugations, other oral manifestations of HIV disease (e.g. pseudomembranous candidosis), most commonly lateral border of tongue. Asymptomatic.
- Tests: biopsy plus in situ hybridization for Epstein–Barr virus, cytology smear to exclude candida.
- Treatment: consider referral for HIV testing. If patient concerned as to appearance, consider antivirals (acyclovir, valacyclovir) (see Appendix 5).

If lesion solitary and with rough surface characteristics

Consider a fungal etiology (e.g. hyperplastic candidosis, histolasmosis):

- History: immunosuppression.
- Clinical signs: solitary lesion with hyperplastic appearance.
- Tests: culture. Biopsy if hyperplastic.
- Treatment: topical antifungals for hyperplastic candidosis. Systemic antifungals used most commonly for non-candidal infection (see Appendix 3). Identify underlying systemic cause (e.g. diabetes, HIV disease).

If none of the above

Consider leukoplakia (histologic range: epithelial hyperplasia to invasive squamous cell carcinoma):

- History: tobacco (to include snuff, chewing tobacco), with or without alcohol use.
- Clinical signs: homogeneous or speckled white patches.
- Tests: biopsy.
- Treatment: observation, incisional biopsy of suspicious lesions. Referral to appropriate clinician for management of squamous cell carcinoma. Excisional biopsy should only be performed by the surgeon who will provide definitive treatment.

Erythematous lesions

Erythematous lesions present as redness with or without other pathology. They can be patchy, restricted to the palate or tongue, or generalized (Fig. 3.2).

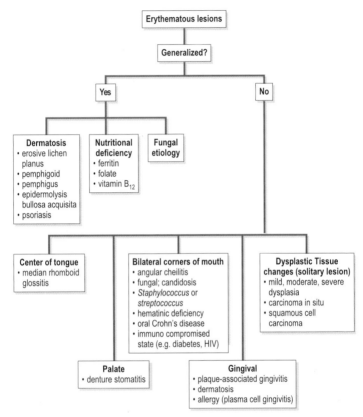

Fig. 3.2 Erythematous lesions.

If lesion is associated with other mucosal lesions

Establish the diagnosis (e.g. candidosis or vesiculobullous – see 'Ulcerative lesions' below):

- History: sensitivity and roughness of mucosa.
- Clinical signs: associated white patches or striae.
- Tests: mycology or biopsy

If clinically atrophic mucosa

Consider nutritional deficiencies:

- History: sensitivity to hot, spicy foods.

- Clinical signs: patchy erythema, associated angular cheilitis, recurrent oral ulceration.
- Tests: full blood count – check the hemoglobin and MCV. Serum ferritin, folate and vitamin B_{12}.
- Treatment: Replacement therapy; investigation of systemic causes for deficiency.

If lesion is generalized with no obvious cause

Consider erythematous candidosis:
- History: immunosuppression or recent antibiotic therapy.
- Tests: swabs, smears for mycology.
- Treatment: antifungals (e.g. topical agents) (see Appendix 3).

If lesion is restricted to the center of the tongue

Consider median rhomboid glossitis:
- History: none, usually smoker or uses steroid inhaler.
- Clinical signs: smooth, erythematous patch in the center of the tongue. Check for a contact lesion on the palate.
- Tests: consider biopsy if etiology in doubt.
- Treatment: identify cause (e.g. smoking, HIV disease, candidosis). Consider topical antifungals (see Appendix 3).

If lesion is restricted to the palate

Consider denture stomatitis:
- History: denture wearer, metallic taste.
- Clinical signs: patchy erythema = type I; diffuse erythema = type II; papilliferous = type III.
- Tests: swabs and smears for mycology, if etiology in doubt.
- Treatment: improve denture hygiene, daily brushing of palate, topical antifungal therapy (see Appendix 3), including soaking the denture in antifungal solution.

If lesion is on the buccal mucosa, palate, or floor of mouth

Consider erythroleukoplakia:
- History: smoking, alcohol
- Clinical signs: speckled leukoplakia inside the commissures if a smoker, but can occur in other intraoral locations.
- Tests: biopsy to determine presence or degree of dysplasia and rule out carcinoma.
- Treatment: stop smoking and drinking. Consider incisional biopsy to establish diagnosis.

Full-thickness gingivitis, red, inflamed and not plaque-related, often aggravated by brushing

Consider desquamative gingivitis.

- If clinical doubt exists and oral hygiene is poor: improve oral hygiene and re-evaluate.
- If associated with oral or skin lesions: consider dermatosis (e.g. lichen planus, psoriasis, vesiculobullous disorder; see 'Ulcerative lesions' below):
  - history: gingival inflammation and bleeding aggravated by brushing
  - clinical signs: may be associated with oral mucosal lesions and/ or associated skin lesions
  - tests: biopsy away from the gingival margin
  - treatment: topical steroids (see Appendix 4).

If no associated features

Consider plasma cell gingivitis:

- History: rapid onset associated with change of habit (e.g. new toothpaste).
- Clinical signs: stinging with toothpastes, foods, etc.
- Tests: patch test for potential allergens.
- Treatment: exclude allergen (e.g. tartar control toothpaste), possible topical steroid therapy.

If bilateral sores at the corners of the mouth, which are weeping or crusted and may persist in the absence of appropriate management

Consider angular cheilitis:

- If associated with intraoral candidosis, consider fungal infection:
  - history: soreness and cracking; persistent weeping or crusted sores at angles of mouth; may bleed; can persist in the absence of appropriate management
  - clinical signs: associated denture stomatitis
  - tests: swabs, smears
  - treatment: topical antifungals (see Appendix 3).

Note: Intraoral infection must also be treated. The condition can be exacerbated in denture patients by a decreased vertical dimension. Dentures might need to be reconstructed to correct.

- If patient dentate: consider infection with staphylococci or streptococci:

- ○ history: recurrent scab formation with or without bleeding
- ○ clinical signs: crusting of the angles of the mouth
- ○ tests: swabs, smears
- ○ treatment: antimicrobials (e.g. miconazole cream or nystatin-triamcinolone acetonide) (see Appendix 3).

If angular cheilitis persists despite treatment, consider microbial resistance, systemic conditions or immunocompromised state.

Hematinic deficiency (e.g. iron, folate or vitamin B_{12} deficiency)

- History: unresponsive to previous local therapy.
- Clinical signs: associated atrophic glossitis, aphthae.
- Tests: investigate cause of deficiency; serum ferritin, folate, vitamin B_{12} levels.
- Treatment: replacement therapy.

Diabetes mellitus

- History: obesity, polyphagia, polyuria, polydipsia ('3 polys'), infections.
- Clinical signs: crusting of angles of mouth.
- Tests: fasting blood sugar.
- Treatment: refer to physician.

HIV infection (angular cheilitis is more common in HIV disease)

- History: known HIV disease or history of high-risk activity for HIV infection.
- Clinical signs: associated pseudomembranous candidosis, hairy leukoplakia, Kaposi's sarcoma.
- Tests: serology, swabs.
- Treatment: antimicrobials (see Appendices 3 and 5).

Oral facial granulomatosis/oral manifestations of Crohn's disease

- History: fluctuating lip swelling with or without GI symptoms.
- Clinical signs: associated lip swelling, cobblestoning, intraoral ulceration, full thickness gingivitis.
- Tests: intraoral biopsy, swabs. Exclude GI tract involvement by screening for underlying malabsorption or chronic blood loss. Angiotensin-converting enzyme (ACE) levels to exclude sarcoidosis.
- Treatment: topical steroids (see Appendix 4). Sulfasalazine.

If angular cheilitis shows chronic fissuring or folding

Consider correction of dentures; refer for surgery if severe.

Ulcerative lesions

May be an end-organ effect of several disease processes. There is therefore a large differential diagnosis (Fig. 3.3).

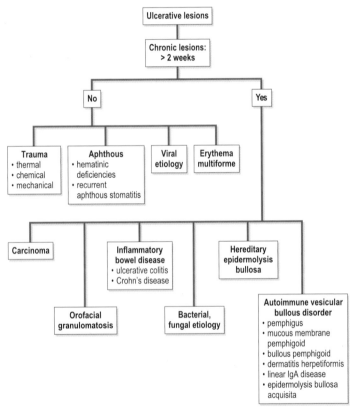

Fig. 3.3 **Ulcerative lesions.**

If single ulcer with no obvious cause

Consider trauma:

- History: pain from local cause, no H/O ulcers.
- Clinical signs: local cause (for example the mid-buccal mucosa at the interocclusal line, and on the lateral borders of the tongue).
- Tests: none.
- Treatment: Remove cause. Follow up for healing.

If single ulcer and long-lasting (more than 2 weeks)

Consider carcinoma:

- History: smoker or smokeless tobacco with or without alcohol.
- Clinical signs: rolled edge, induration, possible regional lymphadenopathy.
- Tests: incisional biopsy after 2 weeks if not resolving from local measures.
- Treatment: if biopsy positive for carcinoma, refer to appropriate surgeon.

If ulcers are recurrent and affect non-keratinizing mucosa

Consider recurrent aphthous stomatitis:

- History: affects only moveable mucosa. Recurrent. Limited duration of about 7–10 days.
- Clinical signs: round or oval, single or crops. Gray, white or yellowish necrotic center with surrounding band of erythema.
- Tests: complete blood count, serum ferritin, folate, and vitamin B_{12} levels to rule out the unusual case of hematinic deficiency.
- Treatment: replacement hematinics with abnormal test above. Although not evidence based, tetracycline mouthwash, chlorhexidine or topical steroids are reported to be effective in some cases (see Appendices 3, 4 and 6).

If there is associated keratosis and striations

Consider lichen planus (see 'White lesions', above).

If there is associated lip swelling and lymphedema

Consider orofacial granulomatosis:

- History: lip swelling, with or without GI symptoms.
- Clinical signs: gingivitis, cobblestoning of mucosa, angular cheilitis, mucosal tags.
- Tests: biopsy. Consider patch testing.
- Treatment: dietary manipulation; consider steroid therapy (see Appendix 4).

If mucosal ulcerations with concomitant GI symptoms (diarrhea, pain, bleeding)

Consider inflammatory bowel disease (ulcerative colitis and Crohn's disease):

- History: chronic recurrent ulcerations.
- Clinical signs: ulcerations, and might have concomitant vitamin deficiency symptoms (e.g. pale mucosa, glossitis). Wide range of oral manifestations for Crohn's disease (cobblestone mucosa to ulcerations). Aphthous appearance for ulcerative colitis.
- Tests: biopsy might be helpful.
- Treatment: control of underlying disease with immunosuppressants, if appropriate (see Appendix 4).

If ulcers are vesicular or there is herpetiform stomatitis

Consider viral infection:

- History: recent onset, unwell.
- Clinical signs: vesicles, fever, lymphadenopathy, malaise.
- Tests: consider serology and viral cultures.
- Treatment: symptomatic, antivirals for herpes virus infections, if severe (see Appendix 5).

If idiopathic

Consider bacterial or fungal ulcers (e.g. tuberculosis, syphilis):

- History: long-standing ulcers, painless.
- Clinical signs: non-specific.
- Tests: biopsy, culture, serology.
- Treatment: antimicrobials (see Appendix 3).

If hereditary

Consider epidermolysis bullosa:

- History: usually diagnosed neonatally.
- Clinical signs: extensive skin involvement.
- Tests: biopsy (immunofluorescence negative).
- Treatment: symptomatic; minimize mucosal trauma.

If ulcers are episodic or there are skin target lesions

Consider erythema multiforme:

- History: recurrent stomatitis lasting 2 weeks.
- Clinical signs: target lesions, especially on hands; bloody crusting of lips.

- Tests: biopsy, consider patch testing.
- Treatment: eliminate cause (medications) if known; corticosteroids; empirical antiviral agents (see Appendices 4 and 5).

If none of the above, and with skin lesions

Consider autoimmune vesiculobullous disorder:

- History: sudden onset of non-healing blisters which ulcerate.
- Clinical signs: often non-specific.
- Tests: biopsy plus direct and indirect immunofluorescence.
- Treatment: see the specific disorders, below.

Pemphigus

- Tests: direct immunofluorescence shows IgG or IgM and/or C3 suprabasally, indirect immunofluorescence positive for intracellular substance antigen (ICSA).
- Treatment: systemic steroids with or without azathioprine (see Appendix 4).

Mucous membrane pemphigoid

- Tests: direct and indirect immunofluorescence shows IgG, IgM and/or C3 linear at basement membrane zone. Indirect may be positive for substance basement membrane antigen (SBMA).
- Treatment: none if mild. Topical steroids with or without systemic steroids (see Appendix 4).

Bullous pemphigoid

- Tests: direct and indirect immunofluorescence shows with or without IgG, IgM and/or C3 linear at basement membrane zone.
- Treatment: topical steroids with or without systemic steroids (see Appendix 4).

Dermatitis herpetiformis

- Tests: direct immunofluorescence shows granular IgA at the basement membrane zone.
- Treatment: gluten-free diet. Topical steroids with or without systemic steroids (see Appendix 4).

Linear IgA disease

- Tests: direct immunofluorescence shows IgA linear at the basement membrane zone.

- Treatment: immunomodulators (consider dapsone, topical steroids with or without systemic steroids) (see Appendix 4).

Epidermolysis bullosa acquisita

- Tests: direct immunofluorescence shows with or without IgG, IgM and/or C3 sub-basilar (antibodies to collagen).
- Treatment: systemic steroids with or without azathioprine) (see Appendix 4).

PIGMENTED LESIONS

Often due to extrinsic substances, such as amalgam or melanotic (intrinsic pigmentation) (Fig. 3.4).

If lesions focal and long standing

Consider amalgam tattoo or intraoral nevus:

- History: extraction or trauma during restoration of tooth versus no etiologic factor.

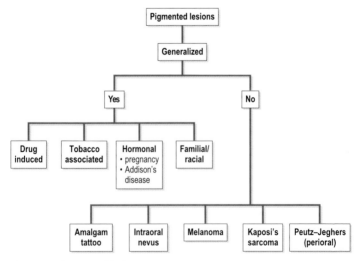

Fig. 3.4 Pigmented lesions.

- Clinical signs: adjacent amalgam or extraction site.
- Tests: radiograph. Biopsy may be positive for metallic fragments.
- Treatment: none.

If lesions focal and recent onset

Consider melanoma or, more likely, Kaposi's sarcoma:
- History: recent change in appearance.
- Clinical signs: enlarging; may be hemorrhagic; color can be blue/black, brown or normal.
- Tests: extreme care with biopsy due to risk of seeding. Refer for HIV workup if suspicious of HIV.
- Treatment: referral to head and neck surgeon if suspicious for melanoma.

If pigmentation is perioral

Consider Peutz–Jeghers syndrome:
- History: lifelong lesions.
- Clinical signs: may have bowel symptoms.
- Tests: barium studies (for premalignant polyposis coli).
- Treatment: observation. Refer to physician.

If pigmentation is diffuse

Consider drug induced (e.g. antibiotics, antihypertensives, oral contraceptives):
- History: drug ingestion; may be some time ago.
- Clinical signs: widespread
- Tests: consider biopsy.
- Treatment: none. May need to change or withdraw drug(s).

If negative drug history and diffuse

Consider tobacco:
- History: smoker.
- Clinical signs: may have leukoplakia.
- Tests: biopsy.
- Treatment: stop tobacco use.

If no drug or smoking history

Consider hormonal causes:

Pregnancy

- History: second or third trimester of pregnancy.

- Clinical signs: none other than mucosal lesion(s).
- Tests: none.
- Treatment: none.

Addison's disease
- History: systemically unwell.
- Clinical signs: sweating, hypotension.
- Tests: adrenal workup.
- Treatment: replacement steroids. Refer to physician.

If no abnormalities detectable
Consider familial or racial.

Pale appearance of mucosa
This can result from anemia (deficiency in production or maturation, or excessive destruction of RBCs). The differential diagnosis includes vitamin deficiency, GI disease, blood loss, sickle-cell anemia, aplastic anemia, hematologic malignancy, hemolytic anemia:
- History: complaint of fatigue in more severe anemia.
- Clinical signs: pallor of mucosa.
- Tests: complete blood count.
- Treatment: management of underlying cause of anemia or blood products when appropriate.

PAIN AND ALTERED SENSATION

Pain and/or altered sensation can be acute or chronic, intermittent or constant. Most causes are readily identifiable but neurologic or neuropathic pain can be difficult to diagnose.

Dental pain

If the pain appears odontogenic (dental) in origin, consider pulpitis, abscess, cracked tooth, or sinus infection. (see Chapter 5):
- History: variable severity and nature of pain. Likely symptomatic with eating and temperature changes.
- Clinical signs: hairline crack on clinical crown, caries, abnormal pocket depths, mobility, regional swelling.

- Tests: radiographs, vitality testing, exploration, percussion, mobility, biting, thermal tests.
- Treatment: restorative, endodontic, surgical as usual.

Perioral pain

If the pain is constant and dental causes have been excluded, consider perioral conditions (e.g. salivary gland infection, ear infection):
- History: short history of constant, severe pain.
- Clinical signs: salivary gland swelling or inflammation of the eardrum.
- Tests: sialography.
- Treatment: referral to appropriate clinician, may require antimicrobial therapy if infectious etiology.

Sinus infection

If the pain is associated with percussion of maxillary posterior teeth and dental causes have been excluded, consider sinus infection:
- History: recent onset of maxillary tooth pain, which is difficult to localize. History of upper respiratory infection in past 2–3 months.
- Clinical signs: pain with percussion of maxillary posterior teeth. (usually premolars and first molar).
- Tests: radiographs – panoramic/CT; if indicated.
- Treatment: referral to appropriate clinician. Might require antimicrobial therapy if infectious etiology. Surgical therapy for tumors.

Neurologic

If the pain is episodic and dental causes have been excluded, consider a neurologic disorder.

Trigeminal neuralgia
- History: sudden onset. Unilateral, intense brief lancinating pain on touching face or eating.
- Clinical signs: lancinating pain with the trigger zone.
- Tests: CT scan, if less than 40 years old, to exclude multiple sclerosis and CNS tumor.
- Treatment: referral to appropriate clinician for consideration of carbamazepine, phenytoin, or neurontin.

Glossopharyngeal neuralgia

- History: sudden onset. Brief lancinating pain with stimulation of pharyngeal tissue (e.g. swallowing).
- Clinical signs: lancinating pain with pharyngeal trigger.
- Tests: none.
- Treatment: referral to appropriate clinician for consideration of carbamazepine, phenytoin, or neurontin.

Migrainous neuralgia

- History: unilateral headaches.
- Clinical signs: associated watering of the eye and nasal stuffiness on the affected side.
- Tests: none.
- Treatment: referral to appropriate clinician for consideration of beta-blockers or ACE inhibitors.

Angina pectoris

- History: exercise-induced jaw pain, usually lower left.
- Clinical signs: none.
- Tests: cardiac function tests.
- Treatment: management of cardiac ischemia, referral to physician.

Sickle-cell disease

If recurrent episodic jaw pain with concomitant extragnathic bone pain, consider sickle-cell disease:

- History: previous history of sickle-cell crisis; may be triggered by hypoxic states (e.g. stress, infection).
- Clinical signs: rule out odontogenic infection. African descent.
- Tests: serology; 90–95% HbS with hemoglobin electrophoresis.
- Treatment: supportive – analgesics, fluids, eliminate sources of infection. Avoid stressful procedures.

Oral soft tissue

If mucosal signs present, consider oral soft tissue disease. (e.g. viral infections, vesiculobullous disorders, recurrent aphthae):

- History: pain on eating or talking.
- Clinical signs: ulcers, vesicles or bullae.

- Tests: serology, consider biopsy.
- Treatment: see 'Ulcerative lesions', above.

If no clinical signs

Consider functional pain.

Temporomandibular dysfunction
- History: fluctuating pain and trismus, not relieved by analgesics.
- Clinical signs: predominantly young females. May have joint clicking, masticatory muscle pain.
- Tests: none.
- Treatment: usually self-limiting. Reassurance, clenching awareness, splint therapy, psychotropic therapy (e.g. dothiepin, amitriptyline; see Appendix 6).

Atypical facial pain
- History: similar to toothache but pain character may be dull/deep. Can be relieved by food. History of unhelpful dental treatment. Females predominate, unresponsive to analgesia, more than 1 month duration.
- Tests: diagnostic local anesthetic block.
- Treatment: reassurance, psychotropic therapy (e.g. dothiepin, amitriptyline; see Appendix 6).

Oral dysesthesia
- History: associated sleep disturbance, diurnal variation, relieved by food. Often perimenopausal female.
- Tests: none.
- Treatment: reassurance, psychotropic therapy (e.g. dothiepin, amitriptyline; see Appendix 6).

Postherpetic neuralgia
- History: history of varicella zoster infection.
- Clinical signs: pain distribution associated with a branch of the trigeminal nerve.
- Tests: diagnostic local anesthetic block.
- Treatment: topical analgesics, EMLA, neurontin.

Temporal arteritis
- History: short history of unilateral, pulsating pain in area of temporal artery.

- Clinical signs: may see dermal erythema. Blindness if untreated. Symptoms can mimic temporomandibular disorder (TMD).
- Tests: sedimentation rate, C-reactive protein, temporal artery biopsy.
- Treatment: prednisone, pain medications (e.g. opioids). Urgent referral to appropriate physician (e.g. ophthalmology) to prevent blindness if untreated.

Burning mouth syndrome

If patient complains of a burning sensation with or without associated taste disorders, pain or mucosal sensitivity affecting the tongue, lips or palate, consider burning mouth syndrome when other etiologic factors have been excluded.

Mucosal disease

If associated with eating hot or spicy foods, look for mucosal disease (e.g. lichen planus, geographic tongue, aphthae, glossitis):
- History: pain on eating, no diurnal variation.
- Clinical signs: mucosal abnormality (e.g. migrating patchy erythema, fissuring, ulceration, plaques or reticular white patches).
- Tests: biopsy or hematological screening.
- Treatment: amitriptyline, dothiepin, clonazepam (see Appendix 6).

Occult organic disease

If clinically normal, exclude occult organic disease (e.g. nutritional deficiency, candidosis, or denture abnormalities):
- History: pain on eating, possible metallic taste.
- Clinical signs: may be none; possible anemia, loss of filiform papillae of tongue.
- Tests: complete blood count, serum ferritin, folate, vitamin B_{12}, fasting blood sugar, mycology.
- Treatment: replacement therapy, antifungal therapy, diabetic referral, prosthodontics referral (see Appendix 3).

Idiopathic

If idiopathic, consider oral dysesthesia.
- History: diurnal variation, relieved by food, sleep disturbance, depression and anxiety.
- Clinical signs: none.

- Tests: none.
- Treatment: psychological counseling, psychotropic therapy (e.g. dothiepin, fluoxetine, amitriptyline) (see Appendix 6).

Paresthesia

- Differential diagnosis: includes recent trauma, malignant infiltrate, nutritional deficiency and multiple sclerosis. Consider recent trauma to facial structures as an etiology.
- History: traumatic damage.
- Clinical signs: displaced bony structures, soft tissue damage in area of trauma, fractured or luxated teeth.
- Tests: intraoral radiographs, CT.
- Treatment: open or closed reduction of facial fractures. Can take over 6 months for nerve regeneration with potential permanent damage.

Malignant infiltrate

Malignant infiltrate might need to be ruled out if the paresthesia is of new onset and is worsening:

- History: previous cancer diagnosis; however, it might be an undiagnosed malignancy.
- Clinical signs: may have soft tissue lesion, swelling.
- Tests: physical examination, MRI/CT, bone scan.
- Treatment: surgery and/or chemotherapy and/or radiotherapy.

Nutritional deficiencies

- History: sensitive to hot, spicy foods.
- Clinical signs: may have anemia.
- Tests: complete blood count, serum ferritin, folate and vitamin B_{12}.
- Treatment: appropriate replacement therapy.

Glossitis

Discomfort of the tongue with or without clinical changes in its appearance. If the tongue appears normal, consider nutritional deficiency or psychogenic causes.

Nutritional deficiencies and psychogenic causes

- History: diurnal variation, sleep disturbance. May have anxiety and depression.

- Clinical signs: none.
- Tests: none.
- Treatment: reassurance, psychotropic therapy (e.g. dothiepin, venlafaxine; see Appendix 6), referral for counseling.

Candidosis

If clinical signs, consider mucosal disease:

- History: may have metallic taste, tongue sensitive.
- Clinical signs: erythema, associated denture stomatitis or angular cheilitis.
- Tests: swabs, smears.
- Treatment: topical antifungals (see Appendix 3).

Geographic tongue

- History: intermittent sensitivity to foods.
- Clinical signs: migrating patchy erythema, usually with a surrounding whitish–yellowish halo, with or without fissuring.
- Tests: none.
- Treatment: reassurance, treatment with psychotropic therapy. Consider topical steroid (see Appendix 4) if inappropriately painful.

Nutritional glossitis

- History: sensitive to hot, spicy foods.
- Clinical signs: loss of filiform papillae.
- Tests: complete blood count, ferritin, folate and vitamin B_{12}.
- Treatment: investigate cause of deficiency, replacement therapy.

Lichen planus

- History: variable sensitivity with or without ulceration.
- Clinical signs: plaques or reticular white patches, on the dorsal and lateral surfaces, or 'half-moon' areas on the lateral sides. May have erosions.
- Tests: biopsy junction of involved and uninvolved tissue.
- Treatment: identification of etiological factors (see lichen planus section), symptomatic therapy including topical steroids (see Appendix 4), monitor for malignant transformation.

Ulceration

- History: pain, especially on eating.
- Clinical signs: lingual ulcer or erosion.

- Tests: see 'Ulcerative lesions', above.
- Treatment: see 'Ulcerative lesions', above.

Median rhomboid glossitis
- History: usually smoker or uses steroid inhaler.
- Clinical signs: central area of erythema associated with loss of papillae. May have associated erythematous candidosis of the palate.
- Tests: biopsy, if clinical doubt
- Treatment: oral rinsing after steroid inhaler, topical or systemic antifungals (see Appendix 3).

Tongue thrusting
- History: anxiety and known habit of thrusting.
- Clinical signs: crenation of borders of tongue, redness of tip.
- Tests: none.
- Treatment: consider splints, psychotherapy, psychotropic therapy (see Appendix 6).

DRY MOUTH

Most commonly a side-effect of medication, radiotherapy, salivary gland disease or dehydration. Symptoms are often more reliable than salivary flow rates.

Drug-induced

If the patient is on medication, consider drug-induced xerostomia (e.g. tricyclic antidepressants, diuretics, cytotoxics or radiotherapy):
- History: onset coincident with medication. Subjectively, often no complaint of dryness when eating a meal.
- Clinical signs: may have frothy saliva, increased incidence of caries.
- Tests: salivary flow rates, serology (e.g. anti-Ro and anti-La).
- Treatment: hydration throughout day, topical salivary substitutes (e.g. mucin or methylcellulose) or systemic (see Appendix 7), oral hygiene, sugar-free candies [sweets] or gum. Discuss with physician if xerostomic medication can be substituted.

Tobacco-induced

If the patient is a tobacco user, consider smoking as a cause:
- History: heavy smoking, bad taste.
- Clinical signs: discolored tongue, tobacco stained teeth.
- Tests: none.
- Treatment: stop smoking.

Dehydration

If patient with a chronic disease state (e.g. diabetic or has renal failure), consider dehydration:
- History: systemically unwell, insulin-dependent diabetes.
- Clinical signs: skin wrinkling, pseudomembranous candidosis.
- Tests: BUN, creatinine, electrolytes, fasting blood sugar.
- Treatment: fluids.

Candidosis

If mucosal erythema, consider candidosis:
- History: denture wearer or history of prolonged antibiotic therapy.
- Clinical signs: mucosal erythema.
- Tests: swabs/smears, culture.
- Treatment: topical antifungals (see Appendix 3).

Systemic disorders

If other etiologic factors have been eliminated, consider systemic disorder, such as Sjögren's syndrome, sarcoidosis, HIV disease.

Sjögren's syndrome
- History: increasing dryness and associated dry eyes.
- Clinical signs: constant or fluctuating salivary gland swelling, systemic disease, increased incidence of caries, candidosis.
- Tests: labial minor salivary gland biopsy or fine-needle aspiration biopsy of salivary gland, serology (e.g. anti-Ro, anti-La), salivary flow rates.
- Treatment: hydration throughout day, salivary substitutes, oral hygiene, fluoride, systemic medications for Sjögren's syndrome (see Appendices 7 and 8).

Dysesthesia

If none of the above, consider dysesthesia:
- History: cyclical problem, associated agitation or depression (see burning mouth).
- Clinical signs: none.
- Tests: none.
- Treatment: counseling and drug therapy, if indicated (see Appendix 6). (*Note*: These drugs may cause xerostomia.)

Previous radiotherapy

If patient has a history of radiotherapy for head and neck cancer and dry mouth complaints, radiation-induced salivary gland dysfunction is likely:
- History: > 4000 cGy radiotherapy affecting major salivary glands.
- Clinical signs: mucosal evidence of dryness, thick/ropy saliva, increased caries, candidosis.
- Tests: confirmation of radiation dose to salivary glands and low salivary flow rates.
- Treatment: hydration throughout day, salivary substitutes, oral hygiene, fluoride, low sucrose diet, systemic medications (see Appendices 7 and 8).

HALITOSIS

The patient might be unaware of the problem or the problems might be inappropriately perceived by the patient but is not apparent on examination.

Periodontal disease

Consider if malodor is detectable:
- History: bleeding on brushing and/or flossing.
- Clinical signs: loss of attachment, pocketing, poor oral hygiene, bleeding on probing, papillary necrosis (acute necrotizing ulcerative gingivitis; ANUG).
- Tests: probing, radiographs, consider microbiologic testing for refractory periodontitis or ANUG.

- Treatment: oral hygiene, scale and polish. Consider antimicrobials (e.g. chlorhexidine; see Appendix 3).

Smoker's halitosis

If periodontal condition satisfactory and patient smokes, consider smoker's halitosis:
- History: smoker, bad taste, dryness.
- Clinical signs: furrowing of the tongue, staining of teeth.
- Tests: none.
- Treatment: stop smoking.

Decreased salivary function

If mouth appears dry, consider decreased salivary function (see 'Dry mouth', above).
- History: drug-induced. Alcohol abuse.
- Clinical signs: dryness, caries, candidosis.
- Tests: salivary flow rates.
- Treatment: oral hygiene instruction, eliminate drug-induced causes.

Sinusitis

Consider if nasal or antral problems present:
- History: nasal stuffiness or discharge with or without antral pain.
- Clinical signs: nasal discharge, pain in upper teeth, especially on leaning over.
- Tests: radiographs (e.g. Water's view, panoramic) or CT of sinuses.
- Treatment: antibiotics (see Appendix 9), decongestant, nasal drops, inhalants.

Systemic disorders

Consider systemic diseases (e.g. cirrhosis, lung infection, renal failure, diabetic ketosis, gastrointestinal disease) or radiotherapy if no oral disease is present.

Psychogenic causes

If not clinically apparent and no systemic disease detectable, consider psychogenic causes:

- History: anxiety or depression.
- Clinical signs: anxiety and depression.
- Tests: none.
- Treatment: reassurance, psychotropic therapy (e.g. amitriptyline, dothiepin; see Appendix 6).

TASTE CHANGES

The etiologic disorders of change in taste sensation can include an olfactory disorder and may be associated with a local or central etiology.

Local etiology

This includes oral and perioral infections, oral appliances, and decreased salivary flow. Elimination of taste complaint with topical anesthetic (e.g. unflavored 1% dyclonine [lignocaine] HCl) on the tongue is suggestive of local etiology.

Infectious cause

It is important to rule out an infectious intra- or perioral etiology, including periodontal disease, odontogenic abscess and fungal and viral infections:
- History: pain, swelling, or bleeding on brushing and/or flossing.
- Clinical sign: periodontal disease (purulence, pocketing, poor oral hygiene, bleeding on probing), periapical abscess (swelling, purulence), viral or fungal (soft tissue lesions).
- Tests: radiographs, probing, KOH smear, culture for candidosis or viral disease.
- Treatment: oral hygiene, for periodontal therapy extraction or root canal therapy for odontogenic abscess, antifungal or anti-viral medication (see Appendices 3 and 5).

Oral appliances

If present, evaluate removable oral appliances:
- History: taste changes temporally related to placement of a new oral appliance.

- Clinical sign: erythema associated with allergy or candidosis.
- Tests: taste assessment after removal of oral appliance, KOH smear, culture for candidosis, allergy patch testing.
- Treatment: if allergy, remake oral appliance with different dental materials; if candidosis, improve hygiene and begin antifungals (see Appendix 3).

Dry mouth

Insufficient saliva decreases the distribution of tastants to the taste buds.

- History: taste changes temporally related to a new medication, radiotherapy for head and neck cancer, diagnosis of Sjögren's syndrome.
- Clinical signs: dryness of oral mucosa with evidence of a thick, foamy saliva.
- Tests: salivary flow, serology (e.g. anti-Ro and anti-La).
- Treatment: elimination of potential causative medications, saliva stimulant medication (see Appendix 7).

Drug metabolites

Drug metabolites in saliva can lead to taste changes:
- History: taste changes temporally related to a new medication.
- Clinical sign: none.
- Tests: none.
- Treatment: elimination of potential causative medications (e.g. captopril).

Upper respiratory infection

Consider upper respiratory infection etiology if symptomatic:
- History: cough, cold symptoms.
- Clinical sign: fever, productive cough.
- Tests: sputum.
- Treatment: referral to appropriate clinician. May require antibiotics if bacterial, symptomatic relief if viral.

Central/systemic etiology

This includes traumatic injury to peripheral nerves or CNS, tumor affecting taste pathway, Bell's palsy, endocrine disorders, gustatory aura with migraine or epilepsy, or aging.

Peripheral nerve damage

This may result from intraoral trauma:
- History: temporal relationship of previous inferior alveolar nerve block or extraction of a lower third molar.
- Clinical signs: none.
- Tests: diagnostic block of affected nerve.
- Treatment: none. Consider surgical correction and/or steroids.

Central tumor

This may affect taste pathways:
- History: recent onset of taste changes with concomitant abnormal CNS symptoms (e.g. headache).
- Clinical signs: abnormal cranial nerve examination.
- Tests: CT with or without MRI.
- Treatment: surgery, radiotherapy, chemotherapy if malignant.

Bell's palsy

Taste disorders can be associated with Bell's palsy:
- History: viral infection, but often idiopathic.
- Clinical signs: unilateral facial nerve dystonia.
- Tests: none, clinically evident.
- Treatment: pulse, high-dose steroids (0.25 to 0.5 mg/kg for days and tapering by 5 mg daily thereafter). Often resolves, but may be permanent.

Endocrine disorders

Taste disorders have been reported with endocrine disorders such as diabetes mellitus, adrenal insufficiency, hypothyroidism and trimethylaminuria:
- History: concomitant symptoms consistent with endocrine disease.
- Clinical signs: none associated with taste abnormalities.
- Tests: laboratory (e.g. CBC, differential, metabolic panel, thyroid scan).
- Treatment: medical control of underlying endocrine disorder.

Migraine headaches or epilepsy

A gustatory aura may be associated with migraine headaches or epilepsy:

- History: migraine headaches or seizures.
- Clinical signs: concomitant autonomic aura (e.g. increased lacrimation), seizure activity.
- Tests: migraine or epilepsy diagnosis with consistent signs and symptoms.
- Treatment: control of underlying condition; prophylactic and therapeutic medications.

OLFACTORY CHANGES

May be primary complaint or the underlying cause of taste change complaints.

Local etiology

May be associated with a local etiology (nasal/sinus disease, upper respiratory infection, smoking, intranasal cocaine, head/neck radiotherapy).

Nasal/sinus disease

Nasal or sinus obstruction/infection and respiratory infection may cause olfactory changes:

- History: frontal headache or congestion for nasal and sinus disease.
- Clinical signs: obstructed nasal passages, discharge.
- Tests: CT/MRI.
- Treatment: appropriate antibiotics for bacterial sinus infection, surgery for nasal obstruction.

Intranasal cocaine

May damage nasal structures:

- Clinical signs: erosion with possible perforation of nasal septum.

Head/neck radiotherapy

May cause limited olfactory changes.

Central/systemic etiology

Head trauma, neurodegenerative disease, medications, chemical exposure, nutritional deficiency, endocrine disease, CNS neoplasm, cerebrovascular accident, olfactory aura, psychiatric, Sjögren's syndrome, lupus and age-related changes.

BLEEDING

Intraoral bleeding may occur from the gingiva or intramucosally in the form of blood-filled bullae, petechiae or ecchymosis.

Periodontal disease

If gingival bleeding occurs, consider periodontal disease:
- History: chronic intermittent bleeding on brushing.
- Clinical signs: erythematous, often swollen gingiva. Loss of attachment, tooth mobility, bleeding on periodontal probing.
- Tests: probing, radiographs, microbiology for suspected ANUG.
- Treatment: oral hygiene under local anesthetic, scale and polish. Consider antimicrobials if systematic signs exist (e.g. fever, enlarged nodes).

If gingival bleeding occurs without periodontal disease, consider a hereditary or acquired bleeding disorder.

Hereditary disorders

For example, hemophilia A and B, von Willebrand's disease:
- History: bleeding with minor trauma. Nose bleeds. Prolonged bleeding from extractions. Usually known H/O hemorrhagic diathesis.
- Clinical signs: associated skin bruising and joint hemorrhages.
- Tests: factor VIII and IX levels, von Willebrand antigen and ristocetin cofactor, PT/INR, APTT.
- Treatment: if abnormal, refer to hematology.

Acquired disorders

Drug induced

Bleeding episodes or risk for bleeding with anticoagulants (e.g. aspirin, NSAIDs, warfarin, heparin and low molecular weight heparinoids), cancer chemotherapeutic agents and ethanol.

NSAIDs

Aspirin and other NSAIDs inhibit thromboxane A, which is required for platelet activation and aggregation:

- History: positive drug history.
- Clinical signs: may predispose to postoperative bleeding from extensive surgery. Significance is unclear from minor surgical procedures (e.g. extractions), but unlikely to be a problem.
- Tests: none.
- Treatment: consider discontinuation of medications prior to extensive surgical procedures or if multiple coagulopathies exist.

Warfarin

Interferes with vitamin-K-dependent clotting factors (II, VII, IX, and X):

- History: positive drug history.
- Clinical signs: may have prolonged bleeding with minor trauma.
- Tests: INR.
- Treatment: minor surgical procedures usually controlled with local hemostatic measures if INR within therapeutic range (i.e. < 3.5). Consider downward adjustment of INR (under supervision of patient's primary care physician) if INR > 3.5 or if a moderate to major surgical procedure is planned.

Heparin

Inhibits thrombin formation:

- History: positive drug history.
- Clinical signs: bleeding from minor trauma.
- Tests: APTT.
- Treatment: discontinuation of heparin (half-life = 4 h) prior to invasive dental procedure.

Alcohol abuse

Can inhibit platelet formation by direct toxicity to bone marrow, folate deficiency or hypersplenism. May have additional coagulopathy from liver disease:

- History: positive drug history.
- Clinical signs: petechiae or ecchymosis.
- Tests: complete blood count, PT/INR.
- Treatment: if abnormal blood tests, may need to consider extra local hemostatic measures or blood products.

Underlying systemic disease

Liver disease

Bleeding episodes can arise from decreased clotting factors from loss of hepatic tissue. Portal hypertension can lead to hypersplenism, which will decrease the platelet count:

- History: may report alcoholism, viral hepatitis.
- Clinical signs: jaundiced appearance of the tissues.
- Tests: PT/INR, platelet count.
- Treatment: local measures to control bleeding episodes. Vitamin K, EACA, systemic desmopressin. Consider blood product replacement with significantly elevated PT/INR and/or severe thrombocytopenia prior to invasive procedures.

Renal disease/uremia

Bleeding episodes can arise from inhibition of platelet adhesion and aggregation from glycoprotein IIb–IIIa defect. Uremia can induce qualitative platelet defect:

- History: chronic renal failure or dialysis.
- Clinical signs: uremic stomatitis can be present with poorly controlled disease.
- Tests: creatinine clearance.
- Treatment: for dialysis patients, invasive dental procedure should be accomplished after the heparin has ceased to cause a significant coagulopathy (2–3 h) and before the patient again becomes uremic (i.e. close to the time of the next dialysis).

Bone marrow failure

Bleeding from deficient platelet production. Loss of hematopoietic bone marrow cells may result from conditions such as hematologic malignancy (e.g. leukemia), suppression from cancer chemotherapy, alcoholism or aplastic anemia:

- History: fatigue, malaise, fever, night sweats, easy bruising, infection, gingival bleeding. Sudden onset, systemically unwell.
- Clinical signs: associated pallor, lymphadenopathy, hepatosplenomegaly.
- Tests: complete blood count with differential.
- Treatment: refer to hematologist.

Idiopathic thrombocytopenia purpura

- History: easy bruising.

- Clinical signs: petechiae, ecchymosis.
- Tests: complete blood count (platelets).
- Treatment: physician referral.

Vitamin deficiency (e.g. vitamin C – scurvy)

- History: malnourishment.
- Clinical signs: weakness, gingival swelling, bleeding.
- Tests: vitamin analysis.
- Treatment: supplement or foods high in vitamin C.

If ulceration(s) are present, consider herpes virus infections, vesiculobullous disorder or trauma (see 'Ulcerative lesions', above).

Vesiculobullous disorders

If mucosal hemorrhage and blisters, consider a vesiculobullous disorder:

Angina bullosa hemorrhagica

- History: infrequent non-troublesome, blood-filled blisters with rapid normal healing.
- Clinical signs: blister formation, especially of soft palate.
- Tests: exclude bleeding disorders/thrombocytopenia.
- Treatment: reassurance.

Other vesiculobullous disorders (e.g. pemphigus)

- History: sudden onset of persistent blisters.
- Clinical signs: non-healing erosions, with or without associated skin lesions.
- Tests: biopsy for immunofluorescence and histopathology. Check platelet count.
- Treatment: see above.

Epstein–Barr virus

If mucosal hemorrhage with petechiae or ecchymosis, consider Epstein–Barr virus infection:

- History: sudden onset, associated malaise.
- Clinical signs: hemorrhages at the junction of the hard and soft palate, tonsil enlargement, pharyngitis, lymphadenopathy, fatigue and mild fevers.
- Tests: monospot.
- Treatment: symptomatic.

Kaposi's sarcoma
- History: known HIV or H/O high risk activity. Elderly males of Mediterranean descent.
- Clinical signs: single or multiple bluish lesions.
- Tests: biopsy.
- Treatment: referral to a physician.

INFECTION

Immunosuppression can predispose to severe infections or to poor healing:
- History: recent onset of infection.
- Clinical signs: erythema (rubor), warmth (calor), pain (dolor), limited movement (functio laesa), and swelling (tumor).
- Tests: aerobic/anaerobic bacterial cultures.
- Treatment: remove source of infection, incision and drainage, and/or antibiotic therapy (see Appendix 9).

ODONTOGENIC/BONY CHANGES ASSOCIATED WITH SYSTEMIC DISEASE

Teeth

Odontogenic manifestations of systemic disease can include increased tooth mobility, malocclusion, discoloration, hypoplastic changes or eruption disturbances:
- Increased tooth mobility differential diagnosis from systemic disease includes: diabetes, AIDS, leukemia, neutropenia, hypophosphatasia, Papillon–Lefevre syndrome, leukocyte adhesion deficiency.
- Malocclusion differential diagnosis from systemic disease includes: Paget's disease, fibrous dysplasia, odontogenic cysts and tumors, hyperparathyroidism, metastatic infiltrate.
- Discoloration differential diagnosis from systemic disease includes: medications (e.g. tetracycline), excessive heavy metal exposure, erythropoietic porphyria, erythroblastosis fetalis, amelogenesis imperfecta, dentinogenesis imperfecta.

- Hypoplastic changes: amelogenesis imperfecta, dentinogenesis imperfecta, ectodermal dysplasia, radiotherapy during tooth development.
- Eruption disturbances: radiotherapy during tooth development, developmental delay, Job's syndrome, cleidocranial dysplasia.

Radiographic changes

Radiographic changes can be the result of systemic disease:
- Lucency differential diagnosis includes: malignancy, multiple myeloma, eosinophilic granuloma, fibrous dysplasia, hyperparathyroidism.
- Opacity differential diagnosis includes: fibrous dysplasia, Paget's disease, hyperparathyroidism, osteomas with Gardner's syndrome.
- Floating teeth differential diagnosis includes: diabetes, malignancy, multiple myeloma, eosinophilic granuloma, Papillon-Lefevre, fibrous dysplasia, Hand–Schuller–Christian, Gaucher's, Paget's, hyperparathyroidism, scurvy.
- Widened periodontal ligament differential diagnosis includes: scleroderma, metastasis, osteosarcoma.

Chapter 4

Consultations

Consultations involve referring patients to another clinician or clinical service for an opinion and/or treatment concerning a specific problem.

REQUESTING AND ANSWERING CONSULTATIONS

Triaging consultations

Consultations (consults) should be prioritized – 'triaged' – on their degree of urgency. For example, trauma, hemorrhage and infection, particularly in immunosuppressed patients, should be considered as true emergencies for a dental service and should be addressed as soon as possible. For non-acute consultation requests, an answer within 24 h is acceptable, but the same day as the request is ideal. This might be specified in the hospital or departmental staff by-laws or policy manual.

The different types of consultations

Whether seeking or responding to a consultation request, keep in mind the different types of consultations:

- Opinion only: you might be seeking or asked to provide only an opinion. For example, you plan an invasive, bacteremia-producing dental procedure for a patient possibly at risk of infective endocarditis; or you might want an opinion or advice from a patient's cardiologist concerning the exact nature of a cardiac murmur. Alternatively, you might be asked to respond to a consultation request concerning the need or desirability for dental treatment for a patient, knowing that on discharge this patient's dental care will be undertaken by the family dentist.
- Opinion and treatment of a specific problem: you might be seeking or asked to provide both an opinion and treatment for a

specific – usually single – problem but not to provide complete, comprehensive care for the patient. For example, you might need an opinion from the hematology service as to the value of desmoplasin [desmopressin] for a patient with moderately severe von Willebrand's disease who needs an extraction and dental scaling.

Requesting consults from other services

Patients admitted to the dental service can benefit from, or need to be seen by, another hospital service. Standard consult request forms exist in most hospitals and should have the following information on them: ● Date. ● Requesting service. ● Service consulted. ● Problem(s) to be addressed. ● Vital information of interest to consultant. ● Questions to be answered. ● Whether you are seeking: an opinion only or a suggested management of a specific aspect of the patient's planned treatment; evaluation and treatment of a specific problem or to transfer the patient and the provision of treatment to another consultant or service.

When consulting physicians concerning the medical management of a dental patient, it might be relevant to include a description of the extent of the dental treatment contemplated with regards to anticipated stress, bacteremia, bleeding and postoperative healing time.

Other clinical services are consulted as dictated by the patients' needs. Services contacted might include allied health/paramedical services, for example:

- Physical therapy: for advice regarding such issues as assistance in transferring a patient between bed, gurney [trolley], wheelchair and dental operatory [surgery], and addressing physical rehabilitation related to TMD management and/or postintermaxillary fixation.
- Occupational therapy: to assist in the selection and fabrication of adjunctive oral health devices for patients with impairment of hands and arms.
- Speech therapy: for appraisal of suspected swallowing dysfunction or other oral motor function (e.g. speech, mastication). Also, to assist in maximizing communication with an aphasic patient.
- Social work: to assist in communicating with a patient's family and other healthcare institutions, social services and health financial services.

- Nutrition/dietary: to assist in nutritional assessment and planning and supplementation (e.g. soft diet) for newly edentulous or wired-jaw patients.

Or medical or surgical services:
- Neurology/geriatrics: for further assessment in the event of suspected dementia.
- Internal medicine: to assist in medical management of patients.
- Anesthesiology: for pre-general anesthesia assessment.
- Specialist surgical services, especially for patients requiring general anesthesia to provide their dental care, but who also need other semielective surgical procedures under general anesthesia.
- Psychiatry or psychology: to assist in behavioral management issues; to address concerns regarding potential interactions with ongoing psychoactive medication regimens and to assess suspected depressive illness.
- Diabetic services: to assist with diet issues and establishing appropriate glycemic control with appropriate diet control.

Answering consult requests from other services

Where are you going to undertake your assessment of the patient?

Does this examination need to take place on the ward or can the patient be transferred to your department, with all the advantages of a dental chair, equipment (lights and mirrors) and access to radiographic equipment? Some patients clearly are not fit to be easily, or indeed safely, transferred. For example, patients with active pulmonary tuberculosis or profound neutropenia should not come into contact with the general population. Intubated patients, those needing ventilator support and those with significant physical impairment are invariably seen on the patient ward. When in doubt, examination should be conducted at the patient's bedside. Patients should almost never be brought to the dental clinic before reviewing the medical chart and seeing them bedside to ensure that there is no risk to the patient or dental clinic staff.

Bedside oral examination

Ensure that you have all the necessary equipment. Most medical/ surgical wards will stock gloves and tongue blades, but not a good source of light (headlight or flashlight [torch] or dental mirrors). For children or minors and intellectually impaired people, consider having a member of the clinical staff of the hospital as a chaperone present for your interview and examination.

Patient transport and escorts

For patients sufficiently healthy and mobile to be seen in your office [surgery], ensure that they are transported in a wheelchair, if appropriate, with their medical chart. Patients in wheelchairs are easier to examine and radiograph than if they are on a stretcher. Prior to their transfer, check if they have any intravenous fluids running, or require continuous oxygen. Patients receiving medication intravenously, such as chemotherapy or antibiotics, or who are in constant need of oxygen, might require a 'nurse escort' both for transportation and for the duration of their visit to dental clinic. This may be mandatory for patients with airways compromise, such as intermaxillary wiring or fixation.

The patient's point of view

A request or problem that might seem mundane to the dentist (e.g. an ill-fitting denture) can be a major concern to the patient, the family or the referring physician. An ill-fitting denture request also provides an opportunity to perform an oral examination on a patient who might not otherwise be seen by a dentist on a regular basis.

Reviewing the patient's records

The patient's records should be reviewed thoroughly. Note significant points in the medical history and hospital course. A concise but thorough note should be written and significant findings and recommendations might need to be discussed with the physician verbally, in addition to their inclusion in the written response. Effort should be made to minimize or eliminate dental jargon or terminology in order to ensure that the reader fully comprehends the response (e.g. 'quadrant', 'ortho', 'endo', and 'apex' mean very different things to physicians and dentists).

Avoid making recommendations that create work for the consulting physician (e.g. ordering/acquiring radiographs, oral debridement of blood clots, arranging appointments with the dental office [surgery]).

Findings and treatment should be discussed with relevant members of the patient's family, if appropriate, and with the family dentist whenever possible.

Clarify who will perform any dental treatment that proves necessary, and who is responsible for follow-up care.

Awareness, availability, promptness and competence often determine both the frequency of consult requests from other services and the quality of consultations, in terms of their appropriateness and interest.

Consult format

The first line of your entry in the record should specify the date and (in some hospitals) the time, your name, your level of appointment and your service.

- Introduction: include ● patient-identifying data ● date of admission ● reason for admission ● reason for consult.
- Chief complaint (CC): the concern for which the consultation was requested.
- History of present illness (HPI) [history of present complaint (HPC)]: brief summary of the development of the admitting diagnosis as well as the hospital course to date. It should be clear to the requesting clinician that the chart has been reviewed and that significant findings were taken into account in making subsequent recommendations.
- Past medical history (PMH): include ● illnesses ● hospitalizations ● operations ● allergies ● medications ● relevant laboratory investigations and any radiology/imaging reports, with dates.
- Past dental history (PDH): relevant information about previous dental treatment, for example, recent extractions and how the patient fared in terms of postoperative bleeding or delayed healing. Such information may be critical to assess the patient's fitness to undergo invasive dental procedures.
- Findings on examination: should include a head and neck and intraoral examination regardless of the reason for the consult, with cranial nerve review, if indicated. Significant negative and positive findings are noted. This section is descriptive rather than diagnostic and should avoid terminology that will not be understood by all concerned (e.g. use 'maxillary right first molar' not 'tooth #3 [6j]').

- Family and social history: include relevant items.
- Impression or assessment: all differential diagnoses should be included in decreasing order of likelihood. Because the reader may not be familiar with the impact of specific dental disease on the patient's medical status, elaboration of the diagnosis and the implications for medical management may be indicated.
- Recommendations or suggestions: the consultant is essentially a guest of the requesting service, as the admitting physician is ultimately responsible for the patient and all treatment rendered. Hence, only recommendations or suggestions are made. No treatment is performed without discussion with the admitting doctor or responsible house officer. It is often helpful for the treating clinicians and the nursing staff, to note in the patient record the date, time, duration and venue for any planned dental treatment. It might also be appropriate to include a brief description of the significance of the problem, to support the recommendations. All findings are addressed, especially the reason for the consultation.
- A statement as to whether or not the patient will be followed by the dental service, followed by: consultant's signature, consultant's printed name and the best way(s) to be contacted (phone/pager number).

EXAMPLES OF CONSULTATION REQUESTS

Most of the following examples are adapted from consults written by general practice residents in dentistry. Some material has been changed to ensure that drugs and procedures are current. They are intended to serve as a guide to format and to illustrate standard approaches to the evaluation and management of typical oral problems of inpatients. Note that although there are a variety of writing styles in these examples, they all address the reason for consultation.

Urgent/acute consultation requests (Figs 4.1–4.7)

Comments on Figure 4.1
- Note that the description of the intraoral findings uses as little dental jargon as possible for the benefit of the physicians and

Fig. 4.1 Dental consult #1: dental trauma following MVA [RTA]; risk of aspiration

Date/Time: ....

Request: Evaluate dental trauma following MVA [RTA]. We plan to deflate the ETT (endotracheal tube) in near future.

Response: Asked by the trauma surgeons to see this 33 yo male admitted (date ......) following MVA with right tib. fib. fracture and facial trauma.

HPI: Struck by a high-speed vehicle, thrown ~ 50 feet. When found by paramedics he had rapid pulse, BP 120/60. His mouth was 'full of blood' and there was no response to verbal commands. Noted large, soft hematoma left scalp. Several anterior teeth noted to be 'unstable'. No skull fracture on CT but positive for diffuse brain swelling. No rhinorrhea or otorrhea. C-spine without fracture. Positive right tib. fib. fracture. During suctioning of mouth earlier this a.m. a nurse suctioned a 'portion of tooth'. Now asked to assess stability of remaining dentition to allow for ETT cuff deflation without risk of aspiration of segments of teeth or subsequent fracture of teeth.

Past medical history: Unknown.

Past surgical history: None.

Past dental history: Unknown.

Labs: (Date ....) WBC 13.4, HCT 31, plts. 101 000

| 132 | 104 | 6 | Sodium | Chloride | BUN |
| 3.7 | 24 | 126 | Potassium | Bicarbonate | Creat. |

Allergy: NKDA (no known drug allergies).
Meds: KCl (potassium chloride), phenytoin, pencillin, Mylanta [Asilone], Tylenol [paracetamol].

Examination:
Extraoral: Lip with laceration, already sutured and with minimal oozing. No deviation with opening of jaw. Maximum opening ~ 30 mm, but patient not very responsive. No tenderness to TMJ areas noted. No mobile segments of mandible. No facial asymmetry, subconjunctival hemorrhage or mobility of maxillary segments relative to zygoma or forehead. Neck supple but exam difficult secondary to obesity.
Intraoral: Extremely limited exam due to patient's immobility and inability to fully open mouth or comply with requests.
1. Hard and soft palate: no lesions.
2. Floor of mouth: minimally observed. However, no ecchymosis or trauma noted.
3. Tongue: much debris, thick secretions.
4. Buccal and labial mucosa: upper lip with large ecchymosis and shallow laceration (poorly visualized). No active hemorrhage noted intraorally.

5. Gingiva: pink, stippled, good contour without hemorrhage, laceration or evidence of trauma, except for max. right ant. region.

6. Dentition: coronal aspect of max. right lateral incisor is missing, possibly avulsed or fractured, cannot visualize a root in the socket. Surrounding gingiva is ecchymotic, with coagulated blood covering the socket. Max. right canine slightly mobile and with vertical fracture through dentin to gingival margin, missing entire facial aspect. Max. central incisors show slight mobility with 'craze' lines in enamel. Max. left lateral incisor with small uncomplicated incisal chip fracture. Lower anteriors with several small incisal chips and hairline fractures. Posterior teeth appear to be grossly intact.

7. Alveolar bone – anteriorly – no mobility of maxilla or alveolus, whole or segmental.

8. Occlusion: no evidence of open bite occlusal disharmony. No step-off occlusion.

9. Oropharynx: not able to observe.

Assessment: 33 yo M following MVA [RTA] with multiple traumatic injuries to the head and facial regions, still with ETT intubation and limited responsiveness. There is no clinical evidence, or by head CT, of Le Forte I or II fracture. Possibility of alveolar fracture unlikely from exam findings. Maxillary right lateral incisor in need of radiographic evaluation to determine if root is still present. Anterior teeth slightly mobile but splinting is not indicated. These teeth should be re-evaluated when his medical condition is stable and before giving solid foods. Maxillary right canine is in need of bonded composite resin coverage of exposed dentin to treat/prevent hypersensitivity. Teeth should not pose aspiration risk during or after deflation of ETT cuff. Intraoral soft tissue trauma requires debridement only.

Recommendations:

1. Suction mouth with soft plastic/rubber tubing, not metal or hard plastic tip.

2. Sodium bicarbonate and water rinse/lavage for oral debridement of accumulations.

3. Soft diet when taking food by mouth.

4. Panoramic radiograph and dental periapical films of anterior teeth – when able to transport to dental clinic – to rule out fracture of alveolus, teeth/roots, condyles, etc.

5. May need extraction/root canal treatment of traumatized teeth in the future.

6. Penicillin should be adequate coverage for oral flora.

Thank you for this consult. We will follow.

Signature: _____

Printed name: _____

Phone/pager #: _____

nurses caring for this patient, but that there is a thorough base-line documentation of significant positive and negative findings.

- Significant negative findings (e.g. lack of jaw deviation, tenderness, occlusal disharmonies, mobile segments) are especially important in the evaluation of the maxillofacial trauma patient.
- The consult addresses the specific reason for the request (i.e. the safety of deflation of the ETT cuff). However, as no other clinical service has addressed the odontogenic trauma, a thorough appraisal of this region is desirable. It must be made clear that only a limited exam could be accomplished and that subsequent clinical evaluations, with radiographs, may reveal additional problems.

Fig. 4.2 **Dental consult #2: persistent hemorrhage following a dental extraction**

Date/Time: ....

Request: Asked to see this 18 yo man who presented 2 h ago with a 3-day history of intermittent but persistent bleeding after extraction of a lower molar tooth by his family dentist [dental practitioner]. No previous history of difficulties with dental extractions.

HPI: Routine dental extraction performed 3 days ago because of advanced 'decay', with pain and mild facial swelling 2 days prior to the extraction. He had some 'mild bleeding' after leaving the dental office, but 2–3 h after the extraction, it 'bled a lot'. He admits to spitting out blood since that time. He returned to his dentist that afternoon and the socket was packed with 'something' and sutures were placed, and he was advised to apply pressure with gauze. Overnight, he awoke to find pillow 'coated in blood'. Bleeding slows with pressure but does not stop and every 3–4 h it starts to bleed more heavily. His mother took him to their family physician, who started antibiotics and also advised to apply pressure with a sponge, but still bleeding. He presented to the Emergency [A&E] Department. BP 120/80, P70, Temp 37.5°C.

PMH/PDH: As per mother and patient – essentially uneventful. Denies any history of easy bruising or problems with bleeding. No previous history of any surgery, including oral surgery or previous dental extractions. Routine dental treatment in the past (e.g. fillings) without problems.

Labs: (Date ....) WBC 11.2, HCT 53, platelets 353 000
Allergy: NKDA (no known drug allergies).
Meds: Amoxycillin [Amoxil] 250 mg three times per day.

FH/SH: Lives with parents. Mother has a history of being a 'bleeder' following dental extractions, as do two of his maternal cousins.

Examination:
Extraoral: Conjunctiva, skin folds, and nail beds of normal coloration; no evidence of anemia. Mild, tender, right submandibular lymphadenopathy; presumedly reactive. Able to open mouth fully with no trismus.
Intraoral: Mild bleeding from the socket of the right mandibular first molar, with a large friable sticky clot present over the socket.
1. Hard and soft palate, buccal and labial mucosa, floor of mouth and tongue without lesions, masses or other abnormalities.
2. Some bruising evident on the buccal and lingual gingiva and alveolar mucosa adjacent to the socket, but no swelling or collection evident.

Assessment: 18 yo M with persistent bleeding but without local factors. His presentation, along with the family history, suggests the possibility of an inheritable bleeding diathesis, most likely von Willebrand's disease.

Recommendations:
1. Will attempt packing of socket with oxidized cellulose, sutures, after attempt at hemostasis with topical thrombin.
2. Start topical tranexamic acid mouthwash/gauze packing.
3. Laboratory investigations for possible von Willebrand's disease.
4. Admit for observation in light of persistent bleeding and concern regarding possible (but rare) bleeding into submaxillary spaces and adjacent parapharyngeal spaces, with resultant risk of airway compromise.
5. Suggest consultation with hematology service.

Thank-you for this consult. We will follow-up with hematology as to result of investigations, and plan any further dental surgery subsequent to their findings.

Signature: _____
Printed name: _____
Phone/pager #: _____

Comments on Figure 4.2

- The first surgical procedure many patients experience involves removal of a tooth, increasingly as part of orthodontic treatment, or as result of complications associated with impacted wisdom teeth. Von Willebrand's disease (vWD) is an uncommon, autosomal dominant disorder with variable penetrance, associated with quantitative and qualitative deficiencies of the von Willebrand factor, which binds platelets to endothelium, as well as stabilizing the factor VIII coagulation factor.

- Patients tend to present with a mix of bleeding derangements: constant bleeding as they fail to form a stable clot complex (vWF) and intermittent bleeding as the clot continuously turns over (absence of factor VIII).

- Patients with mild forms of the disease (types I and II) can usually be satisfactorily managed in the outpatient setting with pre-operative infusions of desmopressin, which induces and increases factor VIII release from the endothelial cells. More severe forms, including some types that are unresponsive to desmopressin, need factor concentrate. Collaboration with the hematology service is vital in determining the safest means of treating the patient.

Fig. 4.3 **Dental consult #3: myeloproliferative disorder and facial swelling**

Date/Time: ....

Request: Left facial cellulitis – please consult for treatment of abscess.

Response: Asked to see this 47 yo M with recently diagnosed myeloproliferative disorder (MPD), admitted (date ....) on an emergency basis for pain and progressive swelling in the left maxillary infraorbital region.

HPI: Patient was in good health until a year ago when he was admitted for venous stripping of lower extremities. Preoperatively found to have increased WBC (12 400) with 5% blasts, decreased platelets and hematocrit, and an enlarged spleen. Bone marrow (BM) biopsy showed hypercellularity with increased granulocytes, promyelocytes and blasts. Referred to cancer institute, initially thought to have early leukemia or CML. Repeat BM biopsy revealed increased megakaryocytes, hypercellularity, 15% blasts with 1–2 prominent nucleoli without Auer rods. Myeloid:erythroid ratio: 4:1. Increased peripheral monocytes. Cytogenetics normal with no Philadelphia chromosome evident. Planned to watch as outpatient biweekly. Recent WBCs stable at 20 000–30 000 with 4–8% blasts, mostly monos. Plts, HCT also stable. Asymptomatic until (date ....) when he developed upper respiratory infection (URI) with a question of viral etiology. Last seen 2 days before admission – reported feeling well. Awoke 1 day ago with tender left facial swelling, T 38.4°C. Relief gained with Tylenol [paracetamol]. Denied nausea and vomiting (N&V), chills, rigors, shortness of breath, leg pain, bone pain, or other

systemic complaint. Myeloproliferative disorder currently characterized as consistent with evolving leukemia, CML versus early AML.
Past surgical history: S/P skin grafts right calf for necrotizing fasciitis (date ....).

PMH: 1. MPD 2. HTN 3. type II diabetes (diet controlled).
Allergies: NKDA (No known drug allergies)

Labs: (Date ....) WBC 50 000, plts 120 000, HCT 42%, peripheral smear 4–8% myelomonocytic blasts with predominant segmented neutrophils.

Meds: Lopressor [Metoprolol], Oxycodone, penicillin (IV).

Habits: 1–2 packs cigarettes per day × 15 years. Positive for alcohol abuse.

PDH: Pt apparently somewhat fearful of dental treatment. Last dental visit 4–5 years ago. No floss or other aids.

Examination:
Extraoral: positive for left submandibular lymphadenopathy, significant left facial swelling suborbitally to nose, over entire left cheek and zygomatic area. Tender to palpation, soft, fluctuant, erythematous and warm to touch, negative for trismus. Right eye with injected sclera.
Intraoral: oropharynx, palate, labial and buccal mucosa, dorsal tongue, floor of mouth, and lips without lesions or abnormalities. Marked soft tissue swelling in left buccal vestibule/canine fossa with fluctuance extending posteriorly from left canine to left second molar region.

- Maxillary gingiva: generally swollen and erythematous, and 1 cm asymptomatic, erythematous, nonraised lesion anterior to left second molar on alveolar ridge.
- Mandibular gingiva: marginal cuff of erythematous tissue with moderate, generalized plaque/debris.
- Maxillary dentition: right second molar – fractured due to caries, missing palatal half of crown, root exposed, positive for furcation involvement, percussion sensitivity, grade 1 mobility. Periapical radiolucency on radiograph with widened periodontal ligament space.
- Maxillary right canine with mesial and distal caries, asymptomatic, without percussion sensitivity or mobility. Radiograph reveals early periapical radiolucency/pathology. Left canine with gross distal caries involving $\frac{1}{2}$ of clinical crown. Positive percussion sens., grade 2 mobility. Radiograph reveals large 1 cm radiolucency at apex, widened periodontal membrane ligament space. Left second molar asymptomatic and without caries.
- Mandibular dentition: All remaining teeth without lesions or symptoms.
- Oral hygiene – poor. Patient wears maxillary prosthesis but did not bring it on this admission. Partial denture is at least several years old.

Assessment: Pleasant, obese, 47 yo M recently diagnosed with MPD (myeloproliferative disorder) presents with emergent left facial swelling from maxillary left canine dentoalveolar abscess. With this degree of swelling a canine space infection is probable, even in a patient with a normal hematologic profile. He suffers from general dental neglect, caries and chronic periodontitis. These should be addressed before myeloproliferative disorder progresses.

Recommendations:
1. Continue IV penicillin but if swelling fails to improve in next 24 h then consider adding metronidazole.
2. Will discuss with you scheduling a more thorough oral exam with radiographs, incision and drainage, and multiple extractions in our clinic while he is still on IV antibiotics.

Thank you for this consult. We will follow.

Signature: _____

Printed name: _____

Phone/pager #: _____

Comments on Figure 4.3

- It is important in cases of facial cellulitis to accurately describe the extent or borders of the swelling, (i.e. anteriorly, posteriorly, superiorly, and inferiorly) for future reference.
- In this patient with evolving leukemia, a delay in dental treatment could be catastrophic. If a patient enters 'blast crisis' with neutropenia and thrombocytopenia, a dental infection might have to be managed medically until the hematologic status allows for surgical intervention.

Fig. 4.4 **Dental consult #4: acute lymphocytic leukemia and oral ulcers**

Date/Time: ....

Request: Please evaluate oral ulcers.

Response: Asked to evaluate this 75 yo M with acute lymphocytic leukemia (ALL) admitted (date ....) with fever, neutropenia, and multiple oral ulcers.

HPI:
Last summer: presented with fatigue, weight loss, splenomegaly, one marrow biopsy consistent with lymphoproliferative disorder.
(Date ....): splenectomy with improvement in symptoms and platelet count.

(Date ....): recurrence of fatigue and weight loss, WBC 200 000, plts 95 K, HCT 27%.

(Date ....): admitted to this hospital with bone marrow biopsy suggestive of ALL, WBC 350 000. Treated with doxorubicin and prednisone with dramatic fall in WBC with subsequent anemia and neutropenia.

(Date ....): WBC 4.5 K, HCT 24%, plts 2000. Complains mainly of fatigue and malaise. Presented to outside hospital (date ....) for platelets, found to be febrile to 39.4°C. Only localized complaints are multiple mouth sores.

PMH: As above.
Allergies: NKDA (No known drug allergies)

Labs: (Date ....) WBC 2.2 (differential pending), HCT 25.6%, plts 9000.

134	103	37	Sodium	Chloride	BUN
4.6	25	1.7	Potassium	Bicarbonate	Creat.

Meds: ceftazidime (IV), tobramycin (IV), nystatin, sodium bicarb. mouthrinses, Colace [Docusate], Tylenol [paracetamol], Benadryl, Mylanta [Asilone], milk of magnesia, allopurinol.

PDH: Last dental visit 2 mos ago for reline of maxillary partial denture. Brushes three times/day. Regular every 6-month care. History of several maxillary and mandibular root canal therapy treated teeth. Has had recent gingival bleeding but no dental abscesses. Mild herpes labialis about one/year. Upper and lower partial dentures, both 3 years old.

Examination:
Extraoral: Left cheek with small 1 × 0.5 cm ecchymotic area, no other lesions. No asymmetry, trismus, lymphadenopathy, tenderness to palpation. Neck supple.
Intraoral:
  1. Soft/hard palate: bilaterally along inner aspect of upper alveolar ridge, patchy 2 cm × 1 cm area of 'curdy' white plaques with no surrounding erythema, removed with cotton tip. Shallow, 1 cm diameter, deep, red ulcerations with debris around margins in hamular notch/tuberosity area bilaterally, without tenderness or hemorrhage. Slight erythema of soft palate. Several scattered petechiae. Small ulcerations on anterior hard palate. No evidence of secondary infection. Oropharynx: generally erythematous, without purulence or exudate.
  2. Tongue: pebbly, grainy appearance to dorsum. No plaques or lesions, sight erythema.
  3. Lips: thin, dry mucosa. No cracking or ulceration.
  4. Buccal mucosa: right posterior buccal mucosa with large, diffuse, non-raised, non-tender 3 × 5 cm semilunar-shaped area of ecchymosis. No break in mucosa.

5. Floor of mouth: supple, no masses, lesions, ecchymosis or debris.
6. Gingiva: multiple large 'liver clot' areas of oozing hemorrhages surrounding upper teeth. No swelling but positive for edema, erythema and debris. Lower anterior teeth with 2–3 mm recession, slight debris, blunt papillae, puffy margins with slight erythema. No bleeding, swelling or purulence.
7. Alveolar ridge: maxilla – generalized diffuse distribution of many small, <1 mm, erythematous, tender ulcerations with many petechiae; mandible – retromolar pad areas with bilateral 1 cm diameter hematomas with slight ulceration.
8. Dentition: all upper remaining teeth have had root canal treatment. All teeth with I–II/III mobility. Sensitivity to percussion maxillary right premolars. Lower teeth with multiple crowns. No caries or sensitivity noted.
9. Prosthesis: upper and lower removable partial worn 24 h/day continuously until (date ....).
10. Vestibules: upper with generalized erythema and several small areas of ulceration.
11. Salivary flow: saliva was expressed from all ducts with grossly normal consistency.

Assessment: very pleasant 75 yo M with fever and neutropenia, about 14 days following chemo. for ALL, now with several mouth problems from longstanding periodontal disease and denture use during chemotherapy.
1. Multiple hematomas, petechiae and ulcers on upper and lower alveolar ridge, palate and buccal mucosa secondary to denture trauma superimposed on friable mucosa and severe thrombocytopenia following chemo. No evidence of secondary bacterial infection at this time.
2. Candidiasis: white material on palate is candida secondary to neutropenia/chronic denture use.
3. Gingival bleeding: bleeding around upper teeth due to thrombocytopenia and long-standing inflammation from periodontal disease. Cannot rule out the possibility of periodontal abscess/severe periodontal disease without dental radiographs and a more thorough and invasive oral examination.
4. Right tooth sensitivity: as all remaining upper teeth have had recent root canal therapy, any of these could be a potential source. The sensitivity to pressure on the upper right could represent a failing root canal or a periodontal abscess, aggravayed by increased forces placed upon the tooth by the denture in function. Radiographs needed to help rule out the possibility of a periapical/periodontal infection. These are a source of chronic bacteremia from his periodontal disease.

Recommendations:

1. Continue current broad-spectrum antibiotics, which should cover the mixed oral flora.
2. Consider fluconazole for control of fungal infection.
3. For pain: 2% viscous xylocaine; or benzydamine HCl [Difflam]; or diphenhydramine/Kaopectate 50:50 rinse for 30 s and spit. Ice chips, sugar-free popsicles [ice lollies].
4. Dentures strictly out of mouth for now. Scrub dentures and denture cup with disinfectant hand soap and warm water. Soak dentures in denture cleaner.
5. Consider antiherpes virus prophylaxis with valacyclovir [valaciclovir].
6. Sodium bicarb. and water 1:3 rinses every 3–4 h, swish/expectorate (as tolerated).
7. Neutral sodium fluoride 5 cc qds swish/expectorate (as tolerated with ulcers).
8. Observe closely for additional secondary infection of hematomas/ulcers.
9. Soft diet.
10. Use care with sublingual thermometers as they can traumatize the thin, dry, friable mucosa.
11. Debridement of all soft and hard tissues with wet 4 × 4 gauze sponges 4 times/day.
12. Will discuss with medical house officer the possibility of obtaining dental radiographs to rule out periapical and periodontal abscesses, but would prefer to do this when WBC increases, as the yield from this test is low and is difficult to accomplish bedside.

Thank you for this consult. We will follow with you.

Signature: _____

Printed name: _____

Phone/pager #: _____

Comments on Figure 4.4

- Neutropenic patients do not have the usual oral manifestations of acute infection that might cause a temperature of 39.4°C. Therefore, swelling, edema, erythema and pain can be muted. The oral cavity in this patient cannot be ruled out as the source of his fever, even though he has minimal signs and symptoms of oral abscess or cellulitis.
- Invasive dental treatment, to include periodontal probing, should be deferred until after the white blood cell counts recover from their nadir, except in the rare situation when a dental abscess is shown to be the source of a fever in a neutropenic patient whose counts are not expected to recover in the next 24–48 h.

Fig. 4.5 **Dental consult #5: endocarditis of possible dental origin**

Date/Time: ....

Request: Poor dentition – rule out as source of infective endocarditis (IE)

Response: Asked to see this 38 yo F who presented to the [Accident and] Emergency Department (date ....) with fever of unknown origin (FUO).

HPI: Pt has history of Marfan syndrome and has been followed for many years by a cardiologist for mitral valve prolapse (MVP) and subsequent mitral regurgitation. She was in good health until (date ....) when she developed fever, chills, sweats, fatigue and eventual temp. to 38.9°C. Admitted to Medicine service with temp. of 40°C. Subsequent blood cultures grew 5/5 (five out of five) positive for Gram-positive cocci. Dental scaling 6 weeks ago. She reports her boyfriend had documented strep. throat approximately 3 wks prior to admission (PTA). She also reports having a sore throat approx. 2 wks PTA. She self-treated with penicillin for 4–5 days. She denies dysuria, pain, skin infections/rashes, chest pain, diarrhea, palpitations, paroxysmal nocturnal dyspnea (PND), edema, cough, orthopnea, or blurred vision. Denies possibility of pregnancy.

PMH:
1. Marfan syndrome with MVP and mitral regurgitation, mild congestive heart failure (CHF).
2. Cervical spondylitis treated by epidural steroid injections.
3. Meningitis @ 12 years.
4. Scarlet fever × 2 as a child.
5. Mononucleosis @ 28 years.
6. Diaphragmatic hernia repair @ 9 months.
7. Pectus excavatum – sternal surgery @ 5 years.
8. Back and leg surgery for scoliosis @ 13 years.

Meds: digoxin, captopril, nafcillin (IV), gentamicin (IV), penicillin (IV), Lasix
Allergy: Sulfa drugs.

Labs: (Date ....) WBC 6800, plts 195 000, HCT 37.8%

136	101	13	Sodium	Chloride	BUN
4.2	24	0.8	Potassium	Bicarbonate	Creat.

SH: Positive H/O tobacco use – 2 PPD × 10 years (20 pack years). Recently quit. Positive EtOH use – social only.

PDH: She reports being followed closely for dental treatment. Last dental scaling was approx. 6 weeks ago. She states that she is 'always careful' to have antibiotic prophylaxis prior to dental treatment. Reports 'boil on gum of tooth' following root canal therapy, and bleeding gingiva when brushing 10–12 days prior to admission. Also reports increased generalized tooth sensitivity to cold in recent weeks. She reports brushing every day but does not use floss or other oral hygiene aids.

Examination:
Extraoral: face and neck without masses, lesions or lymphadenopathy.
Intraoral: soft palate, oropharynx, buccal mucosa, floor of mouth without evidence of abnormality. Bimaxillary micrognathia and high vaulted palate consistent with Marfan.
1. Lips: dry, with slight crusting of blood.
2. Tongue: without lesions but dorsum has an accumulation of yellow plaque.
3. Gingiva: generally dark/dusk color, without noticeable stippling; slightly edematous with puffy interdental papillae, especially in mandibular anterior area. No lesion noted on alveolar mucosa in region of lower incisor where she described a 'boil'.
4. Dentition: generally without sensitivity to percussion, no mobile teeth. Several malpositioned anterior teeth. Poor occlusion. Many large, old amalgam restorations of questionable status.
5. Oral hygiene: fair to poor, with readily visible generalized accumulation of plaque and debris.

Assessment: 38 yo F with Marfan syndrome and endocarditis, with 5/5 Gram-positive cocci blood cultures. The reported 'boil' adjacent to a tooth that received endodontic therapy in the past, as well as her overall dental/oral condition, makes her mouth a possible source. Laboratory identification of the Gram (+) cocci would likely help in this regard. In addition, transient bacteremias are well documented following toothbrushing or any other manipulation of the gingiva. The timing of her probable strep. throat suggests this as a possible portal as well. Cannot rule out a possible dental pathology, associated with a failing root canal therapy or from defective restorations until we can get dental radiographs.

Recommendations:
1. Will discuss with her house officer and arrange for her to be seen in dental clinic for full mouth series of radiographs and a thorough oral exam. When medically stable, she will need dental scaling and possible extractions while still under IV antibiotic therapy.
2. Need for replacement of defective restorations as soon as possible by family dentist or preferably by us while an inpatient and on IV antibiotics.
3. Improve oral hygiene: increase toothbrushing to twice/day with soft, nylon bristle brush. Will have our hygienist teach and encourage flossing.
4. High concentration fluoride rinse 0.04–0.05 stannous fluoride to arrest carious lesions, 5 cc daily at night, swish for 30 s and expectorate (or 1.1% neutral NaFl gel brush-on application or 5000 ppm neutral NaFl toothpaste use once daily).

Thank you for this interesting consult. We will discuss and follow with you.

Signature: _____
Printed name: _____
Phone/pager #: _____

Comments on Figure 4.5

- Note that both the episode of sore throat and the reported evidence of chronic abscess can be temporally related to the endocarditis, that is, within 2 weeks of the onset of symptoms of endocarditis. The history of dental scaling 6 weeks ago is too far removed in time from the onset of her symptoms of IE to be a cause. A further characterization of the species of organisms involved might differentiate it as to odontogenic versus other (e.g. respiratory) origin.

- In general, the best time to provide dental treatment is between the time she becomes medically stable enough to undergo dental treatment and the time that her intensive antibiotic therapy ends. Prophylactic antibiotic coverage is indicated (as per national guidelines) for all invasive dental procedures because she is at high risk for IE in the future. Alternative antibiotics to the agents she is being treated with might be indicated, to lessen the likelihood of a bacteremia with resistant organisms during invasive dental treatment. Keep in mind that the vast majority of cases of IE originating from the oral cavity are likely from chronic bacteremias rather than invasive dental procedures.

Fig. 4.6 **Dental consult #6: Aids with multiple oral problems**

Date/Time: ....

Request: Dysgeusia, dysphagia.

Response: Asked to evaluate this 31 yo M recently diagnosed with *Pneumocystis carinii* pneumonia (PCP). Discharged from hospital (date ....), readmitted (date ....) with persistent fever, and dehydration.

HPI: Diagnosed with HIV 1 year ago. He refuses antiretroviral therapy. Has elevated liver function tests, (+) HBcAb, (–) HbsAg on (date ....). Onset of lymphadenopathy, oral candidiasis, malaise, fatigue, dry cough, about 20 lb wt loss.
(Date ....): admit to this hospital with diffuse bilateral chest infiltrates, transbronchial biopsy was positive for PCP. Treated with Bactrim [co-trimoxazole] for 8 days with improvement. Also had skin biopsy of right arm lesion positive for Kaposi's sarcoma (KS), no treatment.
(Date ....): discharged to home. Subsequently developed fevers, shaking chills, night sweats, dehydration, perirectal pain. Temp. 38.9°C 1 day prior to admission, positive for intraoral candida on admission.

Physical exam: significant for II/VI systolic ejection murmur. Chest film positive for interstitial infiltrates middle/lower lungs bilaterally, worse since (date ....). Decreased oral intake on admission and increasing dysphagia. Afebrile since (date ....). Oral complaints decreased following 3 days of clotrimazole. Noted 'metallic' taste × 10 days, attributed to Flagyl taken recently for perianal pain/abscess. Very dry oral cavity. Feels 'something going on' in region of the right tonsil, like it's 'failing apart' and a 'lump in my throat' when swallowing. No odontogenic pain or complaints. He reports increased viscosity of oral secretions and H_2O_2:H_2O (hydrogen peroxide/water) rinse 'burns'. Also reports alterations in taste since on medications, with subsequent decrease in oral intake.

PMH:
1. As above.
2. Syphilis treated with penicillin, but developed rash.
3. Hepatitis A about 5 years ago.
4. Depression.
Allergy: Penicillin.

Meds: Pentamidine – stopped (date ....), fluoxetine, Metamucil [Fybogel], Colace [Docusate], Nystatin, clotrimazole, H_2O_2:H_2O oral rinse, heparin flush.

Labs: (date ....) WBC 2.2 K (61 P, 22 L), plts 53, HCT 32.5%, afebrile today.

| 139 | 102 | 14 | Sodium | Chloride | BUN |
| 0.1 | 28 | 1.6 | Potassium | Bicarbonate | Creat. |

(Date ....): CD4 count = 40 cells/mm^3; HIV RNA (by PCR) = 394 000 copies/cc.

PDH: He reports every 12 month care. No history of endodontic or periodontal therapy, surgery or trauma. Three times/day oral home care. He reports generalized gingival bleeding with brushing. Uses clotrimazole lozenge after each meal.

Examination:
Extraoral: negative for swelling, trismus, lesions, asymmetry or tenderness.
Intraoral:
1. Soft palate and uvula: heavy mucous secretions. Diffuse erythema with many pinpoint, non-raised, 1 mm, round, localized areas of erythema.
2. Hard palate: bilateral, ecchymotic appearance 2nd premolar region. Right side with distinct, non-tender, raised swelling, ~0.5 cm. Tissue boggy and extremely dry. Much white mucous debris.
3. Oropharynx: generalized, bilateral tonsillar erythema with increased size.

4. Buccal mucosa and floor of mouth: no lesions, abnormalities, debris or erythema noted.
5. Tongue: dorsum with moderate white coating, dry, granular. Localized areas of deep color down midline. Lateral/ventral aspects without lesions.
6. Lips: dry, chapped, with white debris. No lesions noted except erythematous and ulcerated commissures.
7. Gingiva: marginal and papillary erythema, especially posteriorly. Anterior with blunted papillae. Boggy consistency without stippling. Much plaque/debris interproximally.
8. Dentition: 28 teeth present, intact, well restored. Posterior teeth with severe bruxism/abrasion with exposed dentin. No teeth sensitive to hot/cold or percussion. No mobility. Crowding with anterior teeth. Much interproximal staining.
9. Oral hygiene: fair to good.
10. Salivary secretions: decreased flow, increased consistency.

Assessment:
Pleasant 31 yo M with HIV/AIDS, thrombocytopenia, immune suppression and biopsy-proven PCP and KS, with recent admission for persistent fever in setting of neutropenia. Complicated oral picture consistent with AIDS. Generalized erythema of tissue with obvious oropharyngeal candidiasis, likely esophageal candidiasis and clinically suspicious KS of the palate. Many oral problems need to be addressed.

1. Tongue/dysgeusia: possibly secondary to Flagyl and/or chronic hepatitis. However, may also be secondary to changes on dorsum of tongue along with decreased salivary flow/increased viscosity.
2. Dysphagia/N&V: probably due to esophageal or gastric candidiasis. Possibly secondary to Flagyl.
3. Palatal purpura/ecchymosis with right-sided swelling, typical for intraoral KS with respect to location as well as appearance.
4. Right tonsillar mass: differential includes KS. However, benign mucosal polyp, lymphoepithelial lesions and squamous cell cancer cannot be ruled out without a biopsy.
5. Diffuse palatal erythema: possibly secondary to viral syndrome. However, more likely due to chronic candidal involvement of oral mucosa.
6. Lip commissures: angular cheilitis from chronic candidiasis.
7. Xerostomia: from medication, dehydration, or diffuse infiltrative lymphocystis syndrome (DILS)
8. Gingival bleeding: from increased debris and bacterial flora, and decreased platelets.

Recommendations:
1. Suggest otolaryngology (ENT) consult for evaluation of tonsillar growth.
2. Rule out esophageal candidiasis.
3. Discontinue Nystatin and clotrimazole. Add Fluconazole 200 mg now followed by 100 mg qd.
4. Discontinue H_2O_2:H_2O as this is irritating, and substitute sodium bicarb: H_2O or water. Brush with soft nylon toothbrush with fluoride toothpaste 3 times/day. Observe for bleeding if platelets drop below 40 000.
5. Continue 0.12% chlorhexidine rinse, 15 cc twice/day rinse for 30 seconds and spit.
6. Neutral sodium fluoride 5 cc qd swish and expectorate after 30 seconds if not irritating.
7. Frequent water sips/ice chips to soothe mucosa.
8. Palatal gingival biopsy by us today for KS confirmation.

Thank you for this interesting consult. We will follow.

Signature: _____

Printed name: _____

Phone/pager #: _____

Comments on Figure 4.6

- This is an example of several oral manifestations of AIDS. Oral disease in this patient would be improved if he was placed on highly active antiretroviral therapy (HAART) and was able to comply with the complex drug regimen. Unfortunately, he has refused management of his HIV disease and desires only prophylaxis and management of the many opportunistic diseases that arise in the presence of severe immune suppression.
- Note that all significant findings on exam are addressed in the assessment and recommendations.

Fig. 4.7 Dental consult #7: planned aortic valve replacement and poor dentition

Date/Time: ....

Request: Poor dentition.

Response: Asked to evaluate this 51 yo non-English speaking Portuguese male admitted (date ....) for planned aortic valve replacement (AVR) tomorrow morning. Noted on admission H&P to have poor dentition. Daughter serves as an interpreter.

HPI: Limited medical or dental care during his lifetime. Noted onset shortness of breath (SOB) 2 years ago and chest pain several times since. Now with increasing SOB, 2-pillow orthopnea, and lower extremity edema. Cardiac catheterization 2 weeks prior to admission showed aortic insufficiency (AI) with an ascending aortic aneurysm. Now admitted for AVR with question of disposition of patient's poor dental status.

PMH:
1. As above.
2. Hypertension (HTN).
3. Rheumatic heart disease as a child.
Allergy: NKDA (No known drug allergies)

Meds: captopril, digoxin, Lasix, Benadryl.

Labs: WBC, plts, HCT, lytes pending: PT 12.5/10.4 sec; PTT 24.2 sec.

PDH: No visit to a dentist during his lifetime. Daughter cannot recall that he ever brushes his teeth. Currently without oral complaints. No recent history of facial swelling or pain.

Examination:
Extraoral: Without masses, lesions, swelling, asymmetry. No TMJ trismus, crepitus. Without tenderness to palpation. Neck supple, without lymphadenopathy. Thyroid palpable.
Intraoral: Positive for fetor oris. Hard/soft palate, lips, tongue, buccal mucosa – all without lesions or abnormalities.
1. Oropharynx: diffuse erythematous appearance without tonsillar enlargement. No evidence of purulence or exudate.
2. Floor of mouth: supple to palpation, without lesions, abnormalities.
3. Gingiva: generalized severe edema with erythematous appearance and overgrowth of tissues in posterior areas. No evidence of chronic sinus tracts.
4. Dentition: 31 of 32 teeth present with missing maxillary right 1st molar. Mandibular left 1st and 2nd molars and 2nd premolar are decayed root fragments. Remainder of dentition with multiple small carious lesions, especially posteriorly. Much mature plaque and calculus, especially posteriorly. Much mature plaque and calculus, especially posteriorly in both arches, covering much of the tooth surfaces. No mobility or percussion sensitivity. No palpable alveolar swellings.
5. Oral hygiene: poor.

Assessment: 51 yo Portuguese, non-English speaking man with thoracic aneurysm and HTN, awaiting AVR, and in need of eradication of oral infection prior to valvular surgery. As discussed with Dr. Smith by phone today, his mouth is clearly a source of chronic bacteremia, which could seed his prosthetic valve, and he might not be adequately covered with antibiotics alone perioperatively. As a result of his gingival disease and heavy accumulation of plaque, any manipulation of the soft tissues (e.g. mastication, oral hygiene) will cause frequent oral bacteremia with a wide variety of oral pathogens. The grossly decayed mandibular posterior teeth probably have areas of chronic periapical disease as well. Full series of dental radiographs will likely support this. A thorough dental scaling should be performed prior to thoracic surgery, under adequate antibiotic cover, to decrease the bacterial load and to improve the integrity of the oral soft tissues. All hopelessly carious teeth should be extracted as well. He is also in need of oral hygiene instruction.

Recommendations:

1. As discussed with cardiothoracic surgeon, consideration is being given to accomplishing both dental and thoracic surgery during one general anesthetic, otherwise the cardiac surgery will be postponed until after dental needs are resolved. He is scheduled to be seen by the dental service at 08:00 tomorrow for radiographs and treatment planning.
2. Antibiotic prophylaxis: amoxicillin 2 g [3 g in UK] PO 1 h before sending to the dental clinic.
3. Consider diazepam 10 mg by mouth for apprehension prior to dental appointment.
4. Brush teeth three times/day with soft nylon bristle brush using fluoride dentifrice. Fluoride rinse 5 cc rinse (30–60 s) and expectorate.

Thank you for this consult. We will contact you after his clinic visit tomorrow morning.

> Signature: _____
> Printed name: _____
> Phone/pager #: _____

Comments on Figure 4.7

Ideally, all dental disease and infection should be addressed prior to cardiac valve surgery to minimize exposure of a prosthetic valve to chronic bacteremia. However, the ability of the patient to tolerate such stressful dental procedures before cardiac surgery must also be considered. In some situations, dental treatment should be carried out in the operating room [theatre] with IV sedation and anesthesia 'standby'. In the case of severe cardiac compromise, dental treatment might have to be deferred until after cardiac surgery. A case can be made for treating some acutely ill cardiac patients in the operating room [theatre] under general anesthesia immediately prior to thoracic surgery and with IV antibiotic coverage. The only alternatives are postponing thoracic surgery and treating the patient in the dental clinic or in the OR [theatre] under a separate general anesthetic, which poses an increased risk to the patient as well as added financial burden. Each case must be evaluated carefully with consideration for the urgency of dental treatment and severity of cardiac compromise. Close consultation with the cardiac team is required.

Non-urgent consultation requests (Figs 4.8–4.13)

Fig. 4.8 Dental consult #8: newborn infant with masses on alveolar ridge and large lingual frenum

Date/Time: ....

Request: Please evaluate gingival masses and 'tongue-tie'.

Response: Asked to see this ~24-h M newborn for evaluation of masses on mandibular alveolar ridge and a lingual frenum.

HPI: Healthy child born to healthy 14 yo, who has not yet breast-fed.

PMH: N/A.
Allergy: None known.

Labs: None.

Meds: None.

Examination:
Extraoral: No abnormalities.
Intraoral: Hard and soft palate, oropharynx, buccal mucosa, tongue, floor of mouth, lips all without abnormalities or lesions.
1. Gingival/mand. alveolar ridge with several bilateral sessile nodules in region of eventual canine teeth, ~6–8 mm in height, ~5 mm diameter. Rubbery consistency. Yellow translucent membrane, with apparent straw-colored fluid inside. Vessels visible on membrane. Prominent lingual frenum almost to tip of tongue.

Assessment: Newborn male infant with benign, bilateral sessile mandibular nodules, most likely dental lamina cysts of the newborn, also commonly referred to as gingival cysts, 'Epstein's pearls' or 'Bohn's nodules', depending on histology. Histologically, they are true cysts with an epithelial lining, filled with desquamated keratin. As in this case, they are usually displaced lingually when in the canine region. A lingual frenum of this size can interfere with breast-feeding, and if so, it can be shortened surgically in the newborn nursery. If lactation consultant [midwife] observes problems, we will return to 'clip' the frenum if deemed necessary.

Recommendations: No treatment is required as these cysts almost invariably open on to the surface mucosa. Will discuss with mother.

Thank you for this interesting consult.

Signature: _____
Printed name: _____
Phone/pager #: _____

Comment on Figure 4.8

This is a good example of the opportunity that consults provide to teach other services about dental disorders. The issue of when to surgically 'clip' a lingual frenum is not clear and should be based initially on the infant's ability to breast/bottle feed.

Fig. 4.9 Dental consult #9: type I diabetes, failing renal transplant, and poor dentition

Date/Time: ....

Request: Poor dentition.

Response: Asked to evaluate the dentition of this 34 yo M with long-standing type 1 diabetes mellitus, with a history of end stage renal disease (ESRD), now 8 days following cadaveric renal transplant.

HPI: Type 1 diabetes since age 5 years. Nephropathy, retinopathy and neuropathy manifested by gastroparesis, lower extremity paresthesia and poorly controlled hypertension. Problem with compliance with medications in the past.
(Date ....) began hemodialysis (HD) on T/Th/Sat basis for 4 h. Recent trouble with glucose control and frequent episodes of hypoglycemia. Admitted to endocrine service several months ago for insulin adjustment. Admitted via Emergency [A&E] Department for hypoglycemic reaction (date ....). Received cadaver renal allograft (date ....) with poor functioning since, as he has been anuric for most of the last 8 days. Continues on hemodialysis, most recently (date ....), next planned (date ....). Also with possible GI bleed as HCT has recently dropped. Biopsy of cadaveric renal allograft planned early in the week of (date ....) if no improvement.

PMH:
1. As above.
2. Left arm cimino arteriovenous fistula.
3. History of pneumonia.
4. Left ventricular hypertrophy (LVH) as per cardiac ECHO (date ....) with normal mitral and aortic valves.
5. Laser treatment for DM retinopathy.

Labs: (date ....) WBC 8.7 (without diff), plts 297 000, HCT 29.1

139	106	82	Sodium	Chloride	BUN
3.7	20	7.2	Potassium	Bicarbonate	Creat.

Allergy: NKDA (No known drug allergies)

Meds: prednisone [prednisolone], aspirin, cyclosporine, nifedipine, metoclopromide, ranitidine, Aldomet, NPH Insulin, (PRN Demerol [Pethidine], hydroxyzine, Benadryl, Oxycodone, Compazine [Prochlorperazine]).

Habits: Smoking 3–4 PPD (packs/day) × 'years', now 2 PPD.

PDH: He reports no routine care for past 17 years. Last dental visit 6 years ago for emergency extraction of several anterior teeth. Does not use tooth brush. No oral complaints upon exam. No history of trauma. Positive history of gingival bleeding.

Examination:
Extraoral: yellow/gray complexion with many 0.2–0.4 cm blotchy areas on skin, especially forehead. Bearded, head and neck without masses, lesions or adenopathy, negative trismus, negative asymmetry.
Intraoral:
1. Hard and soft palate, lips, floor or mouth: without lesions or abnormalities.
2. Oropharynx: diffuse pallor.
3. Buccal mucosa: pink, moist with bilateral granular/pebbly texture.
4. Tongue: left lateral border with 0.75 cm diameter shallow, tender ulceration with yellow fibrin-like covering. (He reports that he bit his tongue during anesthesia.)
5. Gingiva: generalized erythema, moderate edema. Anterior gingiva retractable due to severe inflammation, gross accumulations of mature plaque and calculus. Maxillary left canine and left 1st molar areas with submucosal 'bluish' pigmentation in marginal 2 mm of gingiva. Recession anteriorly only. No purulence.
6. Dentition: missing maxillary left anterior teeth and mandibular right and left 1st molars. Periodontal involvement of all mandibular anterior teeth. Central incisors with grade 2 mobility. Several small amalgam

restorations in posterior teeth. Gross caries maxillary right and left 1st premolars. Max right anteriors with gross decay such that only roots remain. No teeth are sensitive to percussion.
7. Vestibules: no swelling or evidence of chronic sinus tracts.
8. Salivary flow: normal amount and consistency.
9. Oral hygiene : poor/non-existent.

Assessment: 34 yo M with ESRD, type I diabetes, now following cadaveric renal allograft with poor subsequent function, and long history of extreme dental neglect.
1. He has severe mand. anterior periodontal inflammation and loss of alveolar bone. These teeth will probably require extraction after radiographic assessment. Several grossly carious maxillary anterior teeth may also need to extracted.
2. The blue-pigmented lesions are consistent with ingestion of heavy metals (lead, bismuth) but are more likely secondary to subgingival calculus visualized through thin mucosa. This will be clarified after calculus removal and possible gingival biopsy with histologic examination for submucosal metal deposition.
3. Left tongue lesion probably secondary to trauma. However, with his history of heavy smoking and the possibility of malignancy, we should observe over the next 10–14 days to assure resolution.
4. He is at high risk for infection, given his immunosuppressed state, especially considering his poor periodontal status and large volume of bacterial plaque. He needs a more thorough dental exam, radiographs and extraction of multiple teeth. It should be noted that with periodontal disease there is a localized shift in the oral flora from Gram positives to Gram negatives.

Recommendations:
1. Will discuss with his house officer and schedule for exam and radiographs in our clinic.
2. Any necessary dental treatment will be scheduled the day after HD, with antibiotic prophylaxis. Will discuss with you the control of his hypertension (190/100 on (date ....)) and the desirability of increasing his steroid dose the day of surgery.
3. Oral hygiene: begin brushing with soft nylon, round-tipped brush twice/day, with fluoride toothpaste. Sodium bicarb. mouth rinses, swish and expectorate four times/day. Neutral sodium fluoride rinse after oral hygiene, 5 cc rinse for 1 min and expectorate.

Thank you for this consult. Will follow.

Signature: _____

Printed name: _____

Phone/pager #: _____

Comments on Figure 4.9

- Note that all significant findings on the patient's examination are addressed in the assessment, even though they might not be directly related to the reason for the consult.
- Considerations for dental treatment for patients on hemodialysis include consideration of antibiotic prophylaxis for arteriovenous fistulae or prosthetic shunts, and treatment the day following hemodialysis. Although there is no evidence-base for the use of antibiotic prophylaxis coverage for an immunocompromised state such as exists with renal transplantation, it has become a standard of care in some hospitals due to the concern for infective endocarditis, if not for the dialysis shunt itself. Steroid supplementation in this setting is also controversial, but depending on the current dose, it might be prudent given the minimal risk involved from a dose to cover the procedure, and perhaps the immediate (12-h) postoperative period.

Fig. 4.10 **Dental consult #10: oral ulcerations of unknown etiology**

Date/Time: ....

Request: Please assess and treat dry mouth and oral lesions.

Response: Asked to see this 57 yo F admitted with history of severe rheumatoid arthritis (RA) since age 21 and possible new onset of secondary Sjögren's syndrome.

HPI: History of non-steroidals, 3-month gold salt therapy, male hormone injections. She denies skin rash, night sweats, fever, weight loss, alopecia, photosensitivity or dry eyes. No problems with eating, swallowing; has bilateral tearing. History of increased dryness for 1 year. She reports a need to drink more liquids while eating. No reported dysphagia. Oral hygiene problems secondary to pain.

PMH: As above.
Allergy: NKDA (No known drug allergies)

Labs: (date ....) WBC 6500, HCT 44.5, Creat. 0.9, Sed. rate 60.

Meds: Soma [Carisoprodol]: 1 month duration, indomethacin: 1 month duration.

Habits: Smokes 40 cigarettes per day since age 18. No EtOH.

Examination:
Extraoral: erosive/crusted lesions on vermillion border of lower lip. No swelling of salivary glands, no lymphadenopathy.
Intraoral:
1. Mouth moderately wet;
2. Floor of mouth, tongue, soft palate and pharynx all benign in appearance.
3. Large, 1×3 cm, velvety red areas with leukoplakic lesion midposterior hard palate.
4. Erosive areas with irregular borders on labial mucosa.
5. Large, diffuse, red and white, flat lesion on left buccol mucosa between Stensen's duct and the commissure.
6. Multiple leukoplakic areas on occlusal line of buccal mucosa.
7. Multiple carious and fractured teeth, calculus, debris, and gingival inflammation/swelling.
8. Generalized gingival bleeding with probing.

Assessment:
1. Erythema multiforme (EM): erosive area of lip most consistent with EM but could be a lichenoid reaction. It is noteworthy that Indocin [indomethacin] has been associated with ulcerative stomatitis as an idiosyncratic reaction. If possible, this drug should be discontinued to rule this out as an additional cause of the widespread stomatitis. Viral etiology is highly unlikely.
2. Leukoplakia/erythroplakia: need to watch to ensure these areas disappear with resolution of this likely drug eruption.
3. With the report of a need to drink additional fluids while eating, secondary Sjögren's may also be a factor, but it is not the etiology of these lesions. Screening serology for SS/A and SS/B antibodies may be of value.
4. Caries: multiple teeth.
5. Poor oral hygiene and gingivitis/periodontitis.

Recommendations:
1. Lips: Kenalog [Adcortyl] in Orabase to dried lip lesions.
2. Immediate institution of oral hygiene:
   a. 4×4 wet gauze on gloved finger to clean mouth, especially along gingival margin.
   b. Sodium bicarb. as a mouth rinse 4 times/day.
3. To dental clinic for:
   a. Panoramic film, extraction of non-salvageable teeth and cleaning of remaining teeth when lesions begin to resolve.
   b. Will wait to see if EM resolves, otherwise will need to consider biopsy of area suspicious for dysplastic change of the palatal and

buccal mucosal lesions in light of significant smoking history. May need to consider stopping/replacing Indocin [indomethacin] if lesions do not resolve.

Thank you for this interesting consult. Will discuss management of EM and need for biopsy with dental attending [staff] in a.m. would like to photograph these lesions for comparison when medications have been altered.

Signature: _____

Printed name: _____

Phone/pager #: _____

Comment on Figure 4.10

This patient has a complex clinical presentation. A detailed and well-described oral exam is necessary for diagnosis and later comparison because changes in the clinical picture will help to determine the diagnosis, and therefore the management.

Fig. 4.11 Dental consult #11: poorly fitting denture on an atrophic ridge

Date/Time: ....

Request: 'Needs lower denture'.

Response: Asked to see this 74 yo F admitted 5 days ago for management of her rheumatoid arthritis (RA). Family requests evaluation for a replacement lower denture.

HPI: RA diagnosed 9 years ago, with painful and progressive loss of joint mobility. Also with history of mental deterioration. She states her lower denture has not fit in over 3 years. However, she has been eating well since then without a lower denture, and says she can eat all foods except nuts. Joints affected include the wrists and elbows bilaterally, resulting in considerable limitation in her hand movements, and therefore her ability to maintain her oral hygiene.

PMH: Significant for type II diabetes (presently diet controlled), cataracts, retinitis pigmentosa, lacrimal atrophy, psoriasis for 50 years, decreased hearing.
Allergy: Gold (rash).

Labs: (date ....)

143	105	23	Sodium	Chloride	BUN
4.2	27	1.3	Potassium	Bicarbonate	Creat.

Meds: Ecotrin [aspirin], Mylanta [antacid], natural tears, prednisone, acetaminophen [paracetamol].

Examination:
Extraoral: no lesions, lymphadenopathy or swelling.
Intraoral: palate, buccal and labial mucosa, alveolar ridges, tongue, floor of mouth and pharynx, and other soft tissues are within normal limits. Patient is edentulous. Maxillary ridge firm and prominent, with good height. Maxillary denture has good retention. Mandibular ridge virtually nonexistent causing poor retention of the mandibular denture.

Assessment: 74 yo F with RA with atrophied mandibular ridge and poorly fitting lower denture.

Recommendations: Since she has no lower ridge for retention of mandibular denture and she is functioning well without one, construction of a new prosthesis is not recommended. To do so would require approximately 5 weeks with 5–6 visits, some of which could be strenuous, and she is happy with the decision not to replace the lower denture. Recommend assessment and review by the Dietetics Service as to the adequacy of her diet. Will discuss with her family.

Thank you.

Signature: _____
Printed name: _____
Phone/pager #: _____

Comment on Figure 4.11

In responding to requests for dentures, it is important to note and consider who is making the request – the family, the patient or the physician. At times, the expectations for dentures may be unrealistic and the patient's oral intake, motor control, mental status, ability to cooperate, ability to withstand anesthesia, and oral status should be assessed to determine the appropriateness of denture fabrication.

Fig. 4.12 **Dental consult #12: cerebral palsy and excessive drooling**

Date/Time: ....

Request: Please evaluate and treat this patient for excessive drooling.

Reponse: This 6 yo F with cerebral palsy has impaired ability to control her saliva. The patient's mother reports that she has to change her daughter's shirt approximately four times per day due to constant drooling. The child is otherwise healthy.

Examination: She has moderate to severe spasticity but can hold her head erect. She is unable to communicate verbally. She is presently drooling thick, ropy saliva. Facial exam reveals no gross abnormalities. Intraoral exam shows no abnormalities. Permanent incisors erupting normally.

Assessment: Excessive drooling secondary to lack of orofacial muscular control.

Recommendations: This patient will benefit from assessment by a multidisciplinary team. Likely treatment will consist of prescription of an oral screen combined with therapy from a speech and language therapist. If this does not achieve sufficient control, the use of a palatal training plate should be considered. Alternatives to this include drug therapy (hyoscine) and, as a last resort, surgery. This patient may benefit from repositioning of the submandibular duct orifices to the tonsillar pillars and simultaneous sublingual sialoadenectomy. As most saliva is produced by the submandibular glands when not consuming a meal, redirecting the flow of saliva from these glands will likely be beneficial in reducing drooling. The sublingual glands are simply removed for access to the submandibular ducts. Because the parotid and minor salivary glands are unaffected by this procedure, it is unlikely that she will have any problems with dry mouth. This surgical procedure takes approximately 1–1.5 h and requires an overnight stay in the hospital.

Thank you for consulting us regarding this patient's problem. Please contact me if you have any additional questions. The patient's mother has an appointment with the oromotor team for presurgical workup.

Signature: _____

Printed name: _____

Phone/pager #: _____

Comments on Figure 4.12

- Therapy starting with the least invasive strategies and progressing as patients' needs dictate, is the favored approach based on an assessment of risk and benefit.
- Consideration needs to be given to immaturity; while it is normal for a child to continue drooling until perhaps 4 years of age, 6 is excessive in most children. Having said that, the drooling may not be excessive. An objective assessment, using Crysdale and White's scale, is advisable for monitoring.
- It is important to refer the patient to an expert multidisciplinary team who have the experience and skills to undertake a comprehensive assessment and follow through the interventions. Depending on the patient's cognitive functioning, behavior modification strategies may be successful.
- Oral screens and palatal training plates, in conjunction with oromotor exercises delivered by an expert speech and language therapist, may achieve significant control of saliva with no

associated morbidity. Drug therapy has side-effects which may be unacceptable and is a costly treatment modality. Radiotherapy is an alternative but it too has significant side-effects.

● Surgery should never be the first option; the morbidity may be unacceptable – not only from the surgery under general anesthesia itself but also from paroxysmal return of drooling, ranula formation when the sublingual glands are involved, and potential sequelae of dry mouth.

Fig. 4.13   **Dental consult #13: tonsil cancer and poor dentition, preradiation therapy**

Date/Time: ....

Request: Preradiation dental evaluation for poor dentition.

Response: Asked to see this 58 yo M admitted (date ....) with newly diagnosed T3 N2b M0 squamous cell carcinoma (SCCa) of the right tonsil. Request for evaluation of dental status prior to planned surgery plus radiation, vs. chemo/radiation alone.

HPI: He presented to his family physician 6 weeks prior to admission complaining of a sore throat. Presumptive diagnosis was tonsillitis. Treated with amoxicillin without resolution. He then reported on (date ....) to the emergency room [casualty] at his community hospital, where ENT consult was obtained and transoral tonsil biopsy was taken and read as SCCa on (date ....). He was referred to the university hospital for evaluation, staging and treatment of tonsil cancer.

PMH:
1. SCCa right tonsil.
2. Hypertension.

PSH: Triple endoscopy and biopsy right tonsil and oropharynx (date ....).

Habits: 1.5 ppd × 40 years cigarettes (60 pack/year); 3 beers or ales/day × 25 years
Allergy: iodine.

Meds: hydrochlorothiazide, atenolol, aspirin.

Labs: (date ....) WBC 7.2 (50 P 35 L 2 B 4 M)

Outside path: moderately differentiated SCCa right tonsil. University pathology report pending. Head and neck CT report pending.

PDH: Patient has never been to a dentist and does not brush his teeth. He does not report pain in any teeth.

Examination:
Extraoral: enlarged right submandibular and deep cervical nodes; TMJ within normal limits; slight trismus (opens 24 mm interincisal distance) with guarding.
Intraoral:
1. 3 × 5 cm exophytic mass of right tonsil extending onto base of tongue
2. Buccal and labial mucosa, vestibules, floor of mouth, lips, and palate are within normal limits. Clear saliva expressed from parotid glands.
3. Gingiva are moderately erythematous and boggy. Generalized gingival recession in the lower anterior quadrant. Heavy plaque and calculus are on all anterior teeth.
4. Of 32 teeth, 29 are present; however 13 (mostly posterior teeth) are grossly decayed or are present only as root fragments. Anterior teeth have 2 plus mobility.
5. The patient has poor oral hygiene. Bilateral mandibular tori measuring to 1.5 cm in greatest diameter in the area of the premolars are present with thin overlying mucosa.

Assessment:
Although bedside exam is limited, it is apparent that this patient with stage IV tonsil cancer has substantial dental neglect, with moderate to severe periodontitis, dental caries, multiple retained root fragments and mandibular tori that may need removal prior to onset of radiation therapy if he is to ever wear a prosthesis.

Recommendation:
1. Will arrange/discuss with ENT house officer concerning the timing of transport to dental clinic for dental radiographs and clinical evaluation.
2. Anticipate patient will need removal of all remaining teeth, alveoloplasty of all 4 quadrants and bilateral mandibular tori reduction in OR [theatre] under general anesthesia prior to radiation, preferably immediately prior to ENT surgery.
3. Will coordinate care with ENT and radiation oncology, pending patient decision between cancer treatment options. The radiation oncology consult note suggests that a minimum of 6500/cGy external beam therapy is planned to the tonsils and bilateral necks to include the parotids and submandibular/sublingual salivary glands. Maxillary and mandibular alveolar bone distal to the canine teeth will be in the primary field of radiation. A minimum of 7 days postextraction healing is desirable prior to beginning radiation therapy.

Thank you for this consult. Will follow.

Signature: _____
Printed name: _____
Phone/pager #: _____

Comments on Figure 4.13

- An oral evaluation and appropriate dental radiographs are recommended so that active and potential sources of infection within the planned fields (ports) of high-dose external beam radiation, or near intraoral implant radiation (brachytherapy), can be identified and removed before the ablative cancer therapy; keeping in mind that the anticipated dry mouth will predispose to severe caries in teeth outside the radiation fields as well.

- Preprosthetic surgical procedures, such as mandibular and maxillary exostosis reduction in a planned radiation field, must be completed prior to radiation, with enough time for at least partial healing. Alveoloplasty or alveolectomy performed at the time of extraction enhances healing by facilitating primary closure of extraction sites and provides an adequate denture-bearing ridge form, without bony undercuts, when bone remodeling is anticipated to be limited by radiation. It is ideal to perform the oral surgery immediately prior to (or after if indicated) the ENT surgery and under the same general anesthesia.

- For patients who are expected to develop xerostomia secondary to radiation therapy, the preradiation consult provides an opportunity to educate them on the oral complications of radiation therapy and the need for life-long daily prescription strength topical fluoride therapy, a sugar-free diet, scrupulous oral hygiene and close professional observation.

Chapter 5

Dental emergencies

The management of dental emergencies in the hospital environment has evolved dramatically over the last 20 years. While once providing management limited to odontogenic problems on a consultation basis only, general and pediatric dentists, as well as oral and maxillofacial surgeons, are now often the primary providers of care and might manage everything from a simple toothache to the most severe maxillofacial and craniofacial injuries. This natural evolution has brought with it many opportunities for both practitioners and residents alike. It also carries with it a new level of responsibility, for now the dentist must be aware not only of the odontogenic emergency but also of all the local and systemic consequences of the patient's current emergency condition, as well as overall medical status.

Emergency department (ED) [A&E] organization varies from hospital to hospital. Smaller hospitals often have a single emergency facility staffed by members of the medical staff on a rotating basis, or by specialists in emergency medicine. Larger academic medical centers often have emergency medicine house officers as the primary staffing, with support by the emergency medicine faculty. These medical centers also commonly have several combined or distinct areas for the specific management of medical, surgical, pediatric, obstetric/gynecologic and non-emergency problems.

Non-critical emergency patients are usually first seen by a secretary or nurse, who obtains demographic data and starts a medical chart [notes]. When necessary, old medical records are requested to facilitate obtaining an accurate medical history. A nurse will then triage the patient. This involves an assessment of the problem, establishment of a priority for care and assignment of the patient to an appropriate member of the medical/dental staff. The initial assignment of the patient varies by hospital. In some institutions, patients with isolated dental/oral or maxillofacial problems may be directly referred to and managed by a dentist. In other facilities, patients are first seen by the emergency physician who, after performing an examination and managing any medical conditions, consults a dentist about treating any oral/facial problem(s). A thorough knowledge of the organizational, triage and treatment protocols in the emergency department will greatly enhance the dentist's ability to provide rapid, appropriate and broadly scoped emergency care.

MEDICOLEGAL ASPECTS OF EMERGENCY CARE

As the provision of emergency care is inherently acute and impersonal in nature, the medicolegal aspects of care are of great importance.

Responsibilities of the doctor

Appointment to a hospital staff obligates an attending or house-staff member to treat patients with emergency needs. Depending on the facility, emergency department care may be provided by dentists on a rotating basis or on an 'as needed' basis by specific consultation. Either way, emergency care should be provided in a timely fashion, both for the patient and for the efficient running of the emergency department [A&E].

Consent

As with any hospital procedure, a signed informed consent for treatment is a prerequisite for emergency treatment. In conscious children or adult patients this is not usually a problem. However, children and adults who are unable to give consent because of unconsciousness, intellectual incapacity, neurological disease (e.g. prior stroke or Alzheimer's disease) or emotional/psychiatric instability must be dealt with by alternative means. In the case of children, a parent or legal guardian can give consent. If an adult patient is unable to give consent, an immediate family member can do so for emergency procedures. When no parent or family member can be contacted, telephone consents are usually acceptable if witnessed by at least one other uninvolved healthcare provider.

Emergency consent

If unable to obtain patient, guardian or family consent, emergency care can be rendered only if:

- the care is necessary to prevent loss of life or limb, or severe disability *and*
- the above is documented by the dentist and at least one other doctor.

Non-emergency care should be deferred. As a last resort, the doctor or a hospital administrator can obtain emergency judicial consent by court order. One should become familiar with individual state and national laws and hospital rules concerning such situations.

Follow-up

It is incumbent on the doctor who renders emergency services to provide patients with information on the need and accessibility for follow-up care. Preferably, this information should be in written form and documented in the medical record.

Outpatient versus inpatient care

Generally speaking, most dental emergencies can be treated in an outpatient environment. However, oral and maxillofacial surgeons, in particular, are commonly faced with situations where admission of the patient is warranted.

General indications for admission to the hospital

- Patients with severe, traumatic injuries requiring skilled nursing care, such as a concurrent head injury.
- Patients who require parenteral antibiotics or analgesics.
- Patients who require parenteral hydration or feeding.
- Patients who require emergency surgery.
- Patients unable to care for themselves under the current circumstances, including children whose parents are deemed a risk.
- Patients with the need for airway management.

EMERGENCY DEPARTMENT MEDICAL RECORDS

Documentation

Nowhere is the mandate for accurate and complete documentation more important than in emergency care:

- Many of these patients will be seen for definitive follow-up care by non-dentists.
- Dental treatment and terminology is often poorly understood by physicians and nurses (hence the need to write 'bleeding in maxillary right first molar region' and not 'bleeding from #3').
- Some emergency department cases can eventually involve legal proceedings or litigation. Therefore, the maintenance of objective, accurate detailed records is paramount to the ability to recollect prior events.

Medical records

The medical records used for emergency care are similar to those used elsewhere in the hospital (e.g. the history and physical examination and the progress notes). These notes are presented in detail in Chapters 2 and 4 but some modifications specific to emergency records are outlined below.

Consultation note

This note is for a patient under the care of another provider who requests a dental opinion regarding a specific problem. Primary care responsibilities remain with the requesting provider and all orders should be confirmed with that provider prior to institution, unless responsibility has been transferred to the dentist. A consult note should be thorough yet concise and include the following information:

- History of present illness (HPI): a detailed history of the current dental problem relating to the consult request. If other conditions exist that brought the patient to the ED [A&E] and are being treated by the primary provider (e.g. long bone injuries accompanying a mandible fracture from a motor vehicle accident), these too should be briefly described.
- Past medical history (PMH): a listing of the pertinent positive and negative findings from the patient's past and current medical

history. Any positive review of systems findings are generally included in this section for consultation notes. All positive findings should include a brief discussion describing the current status of the medical condition.

- Current medications: a list of the patient's medications with the route of administration, dose and interval schedule. If unclear, a family member, the pharmacist or the doctor who wrote the prescription(s) should be contacted.
- Allergies: a list of the patient's known drug allergies and the particular response seen from previous administration (e.g. hives, itching, gastrointestinal upset).

Physical examination (PE)

This section should include an appropriate head and neck examination and a thorough oral examination. In addition, any other examination pertinent to the consultation request should also be performed (e.g. a neurologic examination for a patient with facial injuries). Examination results should be detailed, especially in the specific area mentioned for examination in the consult request.

Radiographic and laboratory examination

Necessary radiographs and/or laboratory tests should be obtained and interpreted. Many radiographs (e.g. periapicals, panoramic) are interpreted by the dental consultant, not by a radiologist or the primary provider and should, therefore, be read comprehensively, not just for the specific complaint. All pertinent laboratory data (e.g. CBC, platelet count, PT/INR, PTT) should be listed and interpreted as well.

Assessment

This is a line-by-line listing of all the positive findings, followed by a brief discussion of its current status and its effect on the patient's care.

Recommendations and treatment

These are recommendations regarding diagnosis and appropriate treatment based on the assessment. Recommendations should be thorough and specific, indicating particular therapies, drugs and dosages. No treatment should be performed without the consent of the primary provider. If any treatment is performed, it should be clearly noted in this section, along with any anesthesia used.

Disposition or discharge information

This is a listing of instructions given to the patient, medications prescribed (with primary provider's permission), follow-up appointments or other plans.

Primary care notes

In some circumstances, the dentist might be the only doctor to see the patient. In these cases, it is even more imperative to consider the patient's overall medical condition and not just the head and neck region. For example, patients with facial injuries might have concomitant cervical or intracranial injuries that often cannot be appreciated by the triage staff. Another example would be oral bleeding. Although there are many local reasons for oral bleeding, the dentist is obliged to consider systemic sources or coagulopathies and order the appropriate tests to make the correct diagnosis, and then obtain appropriate medical consultation. It is important to write complete notes that more closely approximate an admission note. Orofacial trauma might be a result of syncope in the elderly (a common but significant and diagnostically complex syndrome with potential cardiovascular, neurologic, endocrinologic, visual, vestibular and neuromotor implications), or abuse in a child or a dependent older individual. These situations dictate a medical and/or social services consult if abuse is suspected.

Primary care notes differ from consult notes as follows:

- HPI: the history must be comprehensive and include all information relating to the present condition, not just those affecting the head and neck. Traumatic dental or facial injuries, for example, should be detailed as to the time, mechanism and severity of the injury as well as previous traumatic episodes. Specific questions should be directed at ascertaining the likelihood of other systemic injuries (e.g. chest, abdominal, cervical or intracranial).
- The physical examination, while certainly emphasizing the head and neck findings, should nevertheless include a basic examination of any other bodily system that is pertinent to the HPI. Positive findings should indicate the need for appropriate medical consultation.
- Radiology/Labs: appropriate films (e.g. C-spine) and lab data should be obtained (when indicated by the history or PE) to rule out

concomitant injuries and/or possible systemic factors, as well as to diagnose the acute dental or facial injuries.

- Assessment/Plan (A/P): this should reflect the patient's overall condition including the oral findings and any others. When non-dental items are listed, specific medical consultation should be ordered and noted in the medical record.
- Admission notes: these should consist of the primary care note and the following: • Indication for admission. • Name of the attending dentist. • Principal diagnosis. • Place to be admitted. • Condition of the patient. • Immediate treatment plan.

Consultation request notes

Written consultation requests to another service or doctor should be instituted whenever the dentist feels that it is necessary for the comprehensive and appropriate care of the patient. The best practitioners are the ones who know when to ask for assistance in the best interest of the patient. When in doubt, obtain a consult. A consult request should include the following:

- A brief summary of the HPI and treatment to date.
- Any pertinent medical history, physical findings and radiographic or laboratory data.
- A detailed and specific explanation of why the consult is being ordered and what information is desired from the consultant. If any necessary treatment by the consultant is desired, this should also be indicated in the note.
- Direct verbal communication between dentist and consulted physician is encouraged whenever possible.

Follow-up notes

Follow-up notes can be written in the 'SOAP' format as follows:

- Subjective: this includes the patient's chief complaint if there is one, or any comments the patient has regarding the condition, past treatment and so on.
- Objective: this includes the physical examination and the radiographic and laboratory data, if ordered.
- Assessment: a summary of the patient's condition.
- Plan: the consideration for the future management of the patient and any appointments scheduled.

INTRAORAL URGENCIES

Odontogenic pain

General principles

Pain of odontogenic origin is the most common dental emergency seen in the ED [A&E]. Although the etiology and management are usually straightforward, other more serious conditions can present with a similar clinical presentation. Misdiagnosis can have serious ramifications and it is incumbent upon the practitioner to perform a complete diagnostic workup that includes the following:

- History: the history of pain should include duration, location, description (character and intensity on a scale of 1–10) and what exacerbates and relieves the pain. Note the medications taken, dose and duration and how effective or ineffective they have proved to be. Watch for acetaminophen [paracetamol] toxicity in children. Any previous treatment or similar history should be noted.
- Physical examination: the patient should be examined for any tooth that is sensitive to percussion, pressure on biting/mastication and palpation, as well as for mobility, periodontal pocketing, adjacent soft tissue swelling, caries, fractures, integrity of existing restorations and pulp vitality.
- Radiographic and laboratory examination: intraoral and/or panoramic radiographs should be obtained and examined for caries, periodontal disease and periapical changes, fractures or other pathology. Occlusal views may be useful for children. A Water's view might be necessary to examine for sinus disease. Laboratory values such as a CBC and cultures are often useful when infection exists or is suspected.

Management of specific intraoral urgencies

Hypersensitivity of dentin or cementum

- History: positive for localized sensitivity to cold, sweets, acids, tooth brushing, fingernail or metal instrument.
- Examination: usually demonstrates localized areas of exposed cementum or dentin, with or without overlying plaque.

- Tests: may be sensitive to air blast or metal instrument (explorer) at gingival level of tooth surface. Hyper- or traumatic occlusion should be ruled out.
- Treatment: use of fluoride gel or commercial dentin desensitizers following thorough cleaning can help to desensitize.
- Prognosis: symptoms should decrease within days and eventually disappear. The area must be kept clean. Restoration might be required.

Pulpal hyperemia

- History: transient thermal or biting sensitivity. History of recent restorative treatment, upper respiratory infection or flu (with sinus involvement) in the past 6–8 weeks.
- Examination: examine patient for faulty restoration, caries, hyper- or traumatic occlusion or enamel or tooth fracture ('cracked tooth' syndrome).
- Tests: may be sensitive to air blast or cold. Electric pulp test (EPT) positive at low level or normal.
- Prognosis: usually reversible with appropriate treatment.
- Treatment: if possible, the source (e.g. high restoration) should be removed. If indicated, a sedative restoration can be useful. If due to deep caries, an indirect pulp cap should be used only in permanent teeth and when pulp pathology is believed to be reversible (e.g. no periapical pathology, no lingering spontaneous pain that might be worse overnight and stimulated pain of short duration only).

Acute pulpitis (early)

- History: spontaneous, intermittent, sharp, spasmodic pain and cold sensitivity. Pain of longer duration than simple hyperemia but not continuous. Sensitivity to hot and/or cold foods/drinks (e.g. coffee/tea and/or ice cream).
- Examination: usually reveals identifiable source of pulpitis (e.g. caries, deep restoration, fractured restoration or clinical crown). Radiograph might not demonstrate periapical radiolucency.
- Tests: positive electric pulp test at low level. Heat and/or cold may excite. Tooth may be percussion sensitive.
- Prognosis: probably not reversible.
- Treatment: if reversible pulpitis and if all infected caries is removed without exposure, use sedative filling. If carious exposure then:

- ○ permanent tooth (open apex): calcium hydroxide pulpotomy
- ○ permanent tooth (closed apex): pulpectomy
- ○ primary tooth: formocresal pulpectomy or pulpectomy, depending on the stage of root resorption
- ○ extraction as an alternative.

Note: A given tooth might have overlapping symptoms from more than one cause, for example, a molar with pulpal hyperemia in a distal canal and necrotic mesial canals (from mesial caries) might give misleading electric pulp test (EPT) results and the history might suggest symptoms of both a reversible and irreversible situation.

Acute suppurative pulpitis (later stage)

- History: spontaneous, intense, sharp pain lasting longer periods of time. Heat sensitive, cold may soothe.
- Examination: look for a source of pulpitis (e.g. caries, fractured tooth or restoration), which might have referred pain and/or may be of periodontal origin. A radiograph will usually show widening of the periodontal ligament at the apex, or periapical lucency. Regional – particularly submandibular – tender lymphadenopathy on palation.
- Tests: electric pulp test unreliable. Usually percussion and/or heat sensitive.
- Prognosis: irreversible.
- Treatment: extraction or root canal therapy.

Non-vital pulp with periapical inflammation

- History: chronic, unstimulated pain; sensitive to biting. May report a recent history of cold sensitivity with a tooth. Percussion sensitivity. Pain may be referred. In severe cases, patient may be sipping cold water to relieve pain.
- Examination: identify source of pulpal pathology. Regional particularly submandibular, tender lymphadenopathy on palpation.
- Tests: no response to heat, cold or electric pulp test. Positive percussion sensitivity.
- Treatment: pulpectomy and eventual root canal therapy or extraction. With regional or systemic involvement, antibiotics may be indicated (e.g. penicillin VK 500 mg QID, amoxil [amoxicillin] 500 mg tds, or for penicillin-allergic patients, clindamycin 250–300 mg QID).

Acute periapical disease (alveolar abscess)

- History: exquisite, localized pain, throbbing. May have history of facial swelling and/or fever.
- Examination: identifiable source of pulpal disease is almost always found. May be tender on direct finger palpation of the vestibule or may see swelling in the vestibule (that can be fluctuant and painful), inflammation and possibly fever and/or regional lymphadenopathy.
- Tests: positive percussion sensitivity. No response to thermal or electrical stimulation. Radiographic evidence of periapical radiolucency.
- Treatment: antibiotics (e.g. penicillin VK 500 mg QID, amoxil 500 mg tds, or for penicillin-allergic patients, clindamycin 250–300 mg QID), analgesics, establishment of adequate drainage either through the pulp chamber, by incision and drainage of the vestibule or by extraction. If drainage will not require opening fascial planes then extraction should be done as the initial therapy. When fascial planes will be violated by an extraction (e.g. a 'surgical extraction'), the patient should initially be placed on antibiotics, an incision and drainage (I&D) done and the extraction performed when less acute, usually in 1–2 days.

Maxillary sinusitis with referred pain to teeth

- History: unilateral or bilateral pain in maxillary posterior teeth, usually difficult to localize to one tooth and often involves pre-molars and molars with root apices adjacent to sinus. The patient may complain that 'all the teeth hurt' and also of increasing pain upon bending over. Pain may occur several weeks following resolution of 'flu, or upper respiratory infection. Otherwise, the patient presents with typical sinus symptoms.
- Examination: primary dental source should be ruled out. Discomfort when digital pressure is placed infraorbitally on the sinus wall. Transillumination of the sinus by placing a fiberoptic light against the hard palate may reveal an increased opacity on the affected side.
- Tests: percussion sensitivity of multiple maxillary teeth. Sinus (Water's or panoramic) films demonstrate increased radiopacity or an air-fluid level. Electric pulp testing should be normal.
- Treatment: with history of sinus infection, pain, drainage, blockage or dental sensitivity that does not improve in 24–48 h, treatment

with appropriate antibiotics and topical nasal decongestant for 3–5 days is recommended. Chronic or refractory cases should be referred to an otolaryngologist [ENT surgeon].

- Prognosis: excellent. Symptoms usually resolve within several days if due to sinus rather than odontogenic source.

Coronal fracture ('fractured/cracked tooth syndrome')

- History: sharp, intermittent, localized pain, usually with chewing (releasing). May have history of trauma to tooth/jaw, recent restoration, or chewing ice.
- Examination: pain elicited by biting pressure or, classically, with release after biting on a tongue depressor. Fracture is usually evident upon close inspection of a dry tooth with mirror and good lighting. Often occurs on marginal ridges at contact point or lingual/occlusal adjacent to overextended restoration groove. May run over cusp tip or be circumferential.
- Treatment: cusp capping restoration often necessary. Intermediate restoration material (IRM), if necessary using an orthodontic band to stabilize, followed by removal or reduction of the fractured area for several weeks to allow for resolution of symptoms. Possible endodontic therapy or extraction if fracture involves furcation or extends below cementoenamel junction.

Dental pain of other origin

Occasionally, pain that appears to be of odontogenic origin actually originates from other sources. Possibilities for such pain include referral from a myofascial source, myocardial ischemia, otalgia, sickle-cell crisis and adverse effects of medications such as vincristine or vinblastine. These sources must be considered when no odontogenic source is identified.

Soft tissue lesions

Periodontal abscess

- Etiology: ○ Acute exacerbation of chronic periodontitis; unable to drain through gingival crevice. ○ Localized plaque and/or calculus deep in gingival crevice. ○ Foreign body in the gingival crevice. ○ Endodontic abscess. ○ Root fracture.
- Diagnosis: ○ Progressive localized pain and deep isolated pocket formation. ○ Gingival tissues become red, swollen and painful

with possible purulence from gingival crevice. ○ Tooth mobility. ○ Foreign body may be found in crevice. ○ Non-vital pulp possible. ○ Identification of root fracture with deep pocket.

- Treatment: ○ Local anesthesia. ○ Irrigation with saline. ○ Ultrasonic debridement, scaling and root planing. ○ Incision and drainage if fluctuant, with or without a Penrose drain, to obtain drainage through gingival crevice. ○ Antibiotic coverage in presence of systemic signs or symptoms (penicillin VK 500 mg QID for 5–7 days, or amoxil [amoxicillin] 500 mg tds or, for penicillin-allergic patients, clindamycin 250 mg QID). ○ Careful periodontal follow-up.

Necrotizing ulcerative gingivitis or periodontitis

- Etiology: necrotizing ulcerative gingivitis (NUG) and necrotizing ulcerative periodontitis (NUP) are painful, non-contagious bacterial infections of the papillary and marginal gingiva. ○ Usually an opportunistic infection of mixed anaerobic flora, but anaerobic spirochetes and fusiforms commonly predominate. ○ Commonly associated with mild local or systemic immunosuppression that accompanies periods of emotional stress, fatigue, malnutrition, poor hygiene, pre-existing gingivitis and smoking. ○ The periodontitis form has been associated with the systemic immunosuppression resulting from HIV infection.
- Diagnosis: ○ Bleeding, necrosis and blunting of the interdental papillary gingiva with pseudomembrane formation. ○ Gingival pain, usually severe and halitosis. ○ Fever, malaise, cervical lymphadenopathy. ○ Periodontitis form also associated with periodontal ligament attachment loss and alveolar bone destruction.
- Treatment: ○ Saline irrigation using a large syringe and plastic IV catheter. ○ Gross mechanical debridement (ultrasonic or, if possible, scaling and curettage) using local anesthesia. ○ Oral hygiene, dietary and stress counseling. ○ Antibiotic therapy when systemic signs present (clindamycin 250–300 mg QID or metronidazole 250 [200] mg tid for 7 days). ○ Prompt follow-up appointment for oral hygiene. ○ Analgesic medication as needed. ○ Consider HIV testing when periodontitis form is present or if index of suspicion is high.

Herpes simplex infection

- Etiology: infection caused by the herpes simplex type 1 (HSV-1) or herpes virus type 1 (HHV-1) virus or, less commonly, by the herpes simplex type 2 (HSV-2) or HHV-2 virus, which more commonly causes genital lesions. Approximately 80% of the adult population have antibodies following primary infection. The latent virus persists in the trigeminal nerve ganglion innervating the affected area, where it may be reactivated to reappear later, under a variety of conditions, as a recurrent herpes infection.

Primary herpetic gingivostomatitis

- Diagnosis: ○ Usually seen in children, or young adults not previously exposed to virus. May be subclinical or quite severe. ○ Prodrome of fever, irritability, headache, dysphagia and regional lymphadenopathy. ○ A few days later, the patient reports painful gingivitis followed by multiple yellowish, fluid-filled vesicles on the lips, tongue, buccal mucosa and hard palate, which rapidly rupture to form ragged, extremely painful ulcers. These ulcers last 7–14 days, crust over and heal without scarring. ○ Diagnosis is usually clinical, although the virus can be cultured from fluid of an intact vesicle. Must be differentiated from erythema multiforme.

Recurrent herpes

- Diagnosis: ○ Usually seen as an attenuated form of primary infection. ○ Reactivated by trauma, emotional stress, fatigue, menstruation, pregnancy, respiratory infections or prolonged exposure to sunlight. ○ Prodromal symptoms include burning, tingling or pain at the site where the recurrent lesion will appear. ○ May see one or multiple small vesicles, which quickly ulcerate and coalesce, leaving a small red area with or without an erythematous halo and which heal without scarring in 7–14 days.

Treatment

- Primary herpes ○ Adequate hydration and nutrition. In severe cases and with young children, this may require intravenous rehydration and dietary supplementation. ○ Systemic and topical analgesics as required (e.g. viscous lidocaine 2% swished and expectorated prior to meals). ○ Avoid aspirin in young patients. ○ In immunocompromised patients with primary herpetic stomatitis or mucocutaneous herpes simplex infection, consider intravenous acyclovir (5 mg/kg every 8 h, slowly).
- Herpes labialis ○ May benefit symptomatically from topical acyclovir (5% ointment) or penciclovir (1% cream) but only if

given during the prodromal stage. ○ Patients with frequent, recurrent bouts of herpes labialis can benefit from oral acyclovir given at the first sign of recurrence (200 mg five times per day).

Aphthous ulcers

- Etiology: the etiology of aphthous ulcers is not clearly understood but they appear to be autoimmune with many possible contributory mechanisms, including psychic, allergic, microbial, traumatic, endocrine and heredity. Despite some clinical similarities, aphthae are separate and distinct entities from recurrent herpetic lesions.
- Diagnosis: ○ Can occur at any age. ○ Originates as an erythematous macule or papule that undergoes central blanching, necrosis and eventual ulceration. Shallow ulcers range in size from 0.5 (minor aphthae) to 3 cm (major aphthae). Demonstrates gray or yellow necrotic center and an erythematous halo. ○ Although usually singular, they can occur in small groups (herpetiform type) that later become a single or a few confluent ulcers. ○ Almost always occur on non-keratinized, unattached tissue (e.g. vestibule, ventral tongue, labial mucosa, floor of mouth). ○ Pain is moderate to severe.
- Treatment: generally supportive in nature, as the lesions usually disappear in 7–14 days. Particularly severe aphthae and major aphthae might require additional measures. This should include adequate hydration and nutrition. Although there is no proven treatment for aphthae, a number of clinical therapies have been advocated for minimizing pain or shortening the life of the ulcer, including: ○ antibiotics – tetracycline (250 mg in 5 cc sterile water) or chlorhexidine mouthwashes ○ protective topical dressings such as hydroxypropyl cellulose (Zilactin) or Orabase used PRN ○ topical steroids such as Kenalog [Adcortyl®] in Orabase or fluocinonide (Lidex) ointment twice a day ○ analgesics – benzocaine in Orabase applied PRN or benzydamine [Difflam] rinse, if available.

Burns

- Etiology: ○ Chemical – most commonly seen with topically used salicylates (e.g. aspirin), which cause coagulation necrosis. Iatrogenic chemical burns can result from common materials such as eugenol. Occasionally seen with accidental or intentional ingestion of caustic materials (e.g. lye). ○ Physical – can occur in a child biting an electrical cord or a burn from a dental handpiece. Also common from hot food (e.g. 'pizza palate').

- Diagnosis: ○ Mild burns (first degree) manifest as erythema. ○ More severe burns will be mixed red–white areas, or just white areas, indicating tissue necrosis. ○ Electrical wire burns usually occur at the commissures of the mouth. Can cause severe scarring and contraction if left to heal without treatment. Can be complicated by delayed hemorrhage from the facial/labial arteries.
- Treatment: ○ Most mild burns require no treatment and heal spontaneously, although adequate hydration and nutrition must be assured. ○ More severe burns may require debridement of necrotic tissue. Can be accomplished with or without local anesthesia as warranted. ○ Saline rinses and good oral hygiene. ○ Topical (e.g. viscous lidocaine) or systemic analgesics often necessary. ○ For electrical burns, the patient should be referred immediately to a pediatric dentist for splint construction to prevent contracture of the commissures subsequent to healing and fibrous scarring. ○ Swallowed caustics – refer for endoscopy.

Human bites

The usual organisms are *Staphylococcus aureus*, *Streptococcus species* and *Eikenella corrodens*. Anaerobic bacteria such as *Bacteroides*, *Prevotella*, *Fusobacteria* species and others are common. Gram-negative species are less common. *E. corrodens* is especially important because of its unusual antibiotic sensitivity, being sensitive to penicillin and ampicillin but resistant to semisynthetic penicillins and first-generation cephalosporins.

Management

- All bites should receive appropriate tetanus prophylaxis. Treatment then involves thorough cleansing, copious irrigation, debridement and the appropriate use of prophylactic antibiotics. Bites often occur in daycare settings. Child abuse should be suspected in bites with a questionable history.
- Human bites to the face seen within 24 h can be primarily sutured after appropriate cleansing and debridement. Prophylactic antibiotics should be given.
- Hand bites require special treatment because of the possibility of unrecognized penetrating injury to a joint. Human bite injuries to the hand must be irrigated thoroughly and should not be sutured primarily because close follow-up is essential. There is a high

incidence of infection of the soft tissue and joint space (metacarpophalangeal).

- Treatment recommendations for bites other than the hand and face are individualized but always include thorough debridement and irrigation and generally prophylactic antibiotics.
- Broad-spectrum second-generation cephalosporins have been widely recommended for human bites. A combination of penicillin and a penicillinase-resistant penicillin can be used. Amoxicillin plus clavulanic acid (Augmentin) is also widely used.

POSTOPERATIVE EMERGENCIES

Postoperative complications sometimes pose difficulties for dentists because little might be known about the original procedure.

- Acquire a complete history of present illness, including as many details about the original procedure as the patient can remember. The medical records should be obtained, if possible.
- Conduct a thorough physical examination of the involved site.
- Contact the doctor who performed the original surgery, if possible.

Bleeding

This can be a particularly frightening complication to the patient or family. Any amount of blood (as little as 5 or 10 cc) can be considered heavy bleeding by the patient when it originates from the mouth or involves the patient's clothing. Blood will mix with saliva in the mouth, increasing the apparent volume of 'blood' present.

Bleeding is most commonly due to local factors and is rarely a manifestation of an underlying systemic problem.

Bleeding from an extraction or bony surgery site

- Identify the site of origin: ○ A small bleeding vessel within the bony wall of the socket. ○ Brisk bleeding from the apical area indicating possible arterial damage especially if pulsatile. ○ Bleeding emanating from the soft tissue around the socket. ○ Bleeding from granulation tissue left in the socket. ○ Generalized oozing from all areas.

- Etiology: ○ Loss of organized blood clot from smoking, excessive spitting and rinsing or using a straw within 24 h of surgery. Can also be caused by salivary plasminogens. ○ Reopening of a vessel that was tamponaded or vasoconstricted at the time of surgery. ○ Loss of one or more sutures. ○ Excessive highly vascular granulation tissue in the socket (as is often seen in severe periodontal disease). ○ An acquired coagulopathy – most commonly drug related (e.g. warfarin or substances containing aspirin or alcohol). ○ Less frequently, an inherited coagulopathy.

- Management:
  ○ Thorough history and physical examination. Particular emphasis should be placed on current medications (patients are often unaware of medications that may impair coagulation. Also inquire about compliance with postoperative instructions; take care phrasing these questions (e.g. 'Have you had to spit much blood to keep from swallowing it?').
  ○ Ensure the appropriate suction equipment (with a small-diameter stiff suction tip) and lighting (preferably a headlight) is available.
  ○ Examine for obvious bleeding vessels in or around the site. If visualized, electrically coagulate or ligate with resorbable suture, under local anesthesia.
  ○ If the bleeding is noted to be brisk or arterial (pulsatile) in nature, inject local anesthesia with a vasoconstrictor, debride, irrigate the socket and examine closely for specific areas of bleeding. Small bone bleeders may be crushed with a metal instrument or stopped with a small amount of bone wax. Apical or non-isolatable bleeds should be packed with Surgicel, Avitene or Gelfoam. Following this, or if bleeding is coming from the soft tissues, use interpapillary or figure-of-eight 'hemorrhagic' sutures and reinstitute pressure.
  ○ If no obvious vessels are seen, initial management should always be direct pressure. This is accomplished by biting on gauze, under observation, for 20 min. If this fails, a gauze impregnated with liquid topical thrombin or the antifibrinolytic syrup, epsilon aminocaproic acid (Amicar) or 5% tranexamic acid, can be tried for an additional 20 min.
  ○ When local causes have been ruled out, appropriate laboratory tests should be ordered. This includes a complete [full] blood count (CBC) [FBC] with differential and platelet count,

prothrombin time (PT) and international normalized ratio (INR) and partial thromboplastin time (APTT). If abnormalities are detected, medical consultation is indicated.

- Instructions: when the bleeding is controlled, the patient should be given careful verbal, and preferably written, instructions to decrease risk of recurrence.

Bleeding from the gingiva

- Etiology: ○ Severe gingival or periodontal infection, including acute necrotizing ulcerative gingivitis, linear gingival erythema and primary herpes. ○ Trauma. ○ Intrinsic (e.g. hemophilia) or extrinsic (medications) coagulopathy. ○ Other systemic cause (e.g. acute leukemia).
- Diagnosis: history and physical examination should differentiate local from systemic sources. When indicated, obtain appropriate blood tests.
- Management: ○ Injection of local anesthesia with vasoconstrictor into the area. ○ Gauze pressure. ○ Removal of granulation tissue in periodontal conditions. ○ Repair of traumatic injuries. ○ Medical consultation for coagulopathies.

Bleeding from postoperative soft-tissue incisions

- Etiology: ○ Wound margin bleeder. ○ Dead-space hematoma. ○ Arterial or venous bleeding within the wound itself.
- Diagnosis: ○ Examine and palpate the surgical site. Gradual discoloration and swelling at the site usually indicates an underlying hematoma. ○ Brisk, bright red blood usually indicates arterial bleeding. This may be immediate or delayed (from loss of a suture or vascular invasion).
- Management: ○ Wound margin bleeders and slow, venous bleeders can usually be stopped with direct pressure or a pressure bandage, but might require additional sutures. ○ Deep arterial bleeding mandates opening the wound; explore for vessel to be coagulated or ligated. ○ Hematomas should be evacuated by opening a small area of the incision, probing with a hemostat until the hematoma is found and expressing the blood. Direct pressure and a pressure bandage should be used to prevent secondary hematoma formation. If bleeding persists, the wound should be explored.

Postextraction pain

- Etiology: ○ Normal pain due to inflammation. ○ Alveolar osteitis ('dry socket') due to loss of the blood clot within the socket and exposure of sensory nerve endings within the socket. ○ Localized infection (periostitis or alveolar infection). ○ Localized tenderness due to loose bone fragment.
- Diagnosis: a careful review of the history will usually lead to a diagnosis:
  - ○ Normal pain: begins soon after surgery and remains constant or improves slowly with time (varies from patient to patient).
  - ○ Alveolar osteitis: pain remains constant or initially improves after surgery, then suddenly increases after 3 or 4 days. Much more common in the mandible than the maxilla. Often radiates to the ipsilateral ear. The examination will only show loss of the clot from the socket. A foul odor is common.
  - ○ Localized infection: usually presents a few days to a few weeks after surgery. Physical examination reveals signs of inflammation and infection. May see purulence and there might be an elevated white blood cell count and fever. Palpation of the area will be acutely painful, especially with periostitis.
  - ○ Fractured buccal plate: palpation over socket, usually buccal, will reveal tenderness and possibly crepitus.
- Management:
  - ○ Normal pain: reassurance, observation and analgesics as indicated.
  - ○ Alveolar osteitis: gentle irrigation of socket to remove debris and placement of a sedative dressing (e.g. Eugenol on 1" × $\frac{1}{4}$" strip gauze or Alvogyl®). This should be left for 4–5 days. Replacement during that period should be carried out at any time the patient feels the pain return. Analgesics should be prescribed.
  - ○ Localized infection: periostitis is usually treatable with antibiotic therapy (e.g. penicillin VK 250–500 mg QID for 5 days). Socket infections are treated with antibiotics and incision and drainage as necessary.
  - ○ For fractured bone: remove suture, identify and remove bone fragment, irrigate and resuture.

Nausea and vomiting

- Etiology: ○ Swallowed blood. ○ Post-anesthetic effects if IV sedation or general anesthesia used. ○ Drug side-effects (antibiotics, analgesics).
- Diagnosis: ○ Examine for bleeding. ○ Determine type of anesthesia used for surgery. ○ Review medications.
- Management: ○ Control bleeding if present. ○ If medication-induced, discontinue or change medications to ones less associated with nausea (e.g. acetaminophen [paracetamol] instead of codeine or ibuprofen). ○ If no change or if anesthetic related, consider an antiemetic given rectally, IV or IM. For example:
  - ○ Phenergan [Stemetil] = promethazine 25 mg PO, IM, PR, IV
  - ○ Compazine = prochlorperazine 10 mg IV, PO, IM; 25 mg PR
  - ○ Tigan = trimethobenzamide 250 mg PO; 200 mg IM, PR
  - ○ Inapsine = droperidol 2.5 mg IV, IM
- [Ondansetron 4 mg IV]

ODONTOGENIC INFECTIONS

General concepts

Pain from odontogenic infections are the most common problem seen by dentists in the emergency department. In fact, because of their ubiquitous nature, pain, infection and swelling in the face and neck region should generally be assumed to be of odontogenic origin until proven otherwise. When addressed early, complications are rare and minor. When allowed to progress and when a particularly virulent organism is involved, or when the host is immunocompromised, odontogenic infections can lead to serious morbidity or even death.

Diagnosis of infection

History

The patient will commonly have a history of toothache at some point in the past, although a lifetime of pulpal regression might spare people of advanced age this particular antecedent to abscess. Swelling will usually have begun only recently and exacerbated quickly. The pain and swelling might have improved and then worsened again as the infection traverses different spaces. The history should include the duration of the infection as well as any previous treatment and its response.

Physical examination

Swelling
- Fluctuant: fluid-filled area indicating abscess formation.
- Non-fluctuant: some organisms (e.g. streptococci) tend to cause spreading infections rather than abscesses. This is seen as a cellulitis.
- Reactive edema: the tissue surrounding the area of infection may develop moderate to severe secondary edema. Often seen in the periorbital area when associated with maxillary dental infections. Can be differentiated clinically from infection by its soft, non-fluctuant, non-tender nature.

Erythema
- Pain to palpation: an area of infection is usually quite tender. Decreasing tenderness is often indicative of the effectiveness of therapy.
- Trismus: as infections impinge on the muscles of mastication, trismus will become evident.
- Source: the source of an odontogenic infection is usually easily identified as a tooth with carious exposure of the pulp or severe periodontal condition. When an obvious source cannot be isolated, non-odontogenic sources must be considered.
- Drainage: in some cases, spontaneous purulent drainage may be evident. This is often accompanied by bad odor and taste.

Lymphadenopathy

Radiographic data. Clinically evident sources should always be confirmed with radiographic data. This could include a panoramic, periapical or occlusal radiograph (useful for children when other films not possible), or lateral oblique views in less cooperative patients, particularly those with a learning disability.

Medical management of odontogenic infections

Systemic medical evaluation

Infections of odontogenic origin are usually managed before the patient demonstrates systemic manifestations. The presence of fever, chills, shaking and malaise – or of confusion and clouded consciousness ('delirium') in an elderly person – indicates that complete systemic evaluation is warranted. In addition, the spread of infection is related to the virulence of the organism and the state of the host's immune system. As such, patients with rapidly advancing odontogenic infections should be thoroughly evaluated for evidence of diminished immune competence.

Indications for hospitalization

- Systemic involvement: fever, dehydration with orthostasis requiring parenteral fluids and nutrition.
- Evidence of spreading tissue necrosis or cellulitis involving critical areas such as periorbital region and areas with potential airway compromise (sublingual, submandibular and/or parapharyngeal spaces).
- Immune system compromise: HIV, diabetes, steroid therapy, alcoholism, cancer chemotherapy.
- Need for intravenous antibiotics.
- Infections requiring special treatment: fungal infections, osteomyelitis, actinomycosis.
- Patients unable to manage their infections at home due to disability.
- Children who can't, won't or have not eaten, or who have unreliable parents/guardians.

Nutrition

Patients with infection are often unable to maintain their dietary and fluid intake and should receive IV maintenance fluids. Patients unable to eat for longer than 48 h should be considered for nasogastric feeding.

Culture and sensitivity (C&S) testing

In all but the most minor of fluctuant odontogenic infections (and these as well if they are resistant to initial treatment), consider sending cultures for C&S. This may be accomplished by:

- Aspiration: a 3–10 cc syringe is attached to a 14–20 gauge needle, which is then inserted through uncompromised and cleansed tissue into the area of fluctuance. May be used for both aerobic and anaerobic culturing.
- Purulence specimen: a small amount of purulence may be collected on a sterile swab and submitted for culture. This is ineffective for anaerobic infections and is subject to contamination.

- Tissue specimens: a small amount of tissue is excised and sent in a sterile container for testing. This not only allows aerobic and anaerobic evaluation but also quantitative analysis.

Principles of antibiotic therapy

- Initial therapy is usually empirical, based on the likely source and organism involved. When available, therapy should be guided by culture and sensitivity testing results.
- Should be parenteral with severe infections.
- When instituting empirical therapy, always use the least expensive, least toxic and narrowest-spectrum antibiotic that will cover the likely organisms.
- Patients must be asked about a history of drug allergy or current medications that could interact with the antibiotics used (e.g. birth-control pills, warfarin therapy and gastric-ulcer medications such as cimetidine).

Diagnostic imaging

Diagnostic imaging studies can help guide surgical therapy. They are used in cases of deep fascial space infections, rapidly spreading infections and infections impinging on vital structures such as the airway. Studies to be considered include:

- Computerized tomography (CT): useful for determining extent of infection, in both soft tissues and bone. Studies can be done with intravenous contrast, assist in determining extent of hyperemia surrounding infectious site.
- Magnetic resonance imaging (MRI): useful for determining extent of infection, especially within soft tissues. Advantage is lack of ionizing radiation exposure. Disadvantages: more expensive than CT and patients must lie still for lengthy periods because of prolonged delay for image capture.
- Ultrasound: used for locating abscess cavities within soft tissues.

Laboratory data

Aside from culture and sensitivity testing, a few laboratory tests can aid in the diagnosis and management of infections.

- Complete [full] blood count with differential:
  - Leukocytosis (WBC >12 000/mm^3) indicative of infection.
  - A 'shift to the left' (presence of many immature or 'segmented' neutrophils) on differential WBC count is seen with acute

infection. Chronic infections do not have this shift and usually have a marginally increased white cell count.
- Elevated platelet count (> 500 000/mm^3) in some cases.
- Chemistry studies:
  - Blood urea nitrogen (BUN) may be elevated due to dehydration.
  - Hypernatremia (Na$^+$) and hypochloremia (Cl$^-$) may also be seen with dehydration.
  - Albumin levels may drop due to malnutrition or necrotizing infections.
- Urinalysis:
  - Dehydration leads to increase in specific gravity (> 1.025).
  - Severe dehydration can lead to oliguria and acute tubular necrosis and renal failure.
  - Severe infections can demonstrate proteinuria.

Surgical management of odontogenic infections

Diagnosis

Prior to any surgical intervention it is imperative that the offending source be isolated and the specific spaces involved with infection be delineated. This can be done by clinical examination or by diagnostic imaging.

Removal of source

When possible, the offending source of the infection should be removed. In many cases this may be adequate treatment (e.g. a tooth extraction with adequate spontaneous drainage from the socket). Removal of the source may include:
- Extraction of a tooth: contrary to popular belief, the extraction of an acutely infected tooth is not contraindicated. This is the appropriate treatment, except when such removal would open up additional fascial planes and spaces to the infection, for example, removal of an impacted tooth requiring elevation of a flap.
- Pulpectomy or endodontic procedures in permanent teeth.
- Pulpotomy or pulpectomy in primary teeth.
- Removal of foreign bodies (e.g. bullet fragment).
- Removal of necrotic bone.
- Removal of infected sutures (stitch abscess).

Principles of incision and drainage (I&D)

When removal of the source is inadequate for allowing elimination of abscessed areas, surgical access is warranted to promote gravitational drainage, although this is rarely needed in children. The particular areas to be drained or explored should be determined presurgically so that they can be prepped accordingly. Basic principles of surgical drainage are:

- When in doubt, drain. With few exceptions, an I&D will only help the situation and, even when non-productive, will allow for future drainage should it begin after the procedure.
- Prior to I&D, consideration must be given to patients with bleeding disorders, those who are taking anticoagulant therapy or immuno-suppressive agents.
- Extraoral incisions should be placed where they will be cosmetic and allow gravitational drainage with the patient in the supine or upright position.
- All drains should be secured to prevent premature loss.
- All incisions should be designed to prevent injury to important structures (e.g. nerves, blood vessels, ducts).
- Drains should be left in place and monitored until they are no longer productive, generally 1–3 days.

Anesthesia

- Local anesthesia injected into an abscess will usually fail because of the acidic pH of the region.
- Local anesthesia infiltrated into the mucosa or regional block injections are usually successful (e.g. mandibular block or V2 block).
- Care should be exercised to inject around an area of infection, not through it.
- If local anesthesia is not possible, general anesthesia may be necessary, especially for larger or deeper fascial space infections.
- Trismus, a common finding with infections near the muscles of mastication, is a product of pain and subsequent spasm in acute infections (not necessarily true with chronic infections, where fibrosis may have occurred). When a patient is placed under general anesthesia, mouths with acute infections will almost always open without difficulty.

Intraoral I&D (Fig. 5.1)

- Locate the area of maximum fluctuance. Provide local anesthesia with mucosal infiltration or regional anesthesia.

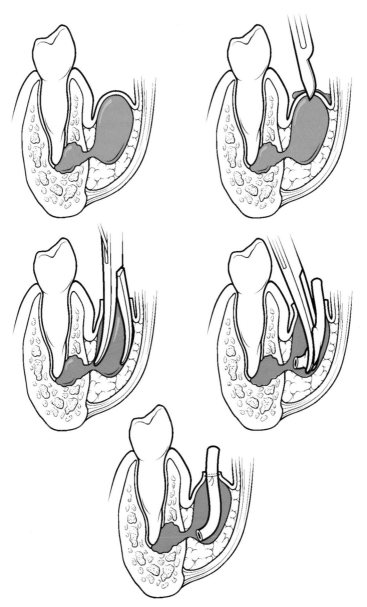

Fig. 5.1 Intraoral incision and drainage.

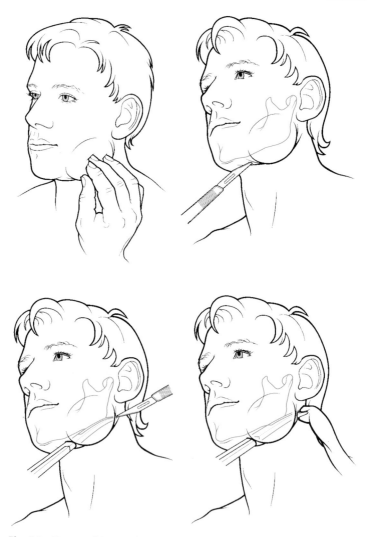

Fig. 5.2 Extraoral incision and drainage.

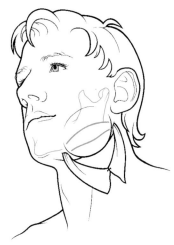

Fig. 5.2 **Extraoral incision and drainage (*continued*).**

- Using a #15 or #11 blade, make a 5 mm incision in the mucosa overlying the area of fluctuance.
- Use a mosquito hemostat to bluntly explore the abscess until purulence [pus] is obtained.
- When all the purulence [pus] has been evacuated and the I&D site irrigated with normal saline, place a small Penrose drain (a hollow latex tube) or other latex material drain well into the abscess cavity and suture it to the end of the wound with a 4-0 non-resorbable suture.
- Leave approximately 1 cm of the drain visible in the mouth.
- Encourage the patient to use saline rinses to keep the drain open.

Extraoral I&D (Fig. 5.2)

- The procedure may be performed under local anesthesia, with IV sedation or under general anesthesia. If local anesthesia is to be used, inject 2–3 cc in the region of the incision and another 2–3 cc in the path of the proposed procedure. Prep area to be drained with an iodine scrub solution and drape in sterile fashion, allowing plenty of room to work. Locate areas of fluctuance, any areas of compromised skin and an area of non-compromised skin that would allow for dependent gravitational drainage and a good cosmetic scar. Ideal places are in skin creases or just below the mandible. Incisions should never be placed in compromised skin due to the lack of healing ability.

- Make a 1-cm incision through the skin and into the subcutaneous tissue. Using a hemostat, bluntly dissect into the abscess cavity. Open the hemostat to allow the purulence [pus] to flow freely.
- When large spaces are to be drained, it is advisable to run a $1/4$" Penrose drain through the space and exit it at the other end of the space, thus creating a 'through and through' drain, which ensures that the drain is in the space and not just folded onto itself under the skin margin.
- Place the drain into the depth of the abscess cavity and suture it to the margin of the incision with any non-resorbable suture. Cover the area with a sterile, non-sticky dressing such as Telfa [Melolin] and gauze.
- A suture can be placed through the ends of the drain to secure placement.

Postoperative care

- Maintain the drain in place for as long as it is productive, generally 1–3 days. Although drains sometimes need to be left in for as long as a week (in severe infections), at some point they become a foreign body and will prolong the drainage. Therefore, removal at the earliest possible time is recommended.
- Change the dressings as often as necessary to keep the wound clean, at least once per day.
- Maintain antibiotics for at least 24 h after the pyrexia has resolved.
- Upon removal of the drain, allow the incision to granulate under a sterile dressing. Intraoral incisions require no dressing.

SALIVARY GLAND EMERGENCIES

Acute parotid infections

Etiology

Acute parotid infections are usually caused by retrograde infection from the oral cavity and are secondary to decreased salivary flow from dehydration or an immunocompromised state. The causative organisms are usually staphylococci or streptococci but many other organisms have also been implicated. Viral acute parotitis is common in children as a bilateral swelling. The most common candidates for acute parotid infection are:

- newborns
- elderly patients
- postsurgical patients
- patients on dehydrating medications (e.g. diuretics, anticholinergics, tranquilizers, antihistamines)
- immunocompromised patients
- patients with primary or secondary Sjögren's syndrome.

Diagnosis

The diagnosis is usually straightforward due to the unique clinical presentation, which includes:

- sudden onset of firm swelling, pain and erythema of the pre-auricular (parotid) or floor of mouth/submandibular region (sublingual/submandibular gland)
- 20% of cases are bilateral
- temperature elevation (not always observed in an elderly person, where the infection is more likely manifested as confusion and disorientation)
- leukocytosis
- thick, purulent discharge from Stenson's duct (opposite maxillary first molar) or Wharton's duct upon milking.

Differential diagnosis

- Sialosis.
- Pneumoparotid: will demonstrate crepitus and will not have the purulent discharge.
- Mumps (bilateral).
- Lymphadenopathy: discrete enlargement without purulent discharge.

Treatment

- Intravenous rehydration is the cornerstone of treatment in most cases. Careful monitoring and control must be exercised with elderly or debilitated patients to prevent fluid overload.
- Discontinuation, if possible, of any medicines associated with xerostomia.
- Empirical antimicrobial therapy with an antistaphylococcal agent with anti-beta-lactamase activity, such as a cephalosporin or

dicloxacillin or cloxacillin. When anaerobic organisms are suspected, as in longer-standing cases, consider metronidazole.

- Culture and sensitivity testing of any purulence.
- In severe, non-responsive cases, surgical drainage may be required. This is accomplished by blunt dissection using a small submandibular or retromandibular incision and placement of a small Penrose drain. Care must be exercised to avoid the facial nerve in cases of suppurative parotiditis.

Obstructive sialadenitis

Etiology

Stones in the submandibular or parotid gland or duct are the major cause. However, ductal stricture from scarring, tumor, foreign bodies or mucous plugs can cause an identical clinical picture. Obstruction leads to back-up of saliva within the gland and a painful enlargement because the glands are bound by a restrictive, fibrous capsule.

Diagnosis

- Pain and swelling of the affected gland, usually just before mealtime.
- Gradual reduction in size within hours to days.
- More common in submandibular gland or duct.
- Milking of duct is either non-productive or produces a thick viscous discharge if the gland is secondarily infected.
- Occlusal, panoramic or facial X-rays will reveal radiopaque stones. Radiolucent stones or mucous plugs can be demonstrated with sialography.

Treatment

- Submandibular stones distal to the mylohyoid flexure (in the floor of the mouth) can be removed by making a small incision over the duct under local anesthesia. The stone is enucleated and the duct left unsutured to fistulate. A silk suture may be passed around the proximal portion of the duct prior to the procedure to prevent accidentally pushing the stone posteriorly.
- Submandibular stones proximal to the flexure or in the gland itself are usually treated by excision of the gland in the operating room [theatre] under general anesthesia.

- Stones in the parotid duct may be located by ultrasonography and enucleated through a 5-mm skin incision or, occasionally, by dilation of the duct.
- Lithotripsy, either extra corporeal or intraductal, may be attempted.

MAXILLOFACIAL TRAUMA

General principles of care

When dealing with multiple trauma, with few exceptions, facial injuries are not usually the first priority of treatment. Nevertheless, when the facial injuries are the most obvious problem, the dentist is often the first healthcare provider to see the patient. It is important to perform an overall assessment before proceeding to examine a specific oral or facial problem. As with all emergencies, the initial evaluator should always do the 'ABCs' first. Establishment of adequate respiratory and cardiac function and determination of neurologic status are paramount. Medical consultation should be obtained immediately for any aberration in the patient's condition. No analgesics, sedatives or anesthetics (or any other drug that could increase intracranial pressure) should be administered until neurologic or other medical complications have been ruled out.

The initial evaluation

Patent airway

The airway is often compromised by facial trauma as a result of fracture displacement, foreign bodies or the inability to maintain forward tongue posture:

- Assure a clear airway and normal rate and depth of breathing. Conscious patients will generally assume the body position that helps airway patency and they should be allowed to do so.
- Remove all foreign objects (e.g. pieces of teeth or restorations) from the oral cavity. Avulsed teeth may be reimplanted and then splinted if the patient is stable after medical assessment; alternatively, they can be stored in saline. Open the airway with a chin thrust, an oral or nasal airway or, if necessary, by cricothyroidotomy, if unable to place an ET tube.

Vital signs

Vital signs can be used to determine adequate circulatory function as well as indicators of intracranial injury:

- Decreased blood pressure and/or increased heart rate may indicate shock.
- Increased intracranial pressure is often associated with a decreased heart and respiratory rate in conjunction with increased blood pressure (Cushing's triad). This situation warrants immediate medical attention.

Neurologic evaluation

Careful examination can provide valuable information regarding both localized facial neurologic and intracranial injuries (see the Glasgow Coma Scale, Chapter 8.) Obtain neurosurgical consult for:

- Lack of spontaneous eye opening.
- Disorientation to verbal questioning.
- Inability to obey verbal commands.
- Rhinorrhea or otorrhea (indicative of cerebrospinal fluid leakage secondary to an anterior or middle cranial fossa fracture). Perform rapid and systematic cranial nerve examination:
  - Eyes: eye movements and sensation are used to evaluate cranial nerves (CN) III, IV, V and VI. If the eyes abduct fully, CN VI is intact. All the other eye movements (tested by having the patient follow finger movements in all four quadrants) indicate the status of CN III and IV. If the pupils are equal, round and reactive to light and accommodation (PERRLA), then CN II is unimpaired. If the patient feels a wisp of cotton on the cornea, CN V is intact. Vision can be tested grossly with a hand-held eye chart.
  - Face: CN V and VII are evaluated by examining the facial musculature and its sensation. A dental explorer or needle can be used to evaluate symmetric sensation to light touch, a function of CN V sensory division. Jaw opening without deviation can be used to evaluate the CN V motor component. However, it must be remembered that a jaw fracture can cause the jaw to deviate upon opening. Symmetry of the facial muscles on grimacing, frowning and eye closing indicates a normally functioning CN VII.
  - Speech and soft palate: if speech appears normal and the soft palate moves normally, CN IX and X are intact.

- Tongue: protrusion of the tongue without deviation from midline is normal for CN XII.
- Hearing: this can be tested by rubbing two fingers gently together, first behind one ear then behind the other. The auditory nerve (CN VIII) can be tested in this manner.
- Bilateral shrugging of the shoulders against pressure indicates normal function of the spinal accessory nerve innervated by CN XI.

Cervical examination

Traumatic facial injuries have a high correlation with neck injuries and it is important to maintain a high suspicion for the presence of associated cervical spine injury. Any significant facial trauma, therefore, mandates the need for a complete C-spine series of radiographs. Normal C-spine films do not completely rule out spinal cord injury; seek medical consultation. Only after ruling out cervical injury should a 'C' collar be removed and the head, neck or facial exams be carried out.

Abdominal examination

The abdomen is often injured in motor vehicle accidents. Examine for distention, tenderness and the presence or absence of bowel sounds.

Indications for immediate emergency treatment

Although facial fractures do not usually require priority emergency management, exceptions include:

- massive arterial bleeding
- airway compromise
- compound fractures should have at least temporary soft-tissue closure.

Diagnosis of facial trauma

Although the diagnosis of facial trauma is usually an obvious one, much information can be gained from a thorough history and physical examination.

History

The patient, or someone at the scene, should be questioned about details including loss of consciousness, seizures or hemorrhage. If any of these are positive, or if the patient has no memory of the incident, suspect intracranial injury and seek appropriate medical consultation.

Ascertain the source (e.g. fists versus baseball bat), direction, number and force of the blows. This can give significant clues to potential fractures or complicating injuries. For example:

- injuries to the midline symphyseal region of the mandible often cause bilateral subcondylar fractures
- injuries to the lateral body can cause a contralateral subcondylar fracture
- bullet wounds can cause delayed tissue necrosis
- stab wounds often cause deep injuries not easily visualized on the surface
- injuries involving high density objects (e.g. baseball bat) should be suspected of comminution.

A tetanus booster will be needed if the wound is clean and the last booster was >10 years ago, or if the wound is dirty and the last booster was >5 years ago; tetanus immune globulin might be needed if no initial tetanus series was ever received.

Question the patient about pre-existing asymmetries, abnormalities or conditions. A change from the pretrauma occlusion often indicates a fracture within the facial skeleton. Also ask about pain, paresthesia or anesthesia, hearing or visual disturbance, breathing difficulty, headache, dizziness, change in occlusion, feeling of crepitus or dysphagia.

Data would suggest that head trauma in children under 2 merits a medical consult. Studies suggest children under 2 years do not react the same as older children and adults.

Head and neck physical examination

The examination should be carried out in a systematic fashion from the cranium to the clavicles.

Inspection

Careful examination for the following:

- Asymmetry or flatness.
- Ecchymosis: if this is seen in the mastoid region (Battle's sign) or periorbital areas bilaterally ('raccoon eyes') without evidence of direct trauma, it is indicative of a basilar skull fracture. Ecchymosis in the floor of the mouth is considered pathognomonic of a mandibular fracture.

- Lacerations that could indicate underlying fractures.
- Obvious proportional changes of facial dimensions. Changes in facial height or width, intercanthal width (normally < 35–40 mm) or apparent ramus height can indicate fracture.
- Examine occlusion carefully for any changes from the preoperative state noted. Broken teeth, steps in the occlusion, tooth mobility and an anterior open bite are all signs of fracture.

Palpation

Whenever possible, palpate in a bilateral, bimanual fashion (placing the area to be examined between one hand or finger and another). This aids in determining small discrepancies:

- Extraoral: palpate all facial bones for 'steps', mobility or crepitus from displaced fractures. Palpation should begin in the frontal region and progress to the orbital rims, zygomatic arch, malar buttress and entire inferior border of the mandible.
- Intraoral: palpate bimanually to feel for steps, hematoma or mobility. Carefully palpate the malar buttress for tenderness or steps, both indicative of a zygoma or maxillary fracture. Examine for maxillary fractures by placing the thumb and index finger of the 'reference hand' on either side of the nasal bridge while the other hand is used to grasp the anterior maxillary ridge above the teeth:
  - movement of the maxilla in the non-reference hand only indicates LeFort 1
  - movement of the maxilla in the reference hand only indicates LeFort 2 or 3
  - movement of the maxilla in both hands indicates multiple fractures of the midface
  - movement at the lateral orbital rim indicates a LeFort 3 fracture or combined fractures with a zygoma fracture.
- Ask the patient to open and close the mandible. Maximum opening between the incisal edges, deviation on opening and joint sounds are noted. The joint is felt by placing two fingers over the preauricular area, or in the ear canals, during excursions. Tenderness, popping, crepitus or clicking can indicate internal trauma to the joint or a condylar fracture.
- Air emphysema in the tissues is manifested by a 'crinkling' feeling and sound and indicates a fracture of a sinus or a laryngeal injury.

Radiographic evaluation

Although careful physical examination is certainly the best diagnostic tool for facial fractures, radiographic imaging can provide confirmation of clinically suspected fractures as well as additional information.

Mandibular fractures

- Right and left lateral oblique views: show the body and angle of the mandible and the position of the condyle.
- Submental vertex ('jug handle') view: shows the inferior border of the mandible and the zygomatic arches.
- Posterior–anterior (PA) view: shows the symphyseal region.
- Towne's view: provides an excellent view of the condyles and condylar necks including their position in the fossa.
- Panoramic: provides an excellent overall view of the mandible. Also provides a slightly better view of the symphyseal region and a good view of the subcondylar and coronoid regions.
- Occlusal view: when a midline fracture or a fracture involving the alveolus is suspected, an occlusal view may be helpful.
- Periapical films: used to show undisplaced fractures of alveolar bone and tooth root fractures.

Maxillary fractures

- Lateral skull: shows the frontal sinus, nasal bones, anterior nasal spine and profile of the anterior maxilla.
- Water's [occipitomental] view: shows the maxilla, maxillary sinus, frontal sinus, orbital rims, zygomatic bones and frontal processes of the maxilla. Give special attention to comparing the volumes of the orbits. Asymmetries indicate orbital fracture. An airfluid level in the sinus indicates a fracture of the sinus wall.
- Panoramic.
- Occlusal and periapical views.
- Posterior–anterior skull.

Zygomatic fractures

- Water's [occipitomental] view.
- Submentovertex view.

Multiple facial fractures
- CT scan: use with 5 mm cuts if frontal bone fractures or multiple facial bone fractures are suspected, as this generally provides more accurate and detailed information than plain films. For even greater detail and information, 2 mm cuts allow three-dimensional reconstruction and computer manipulation.
- Angiography: penetrating injuries, such as a gunshot or knife wound to the region below the inferior border of the mandible, require angiographic determination of the extent of vascular injury. If located between inferior border of mandible and clavicular head, they will also need surgical exploration.

Treatment options for facial fractures

The aim is reduction of the fracture, fixation for an adequate period to allow for bone repair and general supportive and rehabilitative care.

Temporary stabilization
Mobile fractures of the facial skeleton are painful. It is often necessary, for practical or medical reasons, to delay definitive treat-

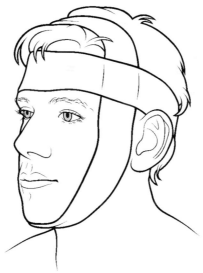

Fig. 5.3 Barton bandage.

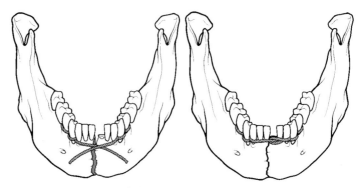

Fig. 5.4 **Risdon wire technique.**

ment for hours or even days. To decrease the discomfort, temporary stabilization may be utilized.

● Barton bandage: a simple bandage wrap composed of 24" gauze that is wrapped first vertically around the head several times and then horizontally around the forehead several times. This bandage is a simple and rapid mechanism for preventing mandibular opening (Fig. 5.3).

● Risdon wire: for anterior mandibular fractures, a 24-gauge wire twisted around each canine and then twisted to each other in the midline will approximate the fracture and prevent localized mobility. This can also be used with the Barton bandage. Alternatively, a single 24-gauge wire can be wrapped around all the anterior teeth and twisted to itself in the midline (Fig. 5.4).

Definitive reduction and fixation

The gold-standard is open reduction with internal fixation with miniplates. When undisplaced fractures occur behind the teeth, or when fractures occur within the dentate segment, closed reduction with intermaxillary fixation (IMF) for 4–6 weeks will often suffice for definitive treatment.

● Closed reduction with Ivy loops: a rapid method of obtaining fixation, used only for short-period IMF (Fig. 5.5). This can easily be performed in the emergency department [A&E] or clinic under local anesthesia.

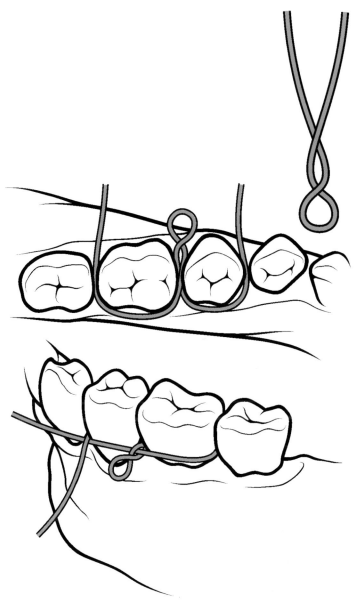

Fig. 5.5   Closed reduction with Ivy loops.

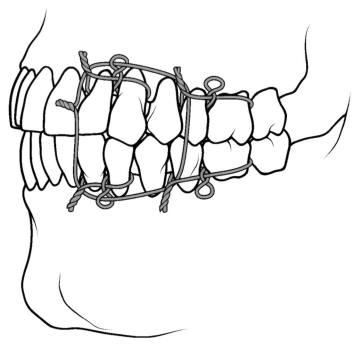

Fig. 5.5 **Closed reduction with Ivy loops** (*continued*).

• Erich arch bar maxillomandibular fixation (MMF): the best and most common way to obtain MMF. A 24-gauge wire is passed around the neck of each tooth using a wire twister. The wire is then twisted down over the arch bar with the lugs facing up in the maxilla and down in the mandible. The lugs can then be used to place interarch elastics or a box-type wire (Fig. 5.6). This procedure can be performed with local anesthesia/IV sedation or general anesthesia.

Dental and dentoalveolar trauma

Traumatic injuries to the teeth and supporting structures are a common ED [A & E] emergency (affecting some 5% of all school age children). A brief but comprehensive assessment of the overall

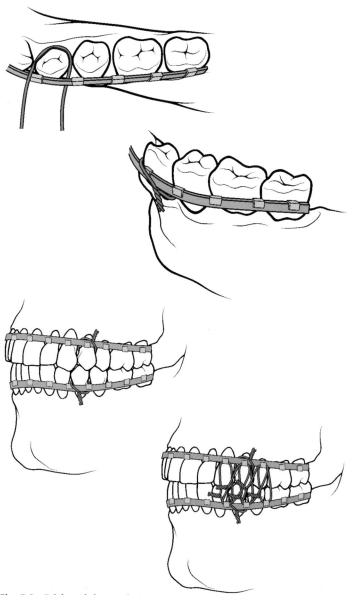

Fig. 5.6 Erich arch bar technique.

patient should be made to rule out other less obvious concomitant injuries. Intracranial, cervical or facial bone injuries often accompany dental trauma and can be overlooked. Although dental trauma is not the first priority for multiply injured patients, successful management of many dental injuries requires proper diagnosis and treatment within a limited period of time.

History and physical examination

A good history is important to determine the nature and time of the injury, the likely dental injuries from that type of trauma, other possible secondary injuries and any pre-existing dental problems (e.g. malocclusion, previous dental trauma). The physical examination should include a rapid, but adequate, general examination as well as detailed head and neck and oral examinations:

- View with suspicion any alteration in dental occlusion from the patient's stated normal as evidence of displaced teeth, dento-alveolar fracture or facial bone fractures.
- Account for all the teeth. Teeth unaccounted for at the scene or on examination should be considered to have been aspirated, swallowed or displaced into the soft tissues or sinuses. Appropriate radiographs (soft tissue neck, PA and lateral skull, chest X-ray and/or flat plate of the abdomen) should be ordered to localize the fragments. Perform a thorough search for any foreign bodies, teeth fragments or debris in the soft tissues of the lips or floor of the mouth. This is a particularly common finding and is associated with a high incidence of infection.
- Perform a careful examination to determine which teeth are traumatized, the presence of mobility, the direction and magnitude of any displacement, presence of crown or root fractures, evidence of pulpal involvement such as bleeding of pulpal tissue and empty sockets. The color of the involved teeth and initial percussion sensitivity should be noted. Pulp testing is of limited value in acute injuries. Differentiate between tooth displacement or fracture and dentoalveolar trauma, where the alveolus itself is also fractured. Grasp the involved ridge between the thumb and forefinger of one hand while grasping an adjacent, unaffected area with the other hand to check relative mobility. There may be mobility of the entire alveolus with teeth intact, one alveolar plate with teeth intact, one or both cortical plates with teeth also mobile within the segment, or just tooth mobility with intact

cortical plates. Examine thoroughly for any mandibular or maxillary fractures.

Radiographic examination

Should include a panoramic radiograph and periapicals of the involved teeth, if possible. In small children, or uncooperative adults, occlusal X-rays are often easier to obtain and are clinically useful. When dental fractures are suspected, a second film from another angle is often useful in diagnosis. When fragments are suspected to be lodged in the lip or floor of the mouth, a soft tissue film (exposure time with KVP turned down to $^1/_4$ normal) might demonstrate the foreign bodies. For dentoalveolar trauma, examine the radiographs for:

- root fractures
- degree of extrusion or intrusion
- pre-existing periodontal disease
- degree of root development
- dimension and location of pulp chamber and root canals
- alveolar or jaw fractures
- foreign bodies (e.g. tooth fragments) lodged in soft tissues.

Classification and treatment (Fig. 5.7)

Crown infraction, craze line or crack

- Does not involve loss of tooth structure.
- No treatment usually necessary.
- Due to propensity for future fracture, should have continued follow-up.

Uncomplicated crown fracture

- Involves enamel or enamel and dentin only.
- Treatment: ○ Account for missing segment (radiograph of soft tissue may be necessary) ○ Smooth off sharp edges.
- Place temporary glass-ionomer cement/compomer bandage or permanent restoration, depending on depth.
- Follow-up important to monitor pulp and periodontal health.
- The tooth should be pumiced, cleaned, dried and etched. The area should be coated and/or built up with a protective restoration such as unfilled resin. Alternatively, reattach the tooth fragment (if available) using composite resin and dentin bonding agents.

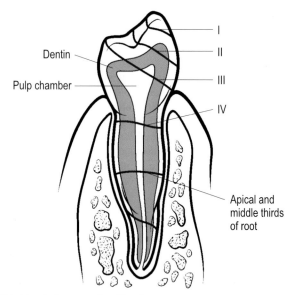

Fig. 5.7   **Tooth fracture classification.**

Complicated crown fracture
- Involves enamel, dentin and pulp.
- Direct pulp cap: calcium hydroxide ($CaOH_2$) is placed on exposed pulp tissue if injury is within 24 h and a very small exposure.
- Careful follow-up of pulp vitality and periodontal health.

Complicated crown–root fracture
- Involves enamel, dentin and pulp.
- If perforation of pulp is < 1 mm and less than a few hours old, $CaOH_2$ can be placed over the exposure and a restoration placed as for a class II fracture.
- If pulpal exposure is larger than 1 mm or more than 24 h old, pulpectomy followed eventually by conventional endodontics.
- With large exposure and open apex, make access to the vital pulp. Amputate 2 mm of pulp and surrounding dentin in teeth fractured from 1 h to 90 days. More amputation might be necessary in the case of a partially necrotic pulp. Direct pressure should be applied to obtain hemostasis and $CaOH_2$ should be applied directly to the

pulp stump. A composite 'sling' is placed over the $CaOH_2$. Copious irrigation should be used. Pulpotomy or pulpectomy of primary teeth can be performed with 5-min application of formocresol for a pulpotomy technique or filling of the root canals, after pulpectomy, with a resorbable paste.

- For primary anterior teeth with a fracture extending into the pulp, a pulpectomy with zinc oxide eugenol is indicated if cooperation is good and provided that there is not significant root resorption, or an extraction if not.

Root fracture

- Fracture apical to the cemento-enamel junction (CEJ) that involves dentin, cementum and pulp.
- If a permanent tooth is injured at or coronal to the crestal bone (e.g. the cervical $1/3$), the coronal portion should be removed and endodontics begun. The endodontic procedure is completed, the restoration is made with a post and core. The root is extruded orthodontically and the crown is fabricated. Alternatively, periodontal surgery may be used for the crown lengthening.
- If the fracture is in the middle $1/3$ of the root, the coronal fragment should be repositioned, if displaced and splinted for 1 month to the adjacent teeth. This allows healing by the formation of calcified tissue, bone, connective tissue or granulation tissue. Pulpectomy and conventional endodontic therapy should be begun within 7–10 days if evidence of pulpal pathology is apparent. Endodontic therapy can be done on the coronal portion only if there is no evidence of periapical pathology. If the fragments are widely displaced or tooth is persistently mobile, extraction should be considered.
- If the fracture is in the apical $1/3$ of the tooth or root, the fragments should be left alone and observed carefully for development of periapical pathology or signs of pulpal necrosis. If the coronal portion is mobile it may need to be removed for patient comfort.
- Fractures of the root in deciduous teeth, with the exception of those in the apical $1/3$, which require only observation, are an indication for extraction. Care must be taken to avoid damage to the developing permanent tooth bud. Small pieces of root can be left behind if their removal would jeopardize the permanent tooth. These injuries should be followed radiographically to confirm resorption of the fragment and eruption of the permanent tooth.

Subluxation

The tooth is in the socket but shows greater than physiologic mobility after trauma.

- If mobility is mild, a soft diet and occlusal adjustment to take the tooth out of occlusion are often sufficient.
- If mobility is moderate to severe, splint to adjacent teeth (one tooth on either side) with non-rigid material (acid-etched composite and thin orthodontic wire or fishing line) for 7–10 days.
- Obtain baseline radiograph, with repeat radiographs at 1, 2, 6 and 12 months post-trauma.
- Perform $CaOH_2$ pulpectomy if external/internal resorption or periapical pathology develops.
- Observe primary teeth with slight mobility radiographically. If the tooth becomes non-vital, treat with pulpectomy or extraction. For moderate to severe mobility, primary teeth should be extracted.

Intrusion

Tooth is pushed further into the socket following trauma. This means that the tooth may have perforated the buccal or palatal plates, or has perforated the floor of the nose or sinus.

- Observe the tooth for re-eruption, but if this does not occur spontaneously, apply gentle orthodontic traction at the rate of approximately 0.3–1.0 mm per week. Surgical repositioning and splinting may be indicated if there is interference with occlusion.
- With moderate intrusion of tooth with open apices, endodontic therapy may be delayed until loss of vitality is suspected. For fully formed roots, start $CaOH_2$ pulpectomy within 7–10 days of injury and fill permanently with gutta percha after 6–12 months if resorption is arrested or non-existent.
- Allow primary teeth that are minimally displaced and that do not appear to be involving the permanent tooth to re-erupt spontaneously. Extract the tooth if gingival infection, ankylosis or permanent tooth bud impingement is suspected.

Partial extrusion

The tooth is partially avulsed or otherwise displaced in the socket.

- Digitally manipulate the permanent tooth back into the socket as soon as possible. Place one finger over the apical region to help prevent lateral perforation. Then splint with a non-rigid material such as monofilament nylon or 28-gauge wire to the adjacent teeth to prevent ankylosis.

- Due to the high probability of pulpal necrosis, perform careful clinical and radiographic evaluation frequently or begin endodontics soon after the injury (7–10 days).
- Extract primary teeth to prevent damage to the permanent tooth and interference with the occlusion.

Avulsion

The tooth has been totally displaced out of the socket. This is a true dental emergency because the treatment and prognosis are extremely time dependent. The success of reimplantation is inversely related to the storage material and the time the tooth is out of the mouth. Teeth reimplanted within 30 min have a good chance of surviving, whereas those reimplanted after 2 or more hours have a more limited survival. The goals of reimplanting teeth are to maintain the viability of periodontal ligament cells and impede resorption of the tooth. Milk, or contact lens solution in an emergency, are satisfactory storage media if the tooth cannot be stored in the patient's buccal sulcus.

- If dirty, the tooth should be grasped by the crown and rinsed gently in saline, tap water or milk at the scene of the injury. Do not scrub off, brush the tooth or handle the root.
- Immediately place the tooth back in the socket and hold in place with light pressure en route to the treating facility. There is no need to physically debride the socket prior to replacement. Gentle saline irrigation will remove debris.
- If the tooth cannot be replaced at the scene, it should be stored in the buccal vestibule or floor of the mouth for transport. If this is not possible, the tooth should be stored in a cup with the Hanks Balanced Salt Solution (HBSS), the patient's saliva, milk, saline or water. Do not wrap tooth in tissue, towel or foil or allowed to dry out.
- Once the tooth is reimplanted in a gently saline-irrigated socket, splint it to the adjacent teeth with a non-rigid or semi-rigid splint for 7–10 days. If a concomitant alveolar fracture is present, maintain the splint for 2–8 weeks. Longer splinting periods are required for more extensive fractures.
- In a permanent tooth with an open apex that has been replanted 2 h after avulsion, radiographs and clinical exam should be

performed in 3–4 weeks to look for evidence of pulpal pathology versus revitalization. If pathosis is noted, root canal therapy should be instituted immediately. The canal should be cleaned and filled with $CaOH_2$ until apexification has occurred (usually 6–24 months). Then obturation with gutta percha is indicated.

- For a permanent tooth with a partially to completely closed apex and less than 2 h dry time, the pulp should be removed in 7–14 days. The canal is cleaned and $CaOH_2$ is placed. The new American Association of Endodontics guidelines recommend only 7–14 days of $CaOH_2$ treatment and immediate obturation of the canal with gutta percha and sealer. These new recommendations to obturate a tooth so quickly after trauma are controversial.
- For permanent teeth with partially to completely closed apices and greater than 2 h extraoral time, root canal therapy can be performed immediately. These teeth will eventually be lost to resorption but may be retained short term and are likely to ankylose. The tooth, once the canal has been extirpated extra-orally can be soaked in sodium fluoride solution to discourage resorption once reimplanted.
- Do not replant primary teeth.
- Consider tetanus prophylaxis and antibiotics (penicillin VK 500 mg QID, clindamycin 150–300 mg QID or erythromycin 250 mg QID) for 7–10 days and place the patient on a soft diet.

Mandibular trauma (Fig. 5.8)

Condylar (intracapsular)

Fractures that occur high on the condylar head (< 8–10 mm from the articular surface). Usually caused by injuries to the symphyseal region (especially bilateral condylar fractures) or contralateral body region. Because the condylar head is a growth site of the mandible, the primary concern for this fracture is eventual ankylosis, especially in children. Treatment is usually confined to careful observation and maintenance of mandibular function to prevent ankylosis.

Subcondylar or condylar (extracapsular)

Fractures that occur below the attachment of the TMJ capsule. The etiology is the same as for intracapsular fractures. Treatment is dependent on the degree of displacement and dysfunction. If the occlusion is normal and there is no deviation upon opening, obser-

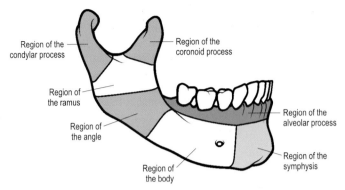

Fig. 5.8 **Regions of mandibular trauma.**

vation is adequate. If dysfunction is moderate, use Ivy loops with guiding elastics for 2 weeks. Open reduction is indicated if there is a foreign body in the joint, displacement laterally or into the middle cranial fossa, or if bilateral and associated with comminuted midfacial fractures.

Coronoid

Fractures of the coronoid process are rare. They are caused by a direct blow to the area when the mouth is in the open position which brings the coronoid below the zygomatic arch. Treatment is usually unnecessary except for associated fractures.

Ramus

Fractures below the condylar neck but above the angle region. The etiology is usually a direct blow to the ramus (often seen with bullet wounds). They may be simple, but are often comminuted. Simple horizontal fractures require only short-term IMF. Displaced fractures require open reduction.

Angle and body

Fractures of the angle region (e.g. distal to the second molar but below the ascending ramus) are very common. They are usually caused by direct injury. Treatment is usually open reduction and fixation with miniplates but the use of IMF versus miniplates varies in different clinical settings and in different geographic locations.

Parasymphysis

The area between the mandibular canines (the symphysis is the midline between the central incisors). Caused by direct injury. Treatment is complicated by muscle effects and, therefore, displaced fractures require either open reduction or closed reduction with a lingual splint to prevent splaying of the inferior border when IMF is applied. Non-displaced and non-mobile fractures can be managed with IMF alone for 4–6 weeks.

Midface trauma

Although isolated midfacial and LeFort injuries do occur, it is common to see multiple fractures that may involve several levels (Fig. 5.9).

LeFort 1

The entire alveolar process of the maxilla up to the floor of the nose, extending from the anterior nasal spine to the pterygoid plates, is fractured in a horizontal manner. If minimal or non-mobile, IMF may suffice as treatment. If mobile, open reduction or suspension wiring in addition to IMF is warranted.

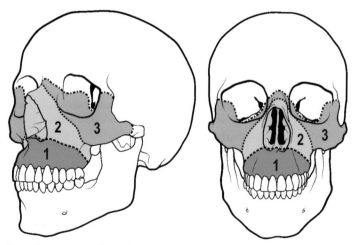

Fig. 5.9 LeFort midface fractures.

LeFort 2

Also called a 'pyramidal fracture' because of its triangular shape, this fracture crosses the maxilla obliquely from the pterygoid plates to the frontonasal area bilaterally. Thus, the maxilla moves at the level of the nasal bridge and infraorbital regions (zygomatico-maxillary suture). If displaced, treatment is open reduction.

LeFort 3

Also called 'craniofacial dysjunction' because of the separation of the midfacial bones from the skull. Begins at the pterygoid plates and involves the lateral orbital rim (frontozygomatic suture), zygomatic arch (zygomatico-maxillary suture), the orbital floor and the frontonasal areas bilaterally. Thus, the entire face will move under the skull at the level of the orbits. Treatment requires open reduction.

Zygomatic arch

Often fractures from a direct blow. Fractures usually occur at the junction of the temporal process of the zygoma and the zygomatic process of the temporal bone. This can create the classic 'W' fracture. Fracture of the zygoma proper will also involve this region but is usually linear and does not produce the 'W'. Treatment usually involves popping the infractured arch out with a long flat instrument via an intraoral or extraoral hairline (Gillie's) incision.

Zygoma

Also called a 'tripod' fracture because of its three clinically evident suture fracture lines (fronto-zygomatic, temporozygomatic and zygomatico-maxillary). Results from a direct blow. The clinical findings are of great importance and include:

- periorbital edema and ecchymosis
- subconjunctival hemorrhage and ecchymosis
- occasional entrapment of muscles with subsequent restriction of movement and diplopia
- occasional displacement of Whitnall's tubercle and the lateral canthus. Treatment begins with an ophthalmologic examination and, if displaced, usually requires open reduction.

Soft tissue wounds

Oral and facial lacerations are a common presentation in the emergency department. Diagnosis and management are usually simple and uncomplicated, but patience and care are needed to ensure good functional and cosmetic results and avoid or minimize damage to vital structures.

Assessment

Because lacerations indicate some form of traumatic injury, perform a complete evaluation with special emphasis on neurologic or cervical damage. Following this, evaluate for the following:

- Magnitude of the laceration: with or without anesthesia, gently probe the wound. Extensive or complicated wounds may often be better managed in an operating room [theatre] if the tissue damage is great, if extensive debridement is needed or if the patient is not, or cannot be, cooperative.

- Appearance of the wound: irrigate and clean dirty or contaminated wounds thoroughly prior to closure. Particulate matter may require gentle scrubbing for removal. Crushed or non-vital edges should be 'freshened' by sharply excising a small amount of tissue from the margins.

- Time sequence: increased time since the injury may increase complications. Unlike lacerations of other areas of the body, the excellent blood supply of the face and oral cavity allows primary closure many hours after injury. In such cases, conservative debridement of the wound margins can often produce a more cosmetic result. In addition, high-velocity wounds (such as a shotgun injury) often undergo delayed tissue necrosis. It is sometimes wise to clean and debride the wound initially and close it a few days later when the extent of tissue necrosis can be better assessed. If closure must be delayed, the wound should be grossly debrided, irrigated and dressed with saline-soaked sponges.

- Damage to vital structures: examine for cranial nerve injury (especially branches of the facial nerve). If the ends of the nerve can be located but not primarily repaired, gently tag with a non-resorbable suture for later identification and grafting. Parotid duct injuries may be seen by direct visualization or by injecting 1 cc of $^1/_2$-strength methylene blue through a 20-gauge catheter passed into Stenson's duct. Dye-filling the wound indicates ductal injury and requires correction and stenting. Tamponade large bleeding vessels until they can be isolated and ligated under proper and optimal conditions (never probe a bleeding wound

with a hemostat searching for a bleeder – you will just as likely grab an adjacent vital structure).
- Cosmetic considerations: carefully evaluate large, jagged wounds that cross flexion creases or traverse critical anatomy (such as the vermillion border or eyelid).

Treatment

Closure may require alteration of the wound (e.g. Z-plasty) and, if extensive, may be better performed in the operating room [theatre] under general anesthesia.

Anesthesia

If local anesthesia is to be used, this should be undertaken first with an anesthetic that is lasting and profound to accomplish good cosmetic and functional results. Lidocaine 2% with 1:100 000 [1:80 000] epinephrine is usually an excellent choice with the exception of the tip of the nose and the pinna of the ear, where caution must be exercised not to cause tissue necrosis secondary to the vasoconstrictor. A sterile dental syringe or a standard 3–5 cc Luer lock and 25-gauge needle can be used to obtain a block injection, infiltration or ring injection. Infiltrations may be performed either by injecting through the skin parallel and adjacent to the wound, or directly into the wound margins. It is usually best to insert the needle and then inject on the way out.

Preparation

When adequate anesthesia has been achieved, remove any obvious, large foreign bodies (e.g. big pieces of glass). Irrigate with large volumes of saline, lactated Ringer's or an antibiotic solution (but not sterile water because of its hypotonicity). The choice of solution is not as important as the volume (250 cc to 1 L, depending on the site of the wound) and the pressure used. Use a 50-cc syringe and an IV catheter (without the needle) placed directly into the wound. A pressure irrigator or water-jet lavage is particularly useful for grossly contaminated wounds. Next, clean the wounds with a surgical soap and irrigate again. Paint the wound with povidone–iodine for an area around the margins of at least 5 cm. Place sterile towels (four, placed in a square fashion or a round hole cut into a disposable paper towel drape) to isolate the wound within the prepped area.

Hemostasis

The initial management for all heavy bleeding should be pressure with sterile gauze until the wound can be examined carefully under sterile, well-lit, well-equipped (e.g. suction available) conditions. Injudicious attempts at clamping vessels prior to this often leads to inadvertent damage to adjacent important structures. Large venous or arterial bleeders may be clamped with a mosquito hemostat and ligated (e.g. 4-0 chromic suture) or electrocoagulated. Intermittent packing of the wound for 5 min with moist gauze will help control profuse bleeding.

Debridement

Examine the wound carefully for any remaining dirt or foreign bodies. Excise any devitalized or necrotic soft or hard tissue. Remember, however, that the excellent blood supply of the face mandates that debridement be conservative. Remove only tissue that is obviously ischemic or necrotic. Also at this time, probe the wound to determine the extent of the injury and look for any unexpected findings such as:

- fractures of the underlying bones
- parotid or submandibular duct transection
- nerve injuries
- cartilage involvement in the ear and nose
- tissue avulsion
- injuries to the canalicular or nasolacrimal system, globe, medial or lateral canthal ligaments, or lacerations that penetrate the tarsal plate of the eyelid.

Abrasions and injuries resulting from being dragged along the ground require special treatment. After thorough examination for embedded foreign bodies, carefully scrub the wound using a soft brush (an operating room scrub brush/sponge works well) and a mild surgical soap solution. Remove all particles from the wound, regardless of size, to obtain good, long-term, cosmetic results.

Primary repair of lacerations

Choice of suture material. There are two basic types of suture material – resorbable and non-resorbable. Resorbable sutures are used for closure of all tissues below the skin, for ligating small vessels and for mucosal closure. Non-resorbable sutures are used for skin closure, for mucosal closure and for ligating larger vessels.

Sutures can also be monofilament or multifilament. Monofilamentous sutures are not generally as strong as multifilamentous but are less likely to convert contamination to infection by tracking bacteria into the wound (see Chapter 8). The choice of suture is based on:
- location of laceration
- desired time for tensile strength
- ability and availability of suture removal.

The choice of suture needle. Four aspects of the suture needle that influence selection.
- Shape: three-eighths circle is the most popular. A half circle is easier to use in confined locations.
- Size: diameter should match the suture size.
- Point: cutting or reverse-cutting (the most popular), which are triangular in cross-section, are used in tough tissue (skin and mucosa). Taper-point needles are used in easily penetrated tissue.
- Method of attachment: swagged needles are the most common in use but controlled-release (or pop-off) needles can be used for single stitches when easy removal of the needle from the operating environment is desired.

Choice of suture technique.
- Simple deep suture: used to close deep layers below the skin or mucosa. This is a simple, interrupted, resorbable suture such as Vicryl, Dexon or gut (Fig. 5.10).
- Inverted simple suture: placed so that the knot is deep to the loop of the suture. It is used to close the subcutaneous tissues so that the knot does not protrude through the wound. This closure is carried out just prior to skin or mucosal closure and is of great importance in obtaining a cosmetic closure (Fig. 5.11).
- Running subcuticular suture: a continuous suture placed in a horizontal fashion just below the epidermis. The ends are carried through the skin just beyond the extent of the wound and either taped down or tied to themselves. This can he used as the final closure if skin sutures are not desired (Fig. 5.12).
- Simple interrupted skin suture: used to close the skin or mucosa. Has the advantage that if an infection ensues, one or two sutures can be removed to allow placement of a drain without dehiscing the entire wound (Fig. 5.13).
- Vertical mattress suture: placed so that there is a deep loop and a superficial loop that everts the skin edge. Most useful when

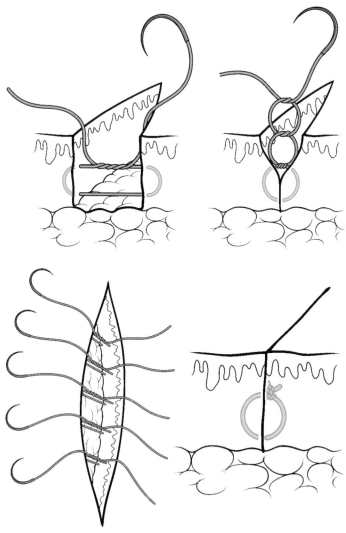

Fig. 5.10 Simple, deep suture.

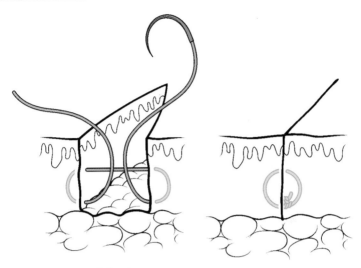

Fig. 5.11 **Inverted simple suture.**

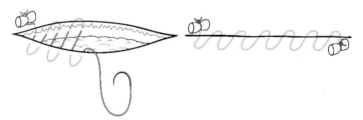

Fig. 5.12 **Running subcuticular suture.**

eversion of skin edges is mandated or for single layer closure of large amounts of tissue (e.g. scalp lacerations) (Fig. 5.14).

- Running epithelial suture: a continuous skin suture used to obtain rapid final closure of the wound edges. Sometimes also called a 'baseball stitch', this technique works well on straight line wounds but is difficult with angled or curved wounds (Figure 5.15).

Standard closure technique for facial lacerations.

- Close deep layers (e.g. periosteum, deep fascia) with resorbable suture (e.g. 3-0 Vicryl, Dexon or chromic gut) using a simple deep

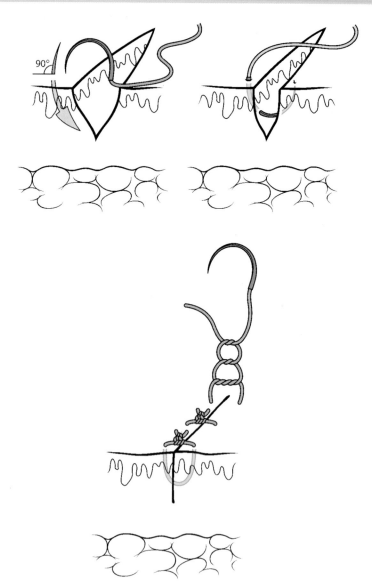

Fig. 5.13 Simple interrupted skin suture.

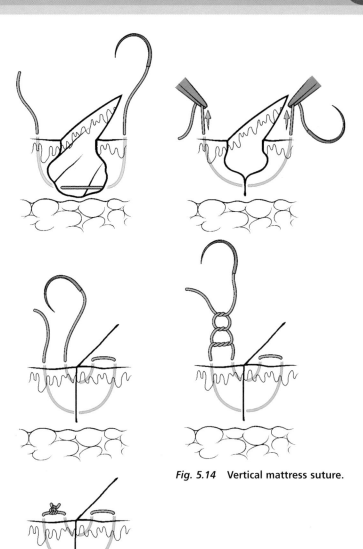

Fig. 5.14 Vertical mattress suture.

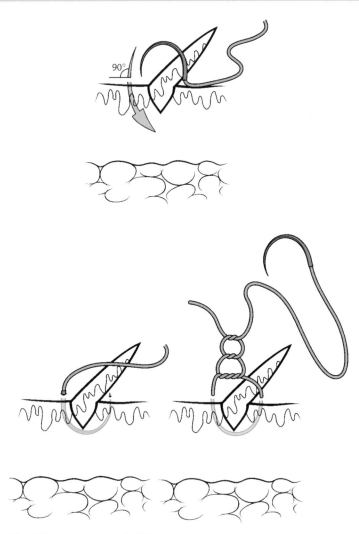

Fig. 5.15 Running epithelial suture.

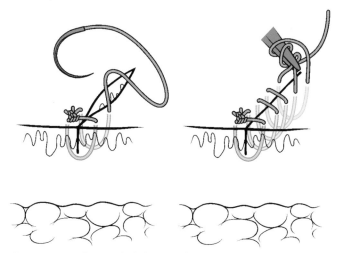

Fig. 5.15 **Running epithelial suture** (*continued*).

interrupted suture. Close muscle by suturing together the fascia layer enveloping the muscle. Eliminate all dead space in layers to prevent hematoma formation (Fig. 5.16).

- Close the subcutaneous layer with a resorbable suture as above but using an inverted simple suture. After tying the knot, pull the knot to one side to place it deep to the suture loop and thus out of the wound margin. The long-term strength of the closure is based on this layer of closure and it is, therefore, imperative to obtain excellent approximation of this layer. A suture that will retain its tensile strength for at least 21 days is also important.
- Close the skin at this point with a running subcuticular suture (e.g. 5-0 non-resorbable suture such as Prolene), a running skin suture (usually 5-0 or 6-0 nylon) or multiple simple interrupted or inverted mattress skin sutures (usually 5-0 or 6-0 nylon). This choice is based on personal preference, except for scalp lacerations, where a 4-0 nylon or Prolene inverted mattress suture is preferred because it will engage the galea layer of the scalp, thereby providing additional strength to the wound closure.

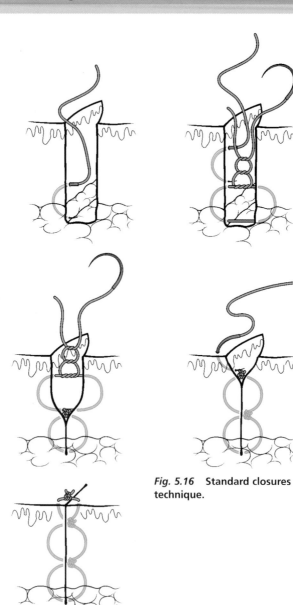

Fig. 5.16   Standard closures technique.

Standard mucosal closure technique.
- Close deeper layers (e.g. periosteum and deep fascia) with resorbable sutures as for the skin closure.
- There is usually no need for submucosal closure in the oral cavity.
- Close mucosa with either a non-resorbable suture (e.g. 3-0 or 4-0 silk or 5-0 nylon) or a resorbable suture (3-0 or 4-0 plain gut, chromic gut, Vicryl or Dexon).

Standard 'through and through' (mucosal–epidermal) closure.
- After initial irrigation as usual, close the intraoral mucosa in routine fashion. A watertight closure should be obtained, if possible.
- Then copiously irrigate the wound again from the extraoral side and prep in the standard sterile fashion for a skin closure.
- Close the deep layers and skin as for a normal skin closure.

Unusual circumstances.
- When closing around lacerated cartilage (e.g. nose or ears), close the tissue deep and superficial to the cartilage to approximate the cartilage, if possible. This is because of the lack of blood supply and therefore healing capacity of cartilage. If absolutely necessary, a few small tacking sutures may be placed in the cartilage to hold the shape of the anatomical area.
- Scalp wounds bleed profusely but will stop quickly once the galea is approximated. This can be done easily by using deep-bite vertical mattress sutures. Staples are very popular for scalp lacerations, especially for children.
- Avoid using electrocoagulation when suturing hair-borne areas (e.g. eyelid, scalp) because this will cause loss of hair follicles. Any incisions made to freshen the edges of the wound should be made very conservatively and along the long axis of the hair follicles (e.g. not necessarily perpendicular to the wound margin) to prevent loss of the follicle.
- Never shave around the eyebrows to better visualize a laceration. Eyebrows do not always grow back!
- Always approximate important anatomical structures first (e.g. eyebrow, commissure or vermillion border of lip). This should be done with tacking sutures even prior to subcutaneous closure to allow for proper alignment.
- Other than scalps and eyebrows, convert beveled wounds to perpendicular margins to avoid raised areas after healing.

- With jagged wounds it is usually better to convert the wounds to several linear portions by conservative excision.
- To obtain primary closure without tension, the wound may be undermined by piercing the deep subcutaneous tissue with a sharp scissor and then opening them as the instrument is withdrawn from the wound. Separation of these layers allows the skin to "slide" on the underlying tissues and aids in easy closure.

Postoperative care.
- Wound dressing: wipe the wound with a saline soaked gauze after final suturing to remove any residual blood, suture material, or iodine. Place a thin layer of an antibiotic ointment on the suture line and cover it with a non-sticky dressing (e.g. Telfa, Xeroform, Melolin). Intraoral wounds require no special dressing.
- Leave skin wounds alone for 48 h. Following this, they should be cleaned gently twice daily with warm water and soap or hydrogen peroxide to remove any crusted blood or other debris. It is important to remove dried blood and debris around the sutures. Follow this with another layer of antibiotic ointment. Rinse intraoral wounds with saline several times per day.
- Antibiotic coverage: as with all infections, the choice of antibiotic therapy should be guided by culture and sensitivity testing. Prophylactic coverage for dirty lacerations, however, may be initiated with the following:
  - Deep or dirty skin wounds: staphylococcal coverage is warranted and provided by either dicloxicillin (500 mg QID) or a cephalosporin (e.g. Keflex 500 mg QID) for 7 days.
  - Intraoral wounds: penicillin VK 500 mg QID or, if penicillin allergic, erythromycin 500 mg QID for 7 days. Older or infected wounds are often colonized by anaerobic organisms and are sometimes better treated by adding metronidazole 200–500 mg tds or QID to the penicillin or switching to clindamycin 150–300 mg QID.
- Tetanus prophylaxis: consider any patient with a laceration of traumatic origin for antitetanus therapy:
  - If clean wound and patient has had initial immunization as a child: give tetanus toxoid booster (0.5 cc IM) if no booster injection within last 10 years.
  - If contaminated or dirty wound and patient has been initially immunized: give tetanus toxoid booster if no booster injection within last 5 years.

○ If patient has not had initial immunization: give toxoid booster (should continue this at 1, 2 and 6 months for immunization) and give 250 U of tetanus immune globulin IM in opposite deltoid muscle.
- Suture removal:
  ○ Remove intraoral, non-resorbable sutures or resorbable sutures that are uncomfortable 5–9 days after placement.
  ○ Skin sutures: these should be removed at different times depending on the thickness of the tissue, type of closure and degree of tissue tension.

In general, nylon facial sutures are removed at 4–6 days. Nylon sutures in the eyelids, ears, nose or other thin tissue should be removed at 3–5 days. Running subcuticular sutures may be left an additional day or two without consequence.

TEMPOROMANDIBULAR JOINT (TMJ) EMERGENCIES

True TMJ emergencies are rare. The most common emergency is condylar trauma, which is covered on p. 242.

Acute condylar dislocation

History
- Sudden inability to close the mouth.
- Precipitating event is usually wide mouth opening, as during a yawn or trauma.
- Can be unilateral or bilateral.
- Often has history of chronic recurrence.
- May or may not be painful.

Examination and diagnosis
- Anterior open bite, which may be asymmetrical if unilateral.
- Panoramic or lateral oblique of mandible shows condyle(s) significantly anterior and superior to eminence.

Treatment
- Stand in front of the patient. Place thumbs bilaterally along external oblique ridges (Fig. 5.17).
- Gently, traction the mandible inferiorly first, then posterior-superiorly until condyle sits in condylar fossa.

(a)

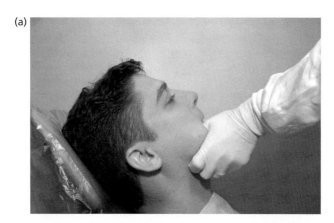

(b)

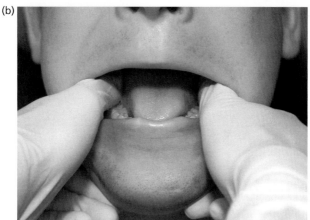

Fig. 5.17 (a) Stand in front of the patient, whose head is against the headrest; (b) place thumbs on the oblique ridges to avoid rapid closure of the teeth against the thumbs.

- If bilateral, do each side separately.
- If unable to reduce, consider injecting 1–2 cc lidocaine without vasoconstrictor near lateral pterygoid muscle to break spasm or premedicating the patient with 2–5 mg of diazepam before trying again.
- Limit function and wide opening of the jaw for 2 weeks.

Acute myofascial pain

History
- Acute but diffuse pain in muscles of face, neck and head.
- Limitation of mandibular motion.
- Difficulty eating.
- Often related to acute stress.

Diagnosis
- No radiographic evidence of joint pathology.
- Pattern of diffuse, non-localized pain
- Pain on masticatory muscle palpation.
- May see mandibular deviation on opening.

Treatment

Generally aimed at breaking muscle spasm, stress reduction and acute pain relief:
- anti-inflammatory agents (e.g. ibuprofen 600 mg QID)
- warm compresses to face 6–8 times per day
- soft non-chewy diet
- consider muscle relaxants (e.g. diazepam 5 mg BID)
- stress reduction
- consider 1–1.5 cc lidocaine without vasoconstrictor injected into trigger areas.

Traumatic hemarthrosis

History
- Recent trauma to mandible.
- Limitation of opening.
- Acute joint pain.
- Patient complains of 'bite' being off.

Diagnosis
- Acute open bite malocclusion on affected side.
- May have swelling in joint region.
- No radiographic evidence of fracture.
- May see increased articular space on radiograph.

Treatment

- Soft diet.
- Ice to the area for first 24 h, then warm compresses 6–8 times per day.
- Anti-inflammatory agents.
- Reassurance and observation for improvement.

Chapter 6

Medical emergencies

True medical emergencies are uncommon in the dental setting but require rapid and appropriate intervention when they arise. Fainting is by far the most common 'emergency' to occur in the setting of dental outpatients or in the dental office [surgery], followed by postural hypotension and hyperventilation. Less common, but of increased significance, are cardiovascular problems such as angina and acute myocardial infarction. Other important problems include grand mal (generalized tonic–clonic) seizures, hypoglycemia, asthma and overdose of local anesthetic.

Please refer to Appendices 10 and 11 at the end of this book for a list of items in a typical emergency kit and for a table of emergency medications.

RESPIRATORY DIFFICULTY

Foreign body

If the patient can speak, cough and breathe
- Do not interfere. Allow the patient to assume the position of maximum comfort.
- If the foreign object is not cleared by coughing, patient should be transported to emergency [accident and emergency] department for further management.

If the patient is unable to speak, cough and breathe (Table 6.1)
- If possible, medical assistance should be sought.
- Heimlich maneuver: five upward abdominal thrusts to the area just above the umbilicus. Repeat until foreign body is dislodged.
- If the patient loses consciousness: place patient supine, head tilted back, jaw lifted to open airway. Sweep oral cavity with

Table 6.1 Relief of foreign body airway obstruction

Adult (8 years of age and older)	Child (1 to 8 years of age)	Infant (less than 1 year of age)
1. Ask 'Are you choking? Can you speak?'	1. Ask 'Are you choking? Can you speak?'	1. Confirm airway obstruction. Check for serious breathing difficulty, ineffective cough, no strong cry.
2. Give abdominal thrusts/Heimlich maneuver or chest thrusts for pregnant or obese victims.	2. Give abdominal thrusts/Heimlich maneuver.	2. Give up to 5 back blows and 5 chest thrusts.
3. Repeat thrusts until effective or victims becomes unresponsive.	3. Repeat thrusts until effective or victim becomes unresponsive.	3. Repeat step 2 until effective or victim becomes unresponsive.
Victim becomes unresponsive	**Victim becomes unresponsive**	**Victim becomes unresponsive**
4. Activate the EMS system.	4. If second rescuer becomes available, have him or her activate the EMS system.	4. If second rescuer becomes available, have him or her activate the EMS system.
5. Perform a tongue–jaw lift followed by finger sweep to remove object.	5. Perform a tongue–jaw lift, and if you see the object, remove it.	5. Perform a tongue–jaw lift, and if you see the object, remove it.
6. Open airway and try to ventilate: if still obstructed, reposition head and try to ventilate again.	6. Open airway and try to ventilate: if still obstructed, reposition head and try to ventilate again.	6. Open airway and try to ventilate: if still obstructed, reposition head and try to ventilate again.
7. Give up to 5 abdominal thrusts.	7. Give up to 5 abdominal thrusts.	7. Give up to 5 back blows and 5 chest thrusts.
8. Repeat steps 5 through 7 until effective.*	8. Repeat steps 5 through 7 until effective.*	8. Repeat steps 5 through 7 until effective.*
	9. If airway obstruction is not relieved after about 1 minute, activate the EMS system.	9. If airway obstruction is not relieved after about 1 minute, activate the EMS system.

*If victim is breathing or resumes effective breathing, place in the recovery position.

During ventilation attempts, use appropriately sized mask or bag-mask as soon as available. Activate resuscitation team as soon as possible. Supplemental oxygen delivery equipment should be immediately available. Consider forceps, cricothyrotomy/transtracheal catheter ventilation (see ACLS text or PALS text).

From: Hazinski M F, Cummins R O, Field J M 2000 Handbook of emergency cardiovascular care for healthcare providers. Reproduced with permission.

© American Heart Association.

index finger to remove any foreign bodies. Seal mouth and nose, attempt mouth to mouth ventilation. If unable to ventilate, straddle the patient's thighs and repeat abdominal thrusts.
- Needle cricothyroidotomy, using a 14-gauge intravenous catheter/needle, may be considered if above measures are unsuccessful and the patient is not moving air.

Asthma

Medical history

Obtain a detailed medical history prior to treatment. Try to determine:
- Age of onset.
- Precipitating factors (recent respiratory infection, seasonal change, allergies, exercise, pollutants, anxiety).
- Frequency and severity: last attack and its duration. The need for the use of a nebulizer as opposed to normal aerosol inhalers (puffers), history of frequent hospitalization, frequent steroid use or intubation implies severe disease.
- Current medications and compliance.
- History of hypersensitivity to aspirin.

Signs and symptoms

- Shortness of breath, tachypnea (Fig. 6.1)
- Pressure on chest.
- Non-productive cough.
- Expiratory wheezes.
- Prolonged expiratory phase (expiration normally twice as long as inspiration).
- Increased respiratory effort (prominent neck muscles, nasal flaring, increased chest and abdominal movement). Usually sitting upright, leaning forward.
- Rapid pulse.
- Apprehension.
- Cyanosis (severe cases).

Prophylaxis

- Bronchodilator aerosol inhaler: the patient should bring the inhaler to the dental office [surgery] and have it accessible to staff. The patient might want to take a puff just before the procedure.
- Oral antiasthmatic medications: the patient should be instructed to take medication as usual, if on a daily dose.

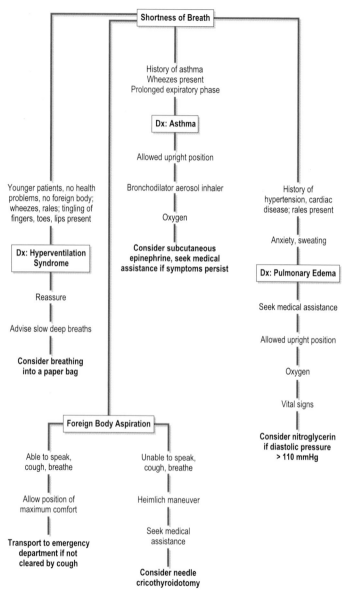

Fig. 6.1   Evaluation of shortness of breath.

Treatment
- Allow the patient to sit upright.
- Several deep breaths from bronchodilator inhaler (if available).
- Oxygen 6–8 L/min by nasal cannula or mask.
- Severe attack: administer epinephrine 1:1000 dilution, 0.3 cc subcutaneously for adults or 0.01 cc/kg subcutaneously for children. May be repeated in 15 min if no response. Transfer for immediate medical evaluation. May cause angina in adults with coronary artery disease.
- Continuation of severe attack:
  - start 0.9% (normal) saline IV
  - seek medical assistance
  - avoid all sedating medications
  - avoid aspirin products and NSAIDs.

CARDIAC AND VASCULAR EMERGENCIES (TABLE 6.2)

Angina pectoris

Signs and symptoms

Effort-related substernal pressure, or sensation of heaviness or weight that can radiate to the throat, jaw, right or left shoulder and/ or arm. Episodes last less than 15 min and can be accompanied by shortness of breath, nausea and sweating. Consistent pattern is easily identified by the patient. Usually responds to nitroglycerin (Fig. 6.2).

Prophylaxis
- History of angina, frequency of occurrence should be obtained.
- Take time to reassure patient and explain treatment.
- Pain control should be obtained.
- Patient should bring nitroglycerin medication to the dental office [surgery], and it should be placed where it will be readily accessible to the staff.
- Pretreatment: one tablet nitroglycerin sublingual.
- Stressful procedures: patient should be scheduled early in the day and oral tranquilizers or other sedation (e.g. nitrous oxide) should be considered.

Table 6.2   **Medical emergencies**

Emergency	Incidence	Stress related	Life threatening	Drug related	Significant medical history
Acute adrenal insufficiency	Rare	+	+	Previous	++
Allergy (rash)	Common	–	–	+	+
Allergy (anaphylaxis)	Rare	–	++	+	+
Angina	Rare	+	Usually not	–	++
Asthma	Unusual	+	+	+	+
Cerebral vascular accident	Rare	+	+	–	+
Drug overdose	Rare	–	+	+	+
Hyperventilation	Common	++	–	–	+
Hypoglycemia	Rare	–	+	+	++
Hypotension (orthostatic)	Common	–	Usually not	+	++
Myocardial infarction	Rare	+	++	–	+
Obstruction of airway	Unusual		++	+	–
Syncope	Common	++	–	–	+
Seizures (epilepsy)	Common	–	+	–	+

Treatment

- Nitroglycerin 0.4 mg sublingual. Tablets should be stored in brown glass bottle. Alternatively, a spray could be used. Check expiration date to assure potency.
- Oxygen 6–8 L/min by nasal cannula or mask.
- Record vital signs.
- If first dose is ineffective and systolic pressure is above 100 mmHg, nitroglycerin dose should be repeated every 5 min for a total of three doses.
- If the angina is new, or it departs from the usual pattern in a patient with chronic angina, the patient should be transported to an emergency facility.
- If angina continues, 0.9% saline IV should be started at minimal rate (KVO) and the patient transported to the emergency [accident and emergency] department. Give one aspirin tablet.

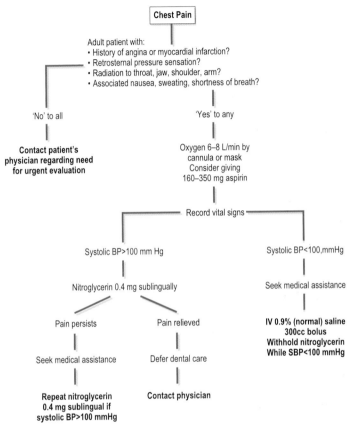

Fig. 6.2 Evaluation of chest pain.

Myocardial infarction

Signs and symptoms

Retrosternal, squeezing pressure or pain that can radiate to the throat, jaw, the right or left shoulder and/or arm. There is often a sense of weakness, impending doom and anxiety. There is often a history of angina. The pain is more severe than angina pain and lasts longer than 15 min. Not relieved by nitroglycerin. Associated signs and symptoms include sweating, nausea, vomiting, pallor and cyanosis.

Treatment
- The procedure should be stopped immediately.
- The emergency medical service should be called immediately.
- Oxygen should be administered, 6–8 L/min by nasal cannula or mask.
- Blood pressure should be monitored; if the systolic pressure is above 100 mmHg, nitroglycerin can be administered sublingually every 5 min until pain is relieved.
- A dose of 160–350 mg aspirin should be given to the non-aspirin allergic patient.
- 0.9% (normal) saline IV should be started at keep open rate.
- Patient should be maintained in the most comfortable position, even if not supine.
- Arrange transportation to the nearest emergency department, via ambulance with paramedics if possible.
- Morphine 3–4 mg IV every 5–10 min as needed for pain (under physician supervision) if no response to nitroglycerin.

Cardiac arrest

Signs and symptoms
Patient is cyanotic, unresponsive, without a carotid pulse and is not breathing.

Treatment
- Seek medical assistance.
- Check breathing first. If absent, give two slow breaths. Then check carotid pulse.
- If both absent, full cardiopulmonary resuscitation (CPR) should be administered in conjunction with use of an automated external defibrillator, if available:
  - Two slow deep breaths with patient's jaw thrust forward to open airway and nostrils pinched together, or via bag valve mask if available.
  - Closed chest massage: the sternal point is located two finger widths above the tip of the xiphoid process:
    - '1 and 2 and ... 15' chest compression count followed by two breaths, if only one rescuer is present.

- '1 one-thousand, 2 one-thousand ... 5 one-thousand' chest compression count followed by one breath if two rescuers are available.
- When medical assistance arrives, advanced cardiac life support (ACLS) procedures should be initiated and the patient transferred to an emergency [accident and emergency] department (Tables 6.3 and Figs 6.3, 6.4).
- Intravenous lines should be started only after cardiopulmonary resuscitation (CPR) is being adequately administered.

Pulmonary edema

Signs and symptoms

Precipitated by high blood pressure, myocardial infarction, arrhythmias or non-compliance with medications. Manifestations include anxiety, dyspnea, sweating, tachycardia and cyanosis. Lethargy is an ominous sign.

Treatment

- Medical assistance should be sought.
- The patient should be allowed to assume the position of maximum comfort.
- Oxygen 10 L/min by oxygen reservoir mask should be administered. Use simple mask or nasal cannula if reservoir mask is unavailable.
- Vital signs should be obtained. Give sublingual nitroglycerin if diastolic blood pressure is above 110 mmHg.

Cerebral vascular accident (stroke)

- Causes: ruptured blood vessel, blood clot or emboli occurring in the brain.
- Symptoms of onset: localized motor and sensory loss, headache, dizziness, vertigo, seizures, coma.

Treatment

- Oxygen.
- Maintenance of airway.
- Medical assistance.

Table 6.3 Basic Life Support for Healthcare Providers

CPR/rescue breathing	Summary of ABCD Maneuvers			
	Maneuver	Adult 8 years of age and older	Child 1 to 8 years of age	Infant Less than 1 year of age
Establish unresponsiveness Activate EMS system or appropriate resuscitation team.	Airway	Head-tilt–chin-lift (If trauma is present, use jaw thrust)	Head-lift–chin-lift (If trauma is present, use jaw thrust)	Head-tilt–chin-lift (If trauma is present, use jaw thrust)
A. Open airway (head-tilt–chin-lift or jaw thrust)	Breathing Initial	2 breaths at 2 sec/breath	2 breaths at 1 to 1½ sec/breath	2 breaths at 1 to 1½ sec/breath
B. Check for breathing (look, listen, and feel for no more than 10 seconds)	Subsequent	10 to 12 breaths/min (approximate)	20 breaths/min (approximate)	20 breaths/min (approximate)
• If victim is breathing or resumes effective breathing, place in the recovery position	Foreign-body airway obstruction	Heimlich maneuver	Heimlich maneuver	Back blows and chest thrusts
• If victim is not breathing, give 2 slow breaths using pocket mask or bag-mask. Allow for exhalation between breaths	Circulation Pulse check*	Carotid	Carotid	Brachial or femoral
C. Check for signs of circulation (breathing, coughing, movement), including pulse for no more than 10 seconds. (Carotid in child and adult; brachial or femoral in infant.)	Compression landmarks	Lower half of sternum	Lower half of sternum	1 finger's width below intermammary line
• If signs of circulation/pulse present but breathing is absent, provide rescue breathing (1 breath every 4 to 5 seconds for adult, 1 breath every 3 seconds for infant or child).	Compression method	Heel of one hand, other hand on top	Heel of one hand	2 or 3 fingers or 2 thumb–encircled hands

Table 6.3 Basic Life Support for Healthcare Providers (cont'd)

CPR/rescue breathing	Summary of ABCD Maneuvers		
• If signs of circulation/pulse absent, begin chest compressions interposed with breaths	Compression depth	1½ to 2 inches	1 to 1½ inches or approximately one-third to one-half the depth of chest	½ to 1 inch or approximately one-third to one-half the depth of chest
• If signs of circulation/pulse present but < 60 bpm in infant or child with poor perfusion, begin chest compressions.	Compression rate	Approximately 100/min	Approximately 100/mn	At least 100/min (newborn: 120/min)
Continue basic life support Integrate procedures appropriate for newborn resuscitation, pediatric advanced life support, or advanced cardiovascular life support at earliest opportunity.	Compression/ventilation ratio	15:2 (Single rescuer or two rescuers. Pause for ventilation with unprotected airway.) 5:1 with protected airway	5:1 (Pause for ventilation until trachea is intubated.)	5:1 (Pause for ventilation until trachea is intubated.) 3:1 for intubated newborn (2 rescuers)
D. Defibrillation Defibrillation using automated external defibrillators (AEDs) is now considered an integral part of adult basic life support by healthcare providers.	Defibrillation AED	Per local EMS protocol	Not yet recommended for use in infants and children.	

*Note: Pulse check if performed by healthcare providers but is not expected of lay rescuers. Lay rescuers are taught to check for *signs of circulation* (e.g. normal breathing, coughing, movement) in response to 2 rescue breaths given to the *unresponsive, non-breathing victim*.

From: Hazinski M F, Cummins R O, Field J M 2000 Handbook of emergency cardiovascular care for healthcare providers. Reproduced with permission.
© American Heart Association.

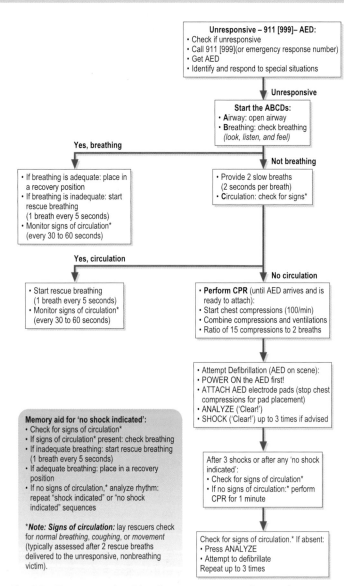

Unresponsive – 911 [999]– AED:
- Check if unresponsive
- Call 911 [999](or emergency response number)
- Get AED
- Identify and respond to special situations

Unresponsive

Start the ABCDs:
- **A**irway: open airway
- **B**reathing: check breathing
  (look, listen, and feel)

Yes, breathing

Not breathing

- If breathing is adequate: place in a recovery position
- If breathing is inadequate: start rescue breathing (1 breath every 5 seconds)
- Monitor signs of circulation* (every 30 to 60 seconds)

- Provide 2 slow breaths (2 seconds per breath)
- **C**irculation: check for signs*

Yes, circulation

No circulation

- Start rescue breathing (1 breath every 5 seconds)
- Monitor signs of circulation* (every 30 to 60 seconds)

- **Perform CPR** (until AED arrives and is ready to attach):
- Start chest compressions (100/min)
- Combine compressions and ventilations
- Ratio of 15 compressions to 2 breaths

- Attempt Defibrillation (AED on scene):
- POWER ON the AED first!
- ATTACH AED electrode pads (stop chest compressions for pad placement)
- ANALYZE ('Clear!')
- SHOCK ('Clear!') up to 3 times if advised

Memory aid for 'no shock indicated':
- Check for signs of circulation*
- If signs of circulation* present: check breathing
- If inadequate breathing: start rescue breathing (1 breath every 5 seconds)
- If adequate breathing: place in a recovery position
- If no signs of circulation,* analyze rhythm: repeat "shock indicated" or "no shock indicated" sequences

Note: Signs of circulation: lay rescuers check for *normal breathing, coughing,* or *movement* (typically assessed after 2 rescue breaths delivered to the unresponsive, nonbreathing victim).

After 3 shocks or after any 'no shock indicated':
- Check for signs of circulation*
- If no signs of circulation:* perform CPR for 1 minute

Check for signs of circulation.* If absent:
- Press ANALYZE
- Attempt to defibrillate
Repeat up to 3 times

Fig. 6.3 Treatment algorithm for emergency cardiovascular care.

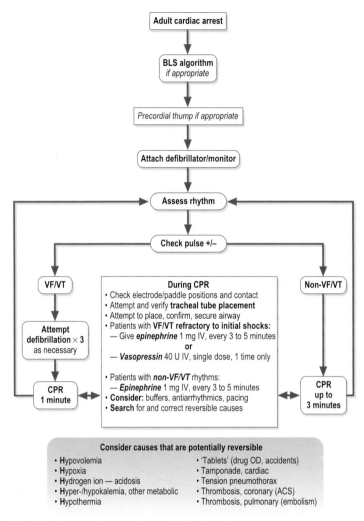

Fig. 6.4   **Universal/international ACLS algorithm.**

ALLERGIC REACTIONS

Immediate hypersensitivity

Signs and symptoms

The allergic reaction begins within minutes of the antigen exposure. Mast cells release several peptides, including histamine, leukotriene and PGD_2 (prostaglandin D_2). Smooth muscle contraction and vasodilation lead to any combination of laryngeal edema, laryngospasm, stridor, wheezing, itching, urticaria, anxiety, hypotension and cardiopulmonary arrest (see Table 6.3 for ACLS protocols).

Most reactions to local anesthetics are not true allergic reactions to the anesthetic itself but are due to inadvertent intravascular injection of solutions containing epinephrine, toxic levels or reactions to preservatives in the local anesthetic solution. A careful history may help prevent occurrence of allergic reactions.

Treatment

Systemic reaction (laryngospasm, stridor, wheezing, tachycardia, hypotension)

- The patient should be placed in supine position with legs elevated.
- Medical assistance should be sought.
- Airway should be maintained. Change in quality of voice or presence of stridor suggests presence of airway edema.
- Oxygen 6 L/min by nasal cannula or face mask should be administered.
- Blood pressure should be recorded.
- An IV should be started, 0.9% (normal) saline or Ringer's lactate if available, flow rate as needed to maintain systolic blood pressure above 90 mmHg.
- Medications: administer:
  - epinephrine 1:1000 dilution, 0.3 cc subcutaneously to adults or 0.01 cc/kg subcutaneously to children. Do not administer epinephrine intravenously except in cases of complete cardiopulmonary arrest.
  - hydrocortisone 200 mg IV to adults or 2.5 mg/kg IV to children.
  - diphenhydramine (Benadryl) 50 mg [chlorpheniramine maleate (Piriton) 10–20 mg] IV over 1 min for adults. Children: 0.5 mg/kg IV over 1 min.

- Be prepared to intubate or perform cricothyrotomy if unable to intubate due to airway edema.
- Be prepared to deliver cardiopulmonary resuscitation (CPR).
- Should be distinguished from vasovagal syncope, which typically produces bradycardia, hypotension and pallor (as opposed to the tachycardia, hypotension and erythema seen in anaphylaxis).

Cutaneous reaction
- Patient has urticaria or itching but no stridor or wheezing. Vital signs are normal.
- Watch for systemic involvement.
- Diphenhydramine 25–50 mg [chlorpheniramine maleate (Piriton) 4 mg] PO every 6 h as needed for adults.

Delayed hypersensitivity (cellular hypersensitivity)

Signs and symptoms

Reaction begins hours after antigen exposure, peaking in approximately 24–48 h.
- Induration and swelling (e.g. positive tuberculin test).
- Contact dermatitis.
- Graft rejection.

Treatment

For a mild systemic reaction, administer diphenhydramine 25–50 mg [chlorpheniramine maleate (Piriton) 4 mg] PO QID to adults; children should be given 0.25–0.50 mg/kg PO QID. Identify and avoid the offending allergen.

BLEEDING

Hemostasis can be altered by extrinsic factors (e.g. medications) or intrinsic abnormalities (e.g. liver disease, hemophilia or thrombocytopenia).

Patient evaluation

History
- Previous bleeding experience (frequency, severity, duration, apparent cause).

- Medications (anticoagulants, dipyridamole, aspirin).
- Presence of severe liver disease, leukemia, recent chemotherapy, hemophilia, thrombocytopenia, alcoholism.

Examination
Look for jaundice, ecchymoses, petechiae or hemarthrosis.

Laboratory tests
Consider deferral of elective surgical procedures or the need for preprocedure medical management in patients with the following:
- platelet count < 50 000
- partial thromboplastin time (APTT) > 2 times normal
- prothrombin time > 2 times normal or INR > 3.0.

Treatment of hemorrhage

Local management techniques
- Pressure to area with gauze for at least 5 min.
- Infiltration with 2% lidocaine with epinephrine (1:50 000 or 1:100 000 [1:80 000]).
- Ligation of vessel or tissue with suture, if brisk bleeding.
- Absorbable cellulose and/or suture to close socket.
- Ice pack to area extraorally (5 min on and 5 min off).
- Crush surrounding bone or pack with bone wax for alveolar bone hemorrhage.
- If bleeding persists, pressure should be applied with gauze soaked in topical thrombin or epsilon aminocaproic acid (EACA 25%, Amicar syrup or 5% tranexamic acid mouthwash).
- Microfibrillar collagen hemostat may be sprinkled on area and, after several minutes, gently flushed with water or used to plug extraction sockets. [Calcium alginate gauze can be applied with pressure to the site or used to plug sockets.]
- Electrocautery.
- Tranexamic acid mouthrinse (2 min QID for 2–7 days) has been suggested in the literature.
- Surgical stents or fibrin glue might be needed in rare cases.

Systemic management techniques
- Physician should be consulted for transfusion with packed red cells (typed and cross-matched) if hemorrhage is severe or for

transfusion of appropriate coagulation factors concentrate in patients with hemophilia, or platelets for thrombocytopenia and fresh frozen plasma in patients with coagulopathy that is primary or secondary to severe hepatic cirrhosis.

- Vitamin K will reverse warfarin effect within 6–10 h. Fresh frozen plasma (200–500 cc) will reverse warfarin effects immediately. Protamine sulfate 25–50 mg IV over 30 min will reverse heparin immediately. Simply turning off heparin will normalize coagulation over 3–4 h.
- Platelet transfusion of 1 unit per 10 kg body weight of random multidonor platelets or one donor apheresis unit in patients with abnormal bleeding and platelet count < 50 000.
- Desmopressin acetate (DDAVP) 0.3 microgram/kg IV or SC can help clotting in von Willebrand's disease, mild–moderate hemophilia A and bleeding due to uremic platelet dysfunction.
- Tranexamic acid (before surgery: 10 mg/kg IV or 25 mg/kg PO TID or QID the day before surgery; after surgery: 25 mg/kg PO TID or QID for 2–8 days) can reduce or prevent hemorrhage in hemophiliacs undergoing oral surgery.

Obtain vital signs and hematocrit if significant blood loss occurs. A medical consult is needed for patients with uncontrolled bleeding, abnormal vital signs or symptomatic acute blood loss, or for suspected abnormalities of APPT, INR, platelet count, bleeding time or hematocrit.

SYNCOPE

Etiology (Fig. 6.5)

Vasovagal syncope

Psychological stress (fear, pain, sight of blood, illness) leads to increased vagal stimulation, venous pooling and bradycardia. The result is decreased cerebral perfusion and loss of consciousness. This is the most common cause of syncope in the dental surgery. Fifty per cent of people have experienced syncope.

Signs and symptoms
- Pallor, flushed feeling, sweating, nausea, vomiting.
- Weakness.

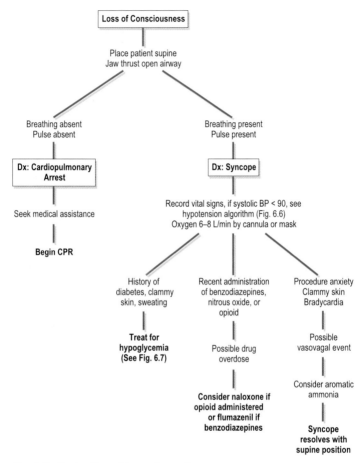

Fig. 6.5   Evaluation of loss of consciousness.

- Light-headedness.
- Dimming of vision.
- Bradycardia.
- Hypotension.
- Brief unconsciousness.

Treatment

- Check for adequate pulse and respirations.
- Patient should be placed in Trendelenburg position (supine with feet elevated and head low). Pregnant females should be placed on their left side.
- Loosen shirt collar to decrease carotid sinus stimulation.
- Oxygen at a flow of 6–8 L/min by mask or nasal cannula.
- Aromatic spirits of ammonia placed into the nostril for 5 sec should elicit a response in patients with vasovagal syncope.
- Blood pressure and pulse should be obtained: if blood pressure is < 90 mmHg systolic, patient should be treated as for shock.
- Syncope should resolve when patient assumes the supine position. Occasionally accompanied by brief (2–3 sec) tonic–clonic movements of the extremities.

Drug reaction

- Oversedation: benzodiazepines, nitrous oxide or opioids.
- Hypotension: antihypertensive drugs (alpha-blockers, beta-blockers, nitrates).

Postural hypotension

Seen in patients with dehydration, diabetes, cardiovascular disease or as a result of drug therapy. Frequently seen following dental care that has been delivered in a supine position but also common after sitting (even upright) for an extended period (Fig. 6.6). Onset just after assuming an upright position.

SHOCK

Definition

Shock is an inadequate blood flow to vital organs or a failure of vital organ cells to utilize oxygen.

Types (See Fig. 6.6)

- Hemorrhagic.
- Cardiogenic.

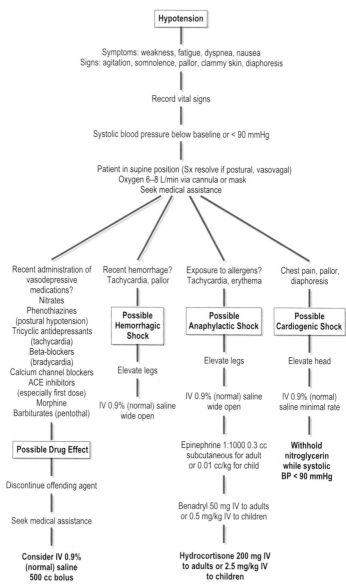

Fig. 6.6 Evaluation of hypotension.

- Septic.
- Anaphylactic.

Signs and symptoms

- Cold, clammy extremities.
- Delayed capillary refill (> 2 seconds at nail bed).
- Tachycardia and tachypnea.
- Hypotension.

Treatment

- Check for adequate pulse and respirations.
- Medical assistance should be sought.
- Patients with hemorrhagic, septic or anaphylactic shock should be placed in Trendelenburg position (supine with feet elevated and head low). Patients with cardiogenic shock should be supine with head elevated.
- Oxygen by mask at a flow of 6–8 L/min.
- An IV drip should be started with 0.9% saline wide open for hemorrhagic, septic or anaphylactic shock, but at sufficient rate to keep open for cardiogenic shock.
- Blood pressure should be obtained. If blood pressure is < 90 mmHg systolic, consider specific therapy:
  - allergic reaction
  - severe hemorrhage.

ADRENAL CORTICAL INSUFFICIENCY

Definition

Adrenal cortical insufficiency is caused by inadequate endogenous steroid production from the adrenal gland due to disease or decreased stimulation.

Recognition

Medical history
History of Addison's disease, pituitary or adrenal surgery, or steroid withdrawal.

Steroid medications

Commonly used in patients with autoimmune, arthritic, or asthmatic conditions and may suppress pituitary function when used chronically.

Signs and symptoms

Weak, tired, chronically nauseated, hyperpigmented skin, hypotensive, abdominal pain, fever and acidosis. In an acute insufficiency, decreased level of consciousness, hypotension or decreased perfusion may be noted.

Treatment

- Medical assistance should be sought.
- The patient should be placed in the Trendelenburg position (supine with feet elevated, head down).
- Vital signs should be monitored.
- Oxygen at 6–8 L/min by mask or nasal cannula.
- For acute insufficiency, hydrocortisone (200–300 mg IV) and intravenous saline wide open.

CONVULSIVE DISORDERS

Definitions

Grand mal

Generalized tonic–clonic. This is the most common type of seizure and is caused by transient alterations in brain function characterized by the abrupt onset of tonic–clonic movements.

Petit mal

Usually seen in children. Consists of 5–10-s lapses of consciousness, staring or blinking usually without movement. Multiple seizures/day.

Psychomotor

Consists of loss of contact with the environment for approximately 1–2 min. The patient tends to stagger, make unintelligible noises, is unable to understand what is said and suffers from amnesia.

Status epilepticus

Consists of repetitive seizures without recovery between episodes.

Cerebral damage, cardiac or renal failure and death can result. This is a medical emergency.

Causes

- Alcohol withdrawal.
- Fever (children aged between 3 months and 5 years).
- Hypoglycemia.
- Hyponatremia.
- Subtherapeutic anticonvulsant levels.
- Local anesthetic toxicity.

Signs and symptoms

- Increased anxiety or depression minutes to hours prior.
- Aura: feeling of impending seizure activity a few seconds prior to seizure onset (an unusual phenomenon).
- Convulsive or ictal phase: consisting of patient falling to floor, 'epileptic cry' as air is expressed, eye deviation, clonic–tonic contractions (high amplitude/frequency movements of all extremities for 3–7 min). Autonomic system discharge with dilated pupils, apnea and cyanosis, ending with respirations returning to normal, urinary and fecal incontinence.
- Postictal phase: patient disoriented and confused with gradual return to fully oriented state over a period of minutes to hours.
- Status epilepticus: continuous or repetitive seizure activity without interval of consciousness. Requires urgent therapy to prevent brain damage.

Treatment

Patient position

- Supine on covered floor, if possible.
- Careful observation of eye and extremity movements helpful for subsequent diagnostic evaluation.

Prevention of self-injury

- Removal of hard objects from area.
- Gentle restraint of extremities from gross movement.
- Soft head rest.

- Removal of dentures or partial dentures, if possible.
- Placement of soft item (e.g. handkerchief, cloth towel, large gauze pads) between teeth, unless already clenching. Do not try to force jaw open.
- Tight-fitting clothes should be loosened.
- Extension of neck or head tilted to side to maintain airway, and in the event of vomiting.
- Oxygen at 6–8 L/min may be administered if cyanotic.
- Vital signs should be monitored.
- When stable, known epileptic patients can be discharged from dental office [surgery] into the care of a responsible adult. For a first-time seizure, medical referral should occur.

Treatment for status epilepticus and seizures over 5 min in duration

- Position patient supine on floor, if possible.
- Airway maintenance.
- Monitoring of vital signs.
- Medical assistance should be sought.
- If possible, an IV drip should be started.

DRUG OVERDOSE AND TOXICITY (FIG. 6.7)

Asymptomatic patient

Lack of symptoms does not guarantee a harmless ingestion.

Treatment

- Consult product label or local poison control center for initial management of specific overdose.
- If ingestion occurred less than 30 min ago and if ipecac [ipecacuanha] is recommended, give 2 teaspoons PO to children 6 months to 1 year of age, 3 teaspoons PO to children over 1 year of age, and 6 teaspoons PO to adults. Follow with 1 glass of tepid water.
- Patient should be transported to the emergency [accident and emergency] department.

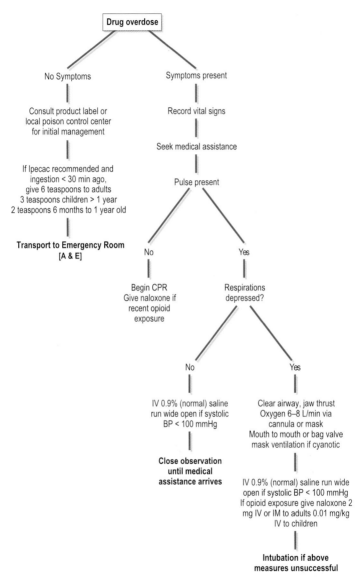

Fig. 6.7 Evaluation of drug overdose.

Symptomatic patient

- Medical assistance should be sought.
- Check for pulse and respirations: cardiopulmonary resuscitation (CPR) as needed (see Table 6.3 and Fig. 6.4).
- Respiratory support: if pulse is adequate but breathing is labored or depressed:
  - airway should be cleared: look for oral foreign body, perform jaw thrust
  - oxygen 6 L/min by nasal cannula or face mask
  - ventilation with mouth-to-mouth or bag valve mask if patient becomes pale or cyanotic. Insertion of nasopharyngeal airway and suction of excess secretions
  - intubation using cuffed endotracheal tube if above measures unsuccessful.
- IV 0.9% (normal) saline may be started at 50 cc/h for an adult. For systolic blood pressure < 80 mmHg, normal saline should be administered at a rate of 200 cc/h.
- Patient should be transferred for medical care, via ambulance if possible.

Opioid overdose

- Check for respirations and pulse: if both absent, full cardio-pulmonary resuscitation (CPR) should be administered:
  - Two slow deep breaths with patient's jaw thrust forward to open airway and nostrils pinched together, or via bag valve mask if available.
  - Closed chest massage: the sternal point is located two finger widths above the tip of the xiphoid process:
    - '1 and 2 and ... 15' chest compression count followed by two breaths if only one rescuer is present.
    - '1 one-thousand, 2 one-thousand ... 5 one-thousand' chest compression count followed by one breath if two rescuers are available.
- When medical assistance arrives, advanced cardiac life support (ACLS) procedures should be initiated and the patient transferred to the emergency [accident and emergency] department (see Table 6.3 and Figs 6.3 and 6.4).
- Intravenous lines should be started only after cardiopulmonary resuscitation (CPR) is being adequately administered.

- Naloxone (Narcan): 2 mg IV, IM or SC for adults or 0.01 mg/kg IV, IM or SC for children.

Benzodiazepine overdose

- Respiratory support: if pulse is adequate but breathing is labored or depressed:
  - airway should be cleared: look for oral foreign body, perform jaw thrust
  - oxygen 6 L/min by nasal cannula or face mask
  - ventilation with mouth-to-mouth or bag valve mask if patient becomes pale or cyanotic. Insertion of nasopharyngeal airway and suction of excess secretions
  - intubation using cuffed endotracheal tube if above measures unsuccessful.
- Monitor vital signs.
- Flumazenil [Anexate] 0.2 mg (2 cc) IV over 15 sec; repeat if needed four times – duration of action is shorter than that of some benzodiazepines and it may require repeat dosing at 20-min intervals.
  Note: Flumazenil can cause seizures in some groups of patients (chronic benzodiazepine dependent, mixed overdose, underlying seizure disorder). Use it only if supportive measures fail (i.e. assisted ventilation, stimulation) as a last resort before intubation.
- Medical assistance should be sought.

Sedative or barbiturate overdose

- Respiratory support: if pulse is adequate but breathing is labored or depressed:
  - airway should be cleared: look for oral foreign body, perform jaw thrust
  - oxygen 6 L/min by nasal cannula or face mask
  - ventilation with mouth-to-mouth or bag valve mask if patient becomes pale or cyanotic. Insertion of nasopharyngeal airway and suction of excess secretions
  - intubation using cuffed endotracheal tube if above measures unsuccessful.
- Monitor vital signs.
- Medical assistance should be sought.

- IV 0.9% (normal) saline at 200 cc/h if systolic blood pressure is < 80 mmHg.

Local anesthetic toxicity

Signs and symptoms

Early (cerebral cortical stimulation)
- Excitement, restlessness, apprehension.
- Increased blood pressure, rapid pulse, rapid respiration.
- Nausea, vomiting, convulsions.

Late (cerebral cortical and cardiovascular depression)
- Depressed blood pressure.
- Weak, rapid pulse or bradycardia.
- Respiratory depression, apnea, cardiac arrest.

Treatment

- Patient position: supine with legs elevated.
- Medical assistance should be sought.
- Oxygen 6–8 L/min by mask or nasal cannula.
- Respiratory support: if pulse is adequate but breathing is labored or depressed:
  - airway should be cleared: look for oral foreign body, perform jaw thrust
  - oxygen 6 L/min by nasal cannula or face mask
  - ventilation with mouth-to-mouth or bag valve mask if patient becomes pale or cyanotic. Insertion of nasopharyngeal airway and suction of excess secretions
  - intubation using cuffed endotracheal tube if above measures unsuccessful.
- An IV drip should be started.
- For convulsions, patient should not be restrained but help should be given to avoid self-injury.
- Avoid barbiturates which will enhance the second stage of depression.
- Be prepared to begin cardiopulmonary resuscitation (see Table 6.3 and Fig. 6.4).
- Monitor vital signs.

DIABETIC EMERGENCIES

Insulin (hypoglycemic) shock

History

Insufficient carbohydrate intake relative to normal or excessive insulin intake. Excessive exercise.

Onset

Sudden (minutes).

Signs and symptoms

- Disoriented behavior, mental confusion.
- Tremors.
- Pale, moist skin.
- Sweating.
- Bounding pulse.
- Convulsions and/or loss of consciousness (see Fig. 6.5).

Treatment

Conscious patient

Foods containing simple sugars (e.g. soda [fizzy drinks], candy [sweets], orange juice, sugar water).

Unconscious patient

The following guidelines are recommended:
- an IV drip should be started
- bolus of one ampule of 50% dextrose IV push should be administered
- monitoring of vital signs
- medical assistance should be summoned
- if cannot gain IV access 1 mg glucagon IM.

Diabetic (hyperglycemic) coma

History

Normal to excessive food intake with insufficient insulin. May be history of infection, non-compliance with insulin.

Onset
   Gradual (usually days).

Signs and symptoms
- Frequent urination.
- Intense thirst.
- Dry skin and mucous membranes.
- Vomiting, often with abdominal pain.
- Acetone odor to breath.
- Low blood pressure with weak, rapid pulse.
- Lethargy, weakness.

Treatment
- Medical assistance should be summoned.
- IV 0.9% (normal) saline 200 cc/hour.
- When in doubt, it is safer to assume insulin (hypoglycemic) shock than diabetic hyperglycemic coma.
- Usual dose of insulin may be administered if hypoglycemia is absolutely ruled out.
- Basic life support if unconscious (see Table 6.3 and Figs 6.3, 6.4).

Chapter 7

Maxillofacial prosthetics

A hospital dental service is quite often called upon by the ENT, radiation therapy, speech pathology, head and neck or plastic surgery services to serve a supporting role in the care of the patient who requires a maxillofacial prosthesis, or to help in determining the treatment options for patients with a variety of intraoral or extra-oral defects. These defects may be either congenital or acquired in their etiology. Similarly, the general dental resident might be called to assist an attending maxillofacial prosthodontist on the staff. As dentists with formal maxillofacial training are not available in most hospitals, the general dental attending and resident staff should be familiar with the more common maxillofacial prosthetic problems and prosthesis.

OBTURATOR PROSTHESIS – TYPES

Surgical obturator

- Sometimes referred to as an 'immediate obturator'.
- Serves as a temporary prosthesis that is usually inserted in the operating room [theatre] immediately following the surgical removal of a portion or all of the maxilla or surrounding osseous structures, including the alveolar bone.
- Functions to separate the oral and nasal cavities that would otherwise communicate with each other following surgery.
- Allows a patient to speak and swallow without the leakage of food and fluids from the mouth into the nasal cavity.
- Usually fabricated from polymethyl methacrylate (PMMA) with wrought wire clasps engaging the remaining teeth for retention.
- In edentulous situations, retention is gained by extension into the tissue undercuts created by the surgical resection.

- Tissue conditioning or reline material and denture adhesives are also useful in improving retention in edentulous resection situations.
- In situations where there is a severe lack of retention, the surgical obturator can be stabilized by transalveolar, piriform aperture, circumzygomatic or temporalis wiring to secure the prosthesis. A palatal screw can also be placed into the residual hard palate.
- Requires frequent modification as the surgical wound heals and changes in dimension.
- Not intended for use longer than 6 months. It is replaced by the interim obturator or, on a long-term basis, by a definitive obturator prosthesis.

Interim obturator

- Replaces the surgical obturator after the completion of initial healing following a maxillary resection, or if no further surgery is required.
- Function is similar to that of the surgical obturator. Separates the nasal and oral cavities, thereby improving a patient's ability to speak and swallow after surgery.
- May have a cast metal framework or be fabricated from PMMA with wrought wire clasps for retention.
- As the margins of the surgical defect become more stable, teeth may be added, although an interim obturator may also require frequent modification.
- Usually used no longer than 12 months and is replaced by a definitive obturator once the resection site has fully healed or no further surgery is anticipated.

Definitive obturator

- Often referred to simply as an 'obturator'. Its function is to separate the oral and nasal cavities to allow the patient to eat and drink without nasal regurgitation. Also reduces the hypernasality of speech following maxillary resection.
- Used to prosthetically rehabilitate all or part of a maxilla and the associated structures removed during surgical resection.
- Usually placed after 9–12 months, once healing is complete.
- Fabricated from a cast metal base (chromium–cobalt or titanium alloy) with cast clasps for retention. PMMA is processed to

obturate the defect and provide soft tissue support. Prosthetic teeth are added for esthetics and speech. Usually, there are light or no occlusal contacts on the resected side of the prosthesis.

- In edentulous patients the undercuts within the defects are engaged for retention. Resilient polymer material may be processed into the undercut areas to improve retention.
- Osseointegrated implants may also be placed into the alveolar bone in the non-resected maxilla for additional retention and stability in the edentulous resection patient.

THE MAXILLARY RESECTION PATIENT

Etiology and incidence

A maxillectomy is often necessary for benign and malignant tumors of the maxillary sinus, hard palate and often the soft palate. The extent of the surgery is dependent upon the size and pathology of the tumor.

It is rare to have a primary tumor of the gingiva covering the hard palate. Palatal tumors most often arise in the sinus and spread inferiorly through the sinus floor:

- squamous cell carcinoma is the most prevalent type (≈ 80%).
- adenocarcinoma
- minor salivary gland tumors.

Suspected etiologic agents/predisposing factors

- Exposure to certain metal powders (chromium), sawdust (furniture workers), chronic snuff use.
- Chronic sinusitis, nasal polyps.

Diagnosis/clinical presentation

- Medial extension (into nasal cavity): nasal discharge, congestion, epistaxis.
- Inferior extension (into oral cavity): palatal swelling, loosening of maxillary teeth, ulceration of mucosa, ill-fitting dentures.
- Superior extension (into orbit): orbital swelling, diplopia, epiphora, proptosis, unilateral fixed glaze.
- Anterior extension: facial swelling, lack of sensation in skin, unilateral pain.
- Posterior extension: otoalgia, trismus.

Rationale for immediate obturation

Function
- Maintain palatal contours after surgery.
- To provide a matrix to hold surgical packing against defect.
- Immediate speech improvement.
- Improve deglutition.
- Improve oral nutritional intake (nasogastric tube may be removed earlier).
- Protect nasal tissues from contents of oral cavity.

Psychology
- Esthetics improved as teeth may be replaced.
- Allows patient to communicate intelligibly.
- Defect is not as readily sensed by patient.
- Provides support and normal contours to soft tissues of face.

Hygiene
Oral and nasal cavities are separated – nasal regurgitation of food and liquids reduced.

Presurgical treatment planning

There is often very little time between the request for a dental consultation and the actual surgical procedure. It is imperative that a proactive working relationship exist between the dental service and the requesting surgical service. This allows for a thorough discussion of the proposed surgical resection, with consideration given to improving the postsurgical prosthetic rehabilitation.

Initial dental evaluation
- Review history of present illness, past medical and surgical history, social history, alcohol and tobacco use for information relevant to condition and prognosis.
- Review prior dental history:
  - hygiene regimen
  - frequency and nature of past dental care
  - prior experience with removable dental prostheses.
- Obtain orthopantomographic and periapical radiographs to evaluate the teeth to be used for abutments, and plan appropriate treatment of carious and/or periodontally involved teeth.

- Obtain intraoral and extraoral presurgical photographs as part of the patient's medical record.
- Fixed dental bridgework may need to be sectioned if it spans a region where a surgical resection will be made.
- Obtain two sets of irreversible hydrocolloid impressions (both maxilla and mandible) and pour both in dental stone. Obtain an interocclusal record:
  - impression trays may require modification with wax or compound to accommodate all landmarks if tumor is extensive
  - one set of casts serve as diagnostic casts
  - one set serve as working laboratory casts.
- Abutment teeth should be identified to retain the surgical prosthesis. Modifications should be made to improve retention if indicated:
  - survey appropriate undercut regions
  - recontour teeth to improve undercuts
  - restorations may be placed to alter undercuts
  - consider dimples, grooves, and rests for additional retention.
- Select and record the appropriate mold and shade of teeth if they are to be included on the prosthesis.
- If a resection of extraoral facial tissues is anticipated, a facial moulage [mould] may also be obtained with irreversible hydrocolloid and plaster backing as a presurgical record for postsurgical prosthetic rehabilitation.

Dental–surgical treatment planning analysis

The member of the dental service responsible for the patient's care should meet with a member of the surgical service performing the maxillary resection to discuss the planned procedure and any possible deviations from the plan that may be anticipated. The articulated diagnostic casts and radiographs should be available for the team to thoroughly discuss the patient's condition and surgical/rehabilitative plan. The definitive rehabilitative plan should be developed before surgery.

The surgeon should outline on the cast the proposed incisions. The dentist should advocate the following points:

- Consideration should be given to retaining as many sound teeth as possible without compromising disease-free surgical margins.
- Osseous structures should be preserved (i.e. anterior hard palate) if possible, again without compromising disease-free surgical margins.

- The incisions should be made through a socket where a tooth has been extracted to increase the support around the terminal abutment tooth.

The need for supplemental retention by transosseous or interdental wire fixation should be discussed for edentulous patients. Transalveolar versus circumzygomatic versus piriform aperture versus interdental versus palatal screw placement.

If postsurgical radiation therapy is anticipated by the surgeon or oncologist, teeth with a questionable prognosis should be removed in time to allow for healing prior to the start of radiation therapy. All carious lesions in teeth deemed to have a fair or better prognosis should be restored.

Immediate surgical obturator

Laboratory procedures

Usually due to time constraints, the fabrication of the actual prosthesis is done at the hospital in the dental laboratory. If adequate time is available prior to surgery, the articulated casts and a detailed laboratory prescription may be sent to a commercial laboratory familiar with the fabrication of obturator prosthesis.

Cast modification

- The teeth in the area of resection are removed and the ridge portion of the cast is contoured to resemble an edentulous alveolar ridge.
- Where the soft palate is also to be resected, the soft palate on the working cast should be reduced to the level of the hard palate, simulating the position of the dynamic soft palate during function, rather than interfering with the function of the tongue.
- Wrought wire clasps are formed to engage the undercuts on the identified abutment teeth and held in place with sticky wax.
- If there is adequate time for flasking and processing with heat-cured methyl methacrylate, the palatal portion should be waxed to a thickness of 2–3 mm across the hard palate and defect area. Teeth may be waxed into place in the anterior region. Care should be taken in designing and fabricating the prosthesis to minimize the adjustment required in the operating room [theatre].
- If there is minimal time prior to surgery, the prosthesis may be directly fashioned by the 'sprinkling method' of adding small

amounts of cold-cure methyl methacrylate powder and monomer liquid directly onto a well-lubricated cast.

- Both the heat-processed and cold-cured prostheses are then trimmed and polished. Recessed holes are drilled with a #8 round bur in a slow speed handpiece in the region where supplemental ligature wires will be needed.
- The completed prosthesis is clearly labeled with the patient's name and sent to the operating room [theatre] along with the instruments necessary for inserting and securing the prosthesis. Ideally, both should be sterilized or decontaminated prior to surgery. Again, if time does not allow for gas sterilization of the prosthesis, it may be delivered to the OR [theatre] and cold-sterilized immediately prior to insertion.
- Instruments required for prosthesis placement:
  - dental mirror, explorer, needle holders (two), wire director (two), wire cutter, band pusher, surgical awl, and multiple pieces of 16 and 18 gauge stainless steel ligature wire
  - hall drill and multiple burs for modifying the prosthesis.

Surgical procedures

Whenever possible, the dentist fabricating the immediate prosthesis should be present in the operating room [theatre] to place or assist in placing the surgical obturator. Following the surgical resection and the placement of a skin graft to line the defect, the prosthesis is inserted.

- Check fit and retention first: there should be no over extension which would place tension across the surgical flap:
  - necessary modifications should be made with the Hall drill away from the surgical field
  - the modified prosthesis is rinsed with sterile normal saline and again fitted to the surgical site.
- If additional retention is required, interdental ligature wires may be placed or transosseous wires or a transpalatal screw placed in the case of the edentulous patient.
- Once the prosthesis is secured to the surgical site, the surgical packing and nasogastric tube is placed by the surgeon and the flap closed to complete the procedure.

Postsurgical care

The patient is seen daily by the dental service while hospitalized:
- Check prosthesis for stability, retention.
- Check patient for comfort, speech quality, ability to swallow, nasal leakage of food and fluids.
- Oral hygiene measures are stressed to the patient and nursing staff.

The immediate prosthesis is removed 7–14 days after surgery, depending upon the patient's healing progress and the extent of the resection. This is often a joint appointment with both the dentist and surgeon present:
- Local anesthetic may be required when removing ligature wires or transpalatal screws.
- Wires should be cut with a bur and/or a wire cutter.
- The prosthesis is carefully removed along with surgical packing and cleaned with an antibacterial soap and water to remove any gross debris. This may be followed by ultrasonic cleansing.
- Reline the defect area of the prosthesis with a soft reline material or tissue conditioner to assist in retention and to obturate the defect. In situations where the defect is large this may require several sequential relines to achieve the necessary obturation.
- Instruct the patient how to insert and remove the prosthesis. The patient should be able to demonstrate the ability to insert and remove the prosthesis before dismissal.
- Upon discharge from the hospital, the patient is directed to return for modification of the prosthesis in 7–10 days.

MANDIBULAR RESECTION PROSTHESIS WITH GUIDE FLANGE

Following a partial resection of the mandible, the lower jaw usually deviates to the resected side upon closure. This prosthesis:
- Uses a guide flange to direct the remaining portion of the resected mandible into a more normal occlusal relationship with the maxilla.
- Provides an improved tooth-to-tooth relationship.
- Improves mastication and deglutition as well as restores facial contour to some degree.
- Consists of a mandibular cast metal framework with a metal guide flange that contacts the buccal aspect of the maxillary teeth on the unresected side.

Prosthetic teeth can be added to the framework if indicated. This prosthesis is most effective when fabricated and delivered as soon after mandibular resection as possible.

SPEECH AID PROSTHESIS

Also referred to as a speech 'bulb' or simply a speech appliance. Can be indicated for both children and adults. Speech aid prostheses are used primarily to improve speech quality in cleft palate patients by obturating a palatal cleft or fistula. They can also assist in improving speech quality in patients with velopharyngeal incompetency (VPI), such as cleft palate patients, stroke patients with neurogenic VPI, or head and neck cancer patients who may have VPI following tumor resection.

They consist of three components.

- A PMMA palatal plate, retained by either wrought wire or cast clasps, is the primary retentive element of the entire prosthesis.
- A stainless steel 0.050" wire extends from the palatal portion to traverse the soft palate and project into the region of the junction of the oro- and nasopharynx.
- An acrylic pharyngeal 'bulb' is fashioned from PMMA to sit at the level of the tubercle of the atlas and close-off the oropharynx from the nasopharynx at appropriate times during speech and swallowing.

The palatal portion and the pharyngeal extension can also be fabricated in a cast framework. Modifications to the bulb are made on a frequent basis because the quality of speech can change, especially in pediatric cleft palate patients.

The pharyngeal extension may be retained by a projection on the major connector of a cast partial denture framework.

PALATAL LIFT APPLIANCE

- CVA is perhaps the most common cause of soft palate incompetency.
- Serves to elevate the soft palate to assist in velopharyngeal closure during speech and swallowing, thereby effectively serving to separate the oro- and nasopharynx at the appropriate times.

- Indicated when the primary deficit in the velopharyngeal mechanism is in the soft palate alone.
- Increased velopharyngeal closure enhances vocal projection and provides a reduction in hypernasality.
- The appliance includes either a cast metal or PMMA hard palatal portion with retention from wrought wire or cast metal clasping. A beaver-tail-shaped elevated portion, fabricated from PMMA, extends from the hard palate section and gently 'lifts' the soft palate.
- The function of the palatal lift can also be achieved with the speech aid appliance.
- If extensive palatal lift is required, retention may be inadequate to use the palatal lift appliance.
- A successful palatal lift prosthesis depends on adequate teeth to retain the prosthesis and counter the downward displacing forces of the soft palate. Edentulous 'palatal lift' prostheses are rarely successful.

PALATAL AUGMENTATION PROSTHESIS

Following a surgical resection of the tongue or after a stroke, the loss of mass and the lack of coordination of the intrinsic muscles of the tongue might not allow the organ to be properly positioned relative to the hard palate, thus compromising speech production and swallowing efficiency. A palatal augmentation prosthesis:

- Allows the palate to be reshaped and improves the tongue-to-palate relationship.
- Improves speech and swallowing by the most efficient contact of the dorsal surface of the tongue with the prosthesis.
- Is made from PMMA and retained by cast or wrought wire clasps around the maxillary teeth.

Low fusing wax is added to the tongue surface of the prosthesis and the patient is allowed to mold the wax to conform to the shape of the dorsum of the tongue. The wax is then processed in PMMA.

CLEFT PLATE MOLDING APPLIANCE

The newborn infant with a cleft palate, whether unilateral or bilateral, suffers from a number of hard and soft tissue deficits in the nasolabial region. With the segments of the maxillary alveolus separated by the cleft, the infant often has great difficulty feeding. Surgery is required to close the defect in the lip and repair the palatal cleft:

- A cleft palate molding appliance resembles a small maxillary denture, which functions to close the palate and separate the oral and nasal cavities and thus allows the baby to create a vacuum by suckling, thereby improving feeding.
- May be modified on a weekly basis as well to mold the alveolar segments closer together as the child grows rapidly.
- When properly molded, the appliance is capable of producing a normal, symmetrical maxillary alveolar arch-form while reducing the size of the cleft. This reduces the extent and complexity of the surgical repair of the cleft of the lip (if present), which is usually performed at approximately 2 to 4 months of age.
- Also reduces the extent of the surgical repair of the palate as well. Palate repair usually is delayed until the first attempt at speech production at 6 to 14 months.
- Fabricated by obtaining an impression of the maxilla and defect with an elastomeric impression material, not alginate, which may easily tear leaving material in the defect that may be swallowed or lodged in the infants airway. The cleft palate molding plate is then fashioned on the recovered stone cast using polymethyl methacrylate.
- The plate is usually self-retentive but may also be retained by palatal pins (Latham appliance) or with adhesive suture strip tape placed across the maxillary lip.

GUNNING (FRACTURE) SPLINT

Allows for the surgical reduction and fixation of fractures of the edentulous maxilla or mandible that are difficult because it is impossible to orient the bony segments properly. The splint can also be fabricated to assist in positioning the jaw segments during orthognathic surgery for edentulous or partially edentulous patients:

- Fabricated from PMMA in a fashion similar to denture fabrication. Arch bars may be incorporated into the PMMA.
- The splints have openings to allow for speech, nutrition, and saliva flow.

- May be fabricated utilizing existing removable prosthesis if the patient has one (or two).

RADIATION CARRIER

A radiation carrier is a device that holds a radiation source in the same position relative to the tumor or tissue intended to receive the radiation dosage. The carrier may be a set of dentures or a denture-like appliance that can hold seeds or needles of a radiation source (i.e. radium, indium, cesium). Also referred to as carrier prostheses, radiation carriers, or radiotherapy prostheses.

EXTRAORAL PROSTHESES

Facial prosthesis

A removable prosthesis used to replace missing or damaged facial structures due to surgery, trauma or congenital absence. The facial prosthesis, sometimes inappropriately referred to as a prosthetic dressing:

- is prescribed when a defect is too large or complex to allow surgical reconstruction of the area or when recurrence of a tumor is a possibility
- allows a patient to function in society on a day-to-day basis by restoring facial form and complexion
- can be fabricated from a variety of prosthetic materials, silicone is the most common, but they can be fashioned from PMMA:
  - materials are colored both intrinsically and extrinsically to simulate the complexion of the surrounding tissues
  - retained by medical-grade silicone adhesives, double-sided tape, extension into the mechanical undercuts of the defect, or trans-cutaneous osseointegrated implants placed into the surrounding facial bones.

Facial moulage 'face mask' impression

Used to record the form and contours of the soft tissues of the face. It produces a negative image of the facial form, from which a 'positive' cast can be obtained. This is especially useful for planning facial plastic surgical procedures and recording a patient's face prior to ablative tumor surgery. Impression is made from irreversible hydrocolloid material. A layer of quickset plaster is then placed over the setting impression material for reinforcement. The impression is then removed and poured in white dental stone or plaster of Paris. The facial moulage may be made of an entire face or be sectional – impressioning only a desired segment of the face.

Auricular prosthesis

Also referred to as an ear prosthesis:
- A removable prosthesis fashioned from elastomeric silicone, polyurethane or latex rubber, or PMMA.
- Replaces all or part of the natural ear that may have been lost to trauma, surgical resection or have been congenitally missing.
- Serves to restore the normal form and contour of the natural ear as well as to collect sound waves for improved hearing. Not purely a cosmetic prosthesis.
- It may be retained with medical-grade skin adhesive, attachment to eyeglasses or through mechanical interlocks or magnets placed on transcutaneous osseointegrated implants.

Ocular prosthesis

Commonly referred to as an 'artificial eye' or 'glass eye':
- Replaces an eye missing as a result of surgical ablation, trauma or congenital absence.
- Does not replace the eyelids, the orbit or the soft tissues surrounding the eye.
- Fabricated from PMMA. In the past, glass was also used to fashion an ocular prosthesis.
- If the extraocular muscles are present, an ocular prosthesis can be placed to allow the movement of the ocular to mimic the movement of the natural eye. If not intact, the ocular will not be capable of animated movement.

Orbital prosthesis

Replaces not only the contents of the orbit with an ocular prosthesis but also the adjacent hard and soft tissues, including skin, muscle and bone that may have been lost due to surgery or trauma. In addition to restoring a normal day-to-day appearance to the orbital region, it also seals the defect from the external environment. This serves to maintain the normal humidity and tissue moisture of the surrounding cavities, the maxillary sinus and the oral and nasal cavities:

- Fabricated from elastomeric silicone, polyurethane or latex rubber to simulate the tissues surrounding the eye, while the eye is simulated by an ocular prosthesis.
- Retained by medical-grade adhesive, double-sided tape or by mechanical undercuts within the defect. Recently, magnets or mechanical interlocks attached to transcutaneous osseointegrated implants have successfully replaced the need for adhesives.

Nasal prosthesis

Replaces those hard and soft tissues that might have been lost as a result of surgical resection, trauma or congenital absence. In addition to restoring the normal day-to-day appearance to the nasal structures and midface region, it also serves to aid in warming and humidifying inspired air before it enters the respiratory system:

- Usually fabricated from elastomeric silicone. Polyurethane, latex rubber and PMMA can also be used.
- Retained by medical-grade adhesive, double-sided tape or mechanical undercuts within the defect. Recently, magnets or mechanical interlocks attached to transcutaneous osseointegrated implants have successfully replaced the need for adhesives.

Cranial prosthesis

Also referred to as a 'skull plate', a cranial implant or a cranioplasty prosthesis:

- A PMMA plate with a reinforcing stainless steel mesh incorporated into the processed PMMA.
- Designed to replace a portion of the skull or cranium and to re-establish a separation of the overlying scalp from the dura. Also protects the exposed brain from trauma and restores the normal contour to the cranium where the bone may have been lost by surgery, infection, trauma or developmental anomalies.
- Fashioned by obtaining an irreversible hydrocolloid impression of the defect area.

- If the segment of bone that is to be replaced is available, it may be invested in plaster, removed and the plate processed in PMMA.
- The plate may also be fashioned from computer-assisted design and computer-assisted manufacturing (CAD–CAM) through the use of a reformatted three-dimensional CT scan of the defect.
- Secured to the surrounding bone with stainless steel surgical wire.
- Historically, cranial prostheses have also been fabricated from surgical stainless steel, tantalum and other biocompatible metals.

Nasal stent

A removable appliance that provides support to the nasal cartilage. Fabricated from PMMA. Returns form to a nose damaged from trauma or surgery which, left untreated, can lead to the collapse of the nasal ala and closure of the nostrils.

Chapter 8

Charts, tables and treatment protocols

ABBREVIATIONS

Clinicians should be careful when using abbreviations because of the possibility of a misinterpretation. There is no universally recognized list of abbreviations and the same abbreviation can stand for two very different words or terms. The following is a partial list of abbreviations to be used to interpret notes in a chart:

A/P	auscultation and percussion	ALB	albumin
AA	active assistive; alcohol abuse	ALL	acute lymphocytic leukemia; acute lymphoblastic leukemia
abd	abdomen; abdominal	ALT	alanine transaminase (SGPT)
ABG	arterial blood gases		
AC	before meals	AML	acute myelogenous leukemia
ACE	angiotensin-converting enzyme	AMY	amylase
ACT	anticoagulant therapy	ANT	anterior
ACTH	adrenocorticotrophic hormone	ANUG	acute necrotizing ulcerative gingivitis
ad lib	as desired	AP & lat	anteroposterior and lateral
AD	right ear		
ADA	American Disabilities Act; American Dietetic Association	AP	anterior–posterior
		APPT	activated partial thromboplastin time
ADH	antidiuretic hormone	AROM	active range of motion
ADM	admit; admission	AS	left ear
AHA	American Heart Association; American Hospital Association	ASA	aspirin (acetylsalicylic acid); American Society of Anesthesiologists
AI	aortic insufficiency	ASD	atrial septal defect
AIDS	acquired immune deficiency syndrome	ASHD	arteriosclerotic heart disease

AST	aspartate transaminase (SGOT)	CABG	coronary artery bypass graft
AV	arteriovenous; atrioventricular	cal.	calorie
		CAP	capsule
AVN	atrioventricular node	CAT	computerized axial tomography
AVR	aortic valve replacement		
AVS	arteriovenous shunt	CATH	catheter(ization); Catholic
AZT	zidovudine (azidothymidine)		
		CBC	complete blood count
BA	brachial artery; blood alcohol	CC	chief complaint
		cc	cubic centimeter
BACT	bacteria	CD	constant drainage; convulsive disorder; Crohn's disease
BaE	barium enema		
BAL	bronchoalveolar lavage		
BE	bacterial [infective] endocarditis	CD4	antigenic marker on helper/inducer T cells
BID	twice daily	CEJ	cementoenamel junction
Bili D	bilirubin direct	cGy	centigray (measure of radiation dose)
Bili T	bilirubin total		
BM	bowel movement; bone marrow; black male	CHF	congestive heart failure
		CHO	carbohydrate
BMB	bone marrow biopsy	Chol.	cholesterol
BMR	basal metabolic rate	CIS	carcinoma in situ
BP	blood pressure	CK	creatinine kinase
BPD	bronchopulmonary dysplasia	Cl	chloride; chlorine
		cl. liq.	clear liquid
BPH	benign prostatic hypertrophy	CML	chronic myelogenous leukemia
BRP	bathroom privileges	CMV	cytomegalovirus
BSAC	British Society for Antimicrobial Chemotherapy	CN	cranial nerve
		CNS	central nervous system
		CO	carbon monoxide; cardiac output
BT	bleeding time		
BUN	blood urea nitrogen	CO_2	carbon dioxide
Bx	biopsy	COPD	chronic obstructive pulmonary disease
C	Celsius; centigrade; complement		
		CP	cold pack; cerebral palsy; cleft palate
c̄	with		
C&B	chair and bed	CR	complete remission
C&S	culture and sensitivity	Creat.	creatinine
C/O	complains of; complaints	CSF	cerebrospinal fluid
C/W	consistent with	CT	computed tomography
Ca	calcium	CVA	cerebrovascular accident
CA	carcinoma; cancer		

CVHD	chronic valvular heart disease	Dx	diagnosis; disease
CVP	central venous pressure	EAC	external auditory canal
CVS	clean voided specimen; cardiovascular system	EACA	epsilon aminocaproic acid
		ECF	extracellular fluid; extended care facility
CXR	chest X-ray		
D	day	ECG	electrocardiogram
D&C	dilation and curettage	EEG	electroencephalogram
d/c	discontinue	EF	erythroblastosis fetalis; ejection fraction
D/S	dextrose/saline		
D10W	10% dextrose in water	EKG	electrocardiogram
D5NS	5% dextrose in normal saline	ELISA	enzyme-linked immunosorbent assay
		Elix.	elixir
D5W	5% dextrose in water	EM	erythema multiforme; early memory; emergency medicine
DAT	diet as tolerated		
DC	discharge; decrease		
DDAVP	desmopressin acetate	ENT	ear, nose, throat
DDC	zalcitabine (dideoxycytidine)	EOM	extraocular movements
		EPT	electric pulp test
DDI	didanosine (dideoxyinosine)	ESR	erythrocyte sedimentation rate
diag.	diagnosis	ESRD	end-stage renal disease
DIC	disseminated intravascular coagulopathy	EtOH	ethyl alcohol
		ETT	endotracheal tube
		eval.	evaluation
Diff.	white blood cell differential	FBS	fasting blood sugar
		Fe	iron (serum)
DIL	dilute	FFP	fresh frozen plasma
disch.	discharge	fl. oz.	fluid ounce
dL	deciliter (100 mL)	FNA	fine needle aspiration
DM	diabetes mellitus; diastolic murmur	FUO	fever of undetermined origin
DNR	do not resuscitate	Fx	fracture
DOB	date of birth	g	gram
DOE	dyspnea on exertion	G6PD	glucose-6-phosphate dehydrogenase
DPT	diphtheria, pertussis, tetanus; dental panoramic tomogram		
		GB	gallbladder series
		GC	gonorrhea; gonococcal
DSD	dry sterile dressing	GFR	glomerular filtration rate
dsg	dressing	GI	gastrointestinal
DTR	deep tendon reflex	Glu.	glucose
DTs	delirium tremens	GM-CSF	granulocyte-macrophage colony-stimulating factor
DVT	deep vein thrombosis		
DW	dextrose in water		

GOT	glutamine-oxaloacetic transaminase (AST)	IgM	immunoglobulin M
GSW	gunshot wound	IM	intramuscular
GU	genitourinary	IMF	intermaxillary fixation
Gy	Gray (radiation unit)	imp.	impression; impacted
GYN	gynecology; gynecologic	INC	incomplete; increase
h	hour	INH	isoniazid
H&N	head and neck	inj.	injection; injury
H&P	history and physical	INR	international normalized ratio
H/O	history of	IPPB	intermittent positive pressure breathing
Hb	hemoglobin		
HBcAb	hepatitis B core antibody	ISG	immune serum globulin
HBO	hyperbaric oxygen	IU	international unit (of hormone activity)
HBsAg	hepatitis B surface antigen		
HBV	hepatitis B virus; hepatitis B vaccine	IV	intravenous
		IVC	intravenous cholangiogram; inferior vena cava
HCT	hematocrit		
HCV	hepatitis C virus	IVDA	intravenous drug abuse
HD	hemodialysis; heart disease	IVP	intravenous pyelogram
		JCAHO	Joint Commission on Accreditation of Healthcare Organizations
HDV	hepatitis delta virus		
HEENT	head, eyes, ears, nose, throat		
		JRA	juvenile rheumatoid arthritis
Hg	mercury		
Hgb	hemoglobin	JVD	jugular venous distension
HIV	human immunodeficiency virus		
		JVP	jugular venous pressure/pulse
HO	house officer		
HPI	history of present illness	K	potassium; thousand
HR	heart rate	kg	kilogram
hr	hour	KS	Kaposi's sarcoma
HS	hour of sleep (bedtime)	KUB	kidneys, ureters, bladder (flat X-ray of abdomen)
ht	height		
HTN	hypertension	KVO	keep vein open
HX	history	K-wire	Kirschner wire
I&D	incision and drainage	L	left; liter
I&O	intake and output	L&W	living and well
IA	intraarterial	LA	lateral; local anesthesia
IDDM	insulin-dependent diabetes mellitus	lab.	laboratory
		LAP	laparotomy; laparoscopy
IE	infective endocarditis	lb	pound
IFA	immunofluorescent assay	LBBB	left bundle branch block
IgA	immunoglobulin A	LDH	lactic dehydrogenase

LE	lupus erythematosus; lower extremity		MRI	magnetic resonance imaging
LFT	liver function test		MS	morphine sulfate; multiple sclerosis
LIG	ligament		MTD	maximum tolerated dose
LLL	left lower lobe		MVA	motor vehicle accident
LLQ	left lower quadrant		MVP	mitral valve prolapse
LOM	loss of motion		N&V	nausea and vomiting
LP	lumbar puncture		N₂0	nitrous oxide
LSB	left sternal border		Na	sodium
LUL	left upper lobe		NAD	no acute distress
LUQ	left upper quadrant		NAS	no added salt
LVH	left ventricular hypertrophy		NED	no evidence of disease
M/E	myeloid–erythroid (ratio)		NG	nasogastric
			NHL	non-Hodgkin's lymphoma
mand.	mandibular		NIDDM	non-insulin-dependent diabetes mellitus
MAO	monoamine oxidase		nil	nothing
max.	maximal; maxillary		NKDA	no known drug allergies
mcg	microgram		NL	normal; nasolacrimal
MCH	mean corpuscular hemoglobin		noc.	night
MCHC	mean corpuscular hemoglobin concentration		NPO	nothing by mouth
			NS	normal saline
			NSAID	non-steroidal anti-inflammatory drug
MCL	midclavicular line		NSR	normal sinus rhythm
MDR	multidrug resistance		NTG	nitroglycerin
mEq	milliequivalent		NUG	necrotizing ulcerative gingivitis
met.	metastasis			
mg	milligram		NUP	necrotizing ulcerative periodontitis
MI	myocardial infarction			
MIC	minimum inhibitory concentration		OD	right eye; overdose
min	minimum; minute		OOB	out of bed
mL	milliliter		OR	operating room [theatre]
MMF	maxillomandibular fixation		ortho.	orthopedic
			OS	left eye
mo	month		OTC	over-the-counter
MOD	moderate		OU	both eyes
MPD	myofacial pain dysfunction; myeloproliferative disorder; maximum permissible dose		oz	ounce
			p̄	after
			P&A	percussion and auscultation
MR	mitral regurgitation		PA	posterior–anterior; periapical

PC	after meals	PTA	prior to admission
PCA	patient-controlled analgesia	PUD	peptic ulcer disease
PCN	penicillin	PVC	premature ventricular contraction
PCP	*Pneumocystis carinii* pneumonia	Q	every (e.g. q2h = every 2 hours)
PDA	patent ductus arteriosus; personal digital assistant	QD	every day
		QH	every hour
PDL	periodontal ligament	QHS	every night at bedtime
PE	physical examination; pulmonary embolism	QID	four times a day
		QOD	every other day
PEG	percutaneous endoscopic gastrostomy	QS	sufficient quantity
		R	right
PERRLA	pupils equal, round, reactive to light and accommodation	R/O	rule out
		RA	rheumatoid arthritis
		RAD	radiation absorbed dose (old term)
PET	positron emission tomography	RAI	radioactive iodine
PH; PHx	past history	RBBB	right bundle branch block
PI	present illness; principal investigator	RBC	red blood cell
plts	platelets	RDS	respiratory distress syndrome
PM&R	physical medicine and rehabilitation	retic.	reticulocyte
PMH	past medical history	RF	rheumatoid factor; rheumatic fever
PMI	point of maximal impulse; past medical illness	RHD	rheumatic heart disease
		RIA	radioimmunoassay
PMMA	polymethyl methacrylate	RL	Ringer's lactate
PMN	polymorphonuclear leukocyte	RLL	right lower lobe (lung)
		RLQ	right lower quadrant (abdomen)
PND	paroxysmal nocturnal dyspnea; postnasal drip	ROM	range of motion
PO	postop; postoperative by mouth	ROS	review of systems
		RUQ	right upper quadrant
PPD	packs per day; purified protein derivative (tuberculin)	Rx	treatment, prescription
		RXN	reaction
		s	without; second
PR	per rectum	S&S	swish and swallow; signs and symptoms
preop.	preoperative		
PRN	as needed	SBE	subacute bacterial [infective] endocarditis
PT	prothrombin time; physical therapy	SC	subcutaneous
pt	patient	SCC	squamous cell carcinoma

SDH	subdural hematoma	TIBC	total iron-binding capacity
SEM	systolic ejection murmur; scanning electron microscopy	TID	three times a day
		tinct.	tincture
SGOT	serum glutamic oxaloacetic transaminase (AST)	TM	tympanic membrane
		TMD	temporomandibular disorder
SGPT	serum glutamic pyruvic transaminase (ALT)	TMJ	temporomandibular joint
		TNM	primary tumor (T), regional lymph nodes (N) and distant metastases (M). Used with subscripts for cancer staging.
SH	social history; surgical history		
SI	International System of Units (SI units)		
SIP	status post		
SK	streptokinase	TO	telephone order
SLE	systemic lupus erythematosus	TP	total protein
		TPA	tissue plasminogen activator
SOAP	subjective, objective, assessment and plan	TPN	total parenteral nutrition
SOB	shortness of breath	TPR	temperature, pulse, respiration
SOC	standard of care		
SOL, soln	solution	tsp.	teaspoon
SOS	only if necessary	TT	thrombin time
sp	species	Tx	treatment; therapy; transplant
SQ	subcutaneous		
SR, sed. rt.	sedimentation rate	U	International unit (enzyme activity)
ss	one-half		
stat.	immediately	UA	urinalysis; uric acid
STS	serologic test(s) for syphilis	UGI	upper gastrointestinal series
SUBL	sublingual	URI	upper respiratory infection
subq.	subcutaneous		
SVCS	superior vena cava syndrome	UTI	urinary tract infection
		VAD	vascular (venous) access device
Sx	symptoms		
T	temperature	VSD	ventricular septal defect
tab.	tablet	W/U	workup
TAH	total abdominal hysterectomy	wk	week
		WNL	within normal limits
TB	tuberculosis	wt	weight
TCDB	turn, cough, deep breath	XRT	radiation therapy
		YAG	yttrium aluminum garnet (laser)
TEE	transesophageal echocardiography		
		yr	year
TIA	transient ischemic attack		

ANTIBIOTIC PROPHYLAXIS, AMERICAN HEART ASSOCIATION (AHA)

Prevention of bacterial endocarditis

The American Heart Association (AHA) first developed guidelines for antibiotic prophylaxis for specific cardiac conditions in 1955.

Box 8.1 Cardiac conditions associated with endocarditis*

Endocarditis prophylaxis recommended
High-risk category
Prosthetic cardiac valves, including bioprosthetic and homograft valves
Previous bacterial endocarditis
Complex cyanotic congenital heart disease (e.g. single ventricle states, transposition of the great arteries, tetralogy of Fallot)
Surgically constructed systemic pulmonary shunts or conduits
Moderate-risk category
Most other congenital cardiac malformation (other than above and below)
Acquired valvular dysfunction (e.g. rheumatic heart disease)
Hypertrophic cardiomyopathy
Mitral valve prolapse with valvar regurgitation and/or thickened leaflets

Endocarditis prophylaxis not recommended
Negligible-risk category (no greater risk than the general population)
Isolated secundum atrial septal defect
Surgical repair of atrial septal defect, ventricular septal defect, or patent ductus arteriosus (without residual beyond 6 mo)
Previous coronary artery bypass graft surgery
Mitral valve prolapse without valvular regurgitation
Physiologic, functional, or innocent heart murmurs
Previous Kawasaki disease without valvular dysfunction
Previous rheumatic fever without valvular dysfunction
Cardiac pacemakers (intravascular and epicardial) and implanted defibrillators

* From: Dajani A S et al 1997 Prevention of bacterial endocarditis – recommendations by the American Heart Association. Journal of the American Medical Association 227:1794–1801. Reproduced with permission.

Like the versions that they supersede, the most recent AHA guidelines suggest that there is still some uncertainty as to which dental procedures and which patients to cover (inside back cover). As the title of the publication suggests, the guidelines are specifically aimed at the prevention of infective endocarditis (Box 8.1, Fig. 8.1 and inside front and back covers). These guidelines are not intended to be used with other medical conditions, such as prosthetic joints. The reader is encouraged to read the sections in the original document that relate to dental practice.

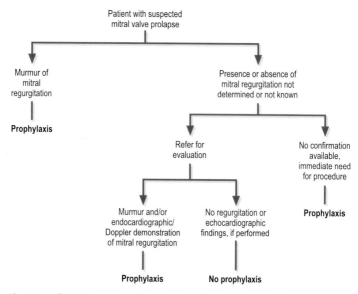

Fig. 8.1 **Clinical approach to determination of the need for prophylaxis in patients with suspected mitral valve prolapse (MVP). For more details on the role of echocardiography in the diagnosis of MVP, see the text and the 1997 American College of Cardiology/American Heart Association guidelines for the clinical application of echocardiography.**

BIOPSY

Types of biopsy

- Excisional removal of a lesion with a margin of normal tissue. This procedure is used when the size of the lesion permits. Not to be done by non-head and neck surgeon if malignancy is expected.
- Incisional or diagnostic biopsy: removal of a section of the lesion and adjacent normal tissue. This procedure is used when the lesion is too large for an excisional biopsy or when the lesion could be malignant.

Procedure

- Make sure all materials (e.g. fixative) are available before starting to perform a biopsy.
- The surface to be biopsied should not be painted with antiseptic or anesthetic but saliva should be wiped from the area with dry sterile cotton gauze.
- When using infiltration anesthesia, anesthetic solution should not be injected into the field from which the specimen will be taken. Rather, infiltrate around the periphery of the lesion to avoid distortion of the specimen.
- Use a sharp scalpel to avoid tearing of tissue. Electrocautery should be avoided because it can cause thermal changes in the tissue.
- A border of normal tissue should be removed with the specimen if possible.
- The specimen should be handled carefully; excessive handling can cause mutilation of the specimen.
- The tissue should be fixed immediately in 10% formalin. If a specimen is thin, it should be placed on a piece of glazed paper and dropped into the fixative; this will prevent curling of the tissue. Immediate fixation will prevent autolysis, distortion, and destruction of the tissue. Immunofluorescence studies (e.g. vesiculobullous disease) require special preservatives (e.g. Michel's solution) instead of formalin, or transport immediately to the laboratory as unfixed specimen over ice.

- When doing incisional biopsy of a larger lesion, samples of every area that demonstrates a different clinical appearance or characteristic should be included.
- The most active and representative areas of the lesion should be sampled. In most cases, the most active portion will be located peripherally; the central portion of many tumors and lesions will demonstrate only necrosis.
- If a biopsy report is inconsistent with the clinical appearance of a lesion and with the history obtained, another biopsy should be performed and submitted to the pathologist. Two or more biopsies might be needed before a definitive diagnosis can be made.
- When temperatures are below freezing, specimens placed in a mailbox [postbox] might freeze. Ice crystals form within the cells of the tissue, disrupting membranes and leading to distortion and artifacts in the specimen, making interpretation of the tissue impossible. This can be avoided by fixing specimens at room temperature in the 10% formalin solution for a period of 2 h before mailing [posting]. In some countries, mailing biological material is prohibited.
- Assure appropriate medical/surgical assessment and management prior to biopsying obviously vascular lesions or lesions in patients with bleeding disorders.

Biopsy request form

- Date of biopsy and your name, address and phone number.
- Patient's name, address and history [case notes] number.
- Age, sex and race of patient.
- Clinical history and location of the lesion.

Reporting

- Tell the patient the biopsy results as soon as possible.
- Malignant findings should be disclosed in person by the appropriate clinician.

COAGULATION AND THE COAGULATION CASCADE (TABLE 8.1, FIG. 8.2)

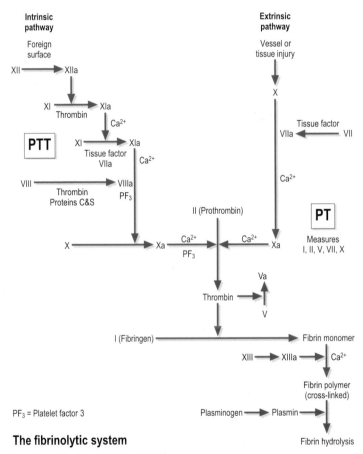

PF$_3$ = Platelet factor 3

The fibrinolytic system

Fig. 8.2 The coagulation cascade.

Table 8.1 **Coagulation**

Bleeding disorder	Bleeding time	Platelet count	INR	PT	APTT	TT
Thrombocytopenia	+	–	0	0	0	0
von Willebrand's	+	0	0	0	0/+	0
Factor VIII, IX deficiency	0	0	0	0	+	0
Vitamin K deficiency and warfarin	0	0	+	+	0/+	0
Chronic liver disease	0	0/–	0	+	+	0/+

0, normal
+, increased
–, decreased

THE GLASGOW COMA SCALE (TABLE 8.2)

Table 8.2 **The Glasgow Coma Scale (GCS)**

Finding	Rating
Eyes	
Open spontaneously	4
Open to loud verbal command	3
Open to pain	2
No response	1
Best motor response	
Follows simple motor commands	6
Pushes away noxious stimulus	5
Moves part of body, but does not remove noxious stimulus	4
Flexion to pain (decorticate)	3
Extension to pain (decerebrate)	2
No motor response to pain	1
Best verbal response	
Alert and oriented	5
Confused, disoriented	4
Talks, but nonsensical	3
Moans, makes unintelligible sounds	2
Makes no noise	1

Minimal score = 3
Maximal score = 15

A GCS of 8 or less has been used as an alternative definition of coma where there is an absence of eye opening to verbal command.

CONVERSION TABLE: FAHRENHEIT/CELSIUS (TABLE 8.3)

Table 8.3 Conversion of Centigrade to Fahrenheit

Centigrade	Fahrenheit
41	105.6
40	104
39.5	103
38.8	102
38.3	101
37.7	100
37.2	99
37	98.6
36	96.8

CONVERSION TABLE: KILOGRAMS TO POUNDS (TABLE 8.4)

Table 8.4 Conversion of kilogram to pounds

Kg	Lb	Kg	Lb	Kg	Lb
40	88	74	162.8	108	237.6
41	90	75	165.0	109	239.8
42	92	76	167.2	110	242.0
43	95	77	169.4	111	244.2
44	97	78	171.6	112	246.4
45	99	79	173.8	113	248.6
46	101	80	176.0	114	250.8
47	103	81	178.2	115	253.0
48	106	82	180.4	116	255.2
49	108	83	182.6	117	257.4
50	110	84	184.8	118	259.6
51	112.2	85	187.0	119	261.8
52	114.4	86	189.2	120	264.0
53	116.6	87	191.4	121	266.2
54	118.8	88	193.6	122	268.4
55	121.0	89	195.8	123	270.6
56	123.2	90	198.0	124	272.8

Table 8.4 continued

Kg	Lb	Kg	Lb	Kg	Lb
57	125.4	91	200.2	125	275.0
58	127.6	92	202.4	126	277.2
59	129.8	93	204.6	127	279.4
60	132.0	94	206.8	128	281.6
61	134.2	95	209.0	129	283.8
62	136.4	96	211.2	130	286.0
63	138.6	97	213.4	131	288.2
64	140.8	98	215.6	132	290.4
65	143.0	99	217.8	133	292.6
66	145.2	100	220.0	134	294.8
67	147.4	101	222.2	135	297.0
68	149.6	102	224.4	136	299.2
69	151.8	103	226.6	137	301.4
70	154.0	104	228.8	138	303.6
71	156.2	105	231.0	139	305.8
72	158.4	106	233.2	140	308.0
73	160.6	107	235.4		

CONVERSION TABLE: METRIC EQUIVALENTS (TABLE 8.5)

Table 8.5 Metric equivalents

Weight

1 kilogram (kg)	= 1000 grams (10^3 g) = 2.2 pounds (1b)
1 gram (g)	= 1000 milligrams (10^3 mg)
1 milligram (mg)	= 1000 micrograms (10^3 mcg or 10 mEq)
60 milligrams (mg)	= 1 grain (Gr)

Volume

1 liter (L)	= 1000 cubic centimeters (cc) of water
	= 1000 milliliters (mL)

Liquid

30 mL	= 1 fluid ounce (oz) = 28.35 grams (g)
240 mL	= 8 fluid ounces (oz)
480 mL	= 1 pint (pt)
960 mL	= 1 quart (qt)

Linear

1 millimeter (mm)	= 0.04 inch (in)
1 centimeter (cm)	= 0.4 inch (in)
2.54 centimeters	= 1 inch (in)
1 meter (m)	= 39.37 inches (in)

DECIMAL FACTORS: PREFIXES (TABLE 8.6)

Table 8.6   Decimal factors: prefixes

Prefix	Symbol	Factor
mega	M	10^6
kilo	k	10^3
hecto	h	10^2
deca	da	10^1
deci	d	10^{-1}
centi	c	10^{-2}
milli	m	10^{-3}
micro	mu	10^{-6}
nano	n	10^{-9}
pico	p	10^{-12}
femto	f	10^{-15}

DIETS

Selection of the appropriate diet is important in many disease states, and is essential in others. A dietician can be consulted to design a diet for specific needs. The goal for any patient is to progress to a normal diet as rapidly as tolerated.

Liquid diet

Clear liquid

Provides only sugar, salt and fluid and is inadequate in protein, vitamins and minerals. It permits such foods as broth, tea, coffee, carbonated beverages and strained fruit juices.

Full liquid

Requires normal gastrointestinal function, although it requires no chewing. It is inadequate in protein, thiamine, niacin, iron and phosphorus. It includes all items in the clear liquid category, as well as milk, ice creams, eggnogs, creamed cereals, gelatins and strained creamed soups.

Low-residue commercial diets

Commercial diets (Sustecal, Meritine) are expensive but valuable for patients who require a long-term, low-residue diet. The amounts of protein, carbohydrate and fats vary by product.

Vitamins

Vitamin supplements are essential for any patient on a long-term liquid diet.

Supplement feedings

Between-meal supplemental feedings are helpful for long-term patients.

Soft diet

The soft diet consists of low-residue foods and is adequate in proteins, vitamins and calories. It often serves as the transition between full liquid to regular diets, containing such easily digested proteins and carbohydrates as ground meats, eggs, cottage cheese, bananas, cooked fruits, apple sauce, white breads and crackers [biscuits], as well as those foods in the liquid diets.

Regular diet

The regular diet permits all foods except those that are exceptionally difficult to digest, such as deep-fried foods.

Special consistency diets

Equivalent to regular diet in nutritional content, special consistency diets are modified to accommodate inadequate dentition, impaired swallowing or patient preference. Examples include:

- Geriatric: cooked (as opposed to raw) vegetables, ground or tender-cooked beef, whole cooked fish or chicken.
- Mechanical: chopped, cooked vegetables, ground meats and chicken, noodle casseroles, canned diced fruits and sauces.
- Pureed: thickened soups, pureed vegetables and meats, cooked and strained fruits.

Special diets

These require special orders:

- Diabetes mellitus: caloric intake should be approximated in kcal/kg. Denoted as '# cal. ADA diet'.
- Chronic renal failure: generally, a diet of 0.05–0.75 g/kg high-quality protein with 3–5 g salt is acceptable.
- Congestive heart failure: salt restriction is important in management. A patient can generally be managed successfully on a diet containing 2 g salt, although a palatable low-salt diet (2.5 g salt, 1.0 g sodium) can be obtained successfully only in the hospital setting; the average diet contains 6–15 g salt. If the addition of salt at the table is restricted, this value can be reduced to 4–7 g; if additional cooking salt is also limited this can be reduced to 3–4 g.

DILUTIONS FOR PARENTERAL DRUGS (TABLE 8.7)

DRUG INTERACTIONS (TABLE 8.8)

DRUGS – FEDERALLY CONTROLLED

Controlled Substances Act – United States

The US Federal Controlled Substances Act of 1970 placed drugs controlled by the Act into five categories, or schedules, based on their potential to cause psychologic and/or physical dependence as well as on their potential for abuse. The schedules are defined in Table 8.9.

When combined with non-narcotic medicinal ingredients, preparations containing certain narcotics can be placed in Schedules III and V. When combined with one or more non-controlled medicinal ingredients, preparations containing Schedule II barbiturates are placed in Schedule III. Suppository forms of these barbiturates are also controlled in Schedule III.

Table 8.7 Dilutions for parenteral drugs

Medication	Common adult dosage	Vehicle solution	Common administration rates	Volume of vehicle solution	Expiration date upon dispensing*
Ampicillin	1 g	NS	Usually over 30 min; dose must be given over at least 15 min	50 cc	24 h
	2 g	NS		100 cc	Less stable in more concentrated solutions
Ampicillin/sulbactam (Unasyn)	1.5–3 g	NS	Usually over 30 min; dose must be given over at least 15 min	50–100 cc	24 h
Cefazolin	1 g	D5W or NS	Over 30 min	50 cc	24 h
Cefoxitin [cefotaxime]	1 g	D5W or NS	Over 30 min	50 cc	24 h
Clindamycin	600 mg	D5W or NS	Usually over 60 min; 600 mg must be given over at least 20 min	100 cc	24 h
Gentamicin	60–80 mg	D5W or NS	Over at least 30 min	50–100 cc	24 h
Nafcillin	1–2 g	D5W or NS	Over 30 min	1 g in 50 cc	24 h
Potassium penicillin	Up to 3 million units	D5W or NS	Over 60 min	50 cc	24 h
Vancomycin	1 g	D5W or NS	Over at least 60 min	250 cc	24 h
Hydrocortisone sodium succinate (Solu-Cortef®)		Reconstitute with sterile water	Over at least 1 min		

*Maximum of 24-h expiration recommended due to sterility concerns. Some products chemically stable longer and have longer expirations if prepared in an LAF hood in a pharmacy or in a ready-to-use form from the manufacturer.

Table 8.8 **Drug interactions**

Drug	Interacting agents	Resulting effect
Acetaminophen [paracetamol]	Ethanol	Increased liver toxicity
Aminoglycosides	Neuromuscular blockers	Enhanced neuromuscular blockade, respiratory suppression
Anesthetics, general	Antidepressants	Hypotension
	Antihypertensives	Hypotension
Anticholinergics (atropine)	Antihistamines	Increased anticholinergic effect
	Levodopa	Increased anticholinergic effect
	Phenothiazines	Increased anticholinergic effect
	Antidepressants, tricyclics	Increased anticholinergic effect
Antihistamines (sedating)	Alcohol	CNS depression
	Phenothiazines	Increased sedation
Anti-inflammatories (NSAIDs)	Anticoagulant	Increased bleeding
	Ethanol	Increased gastric bleeding
	Heart failure medications	Fluid retention, CHF exacerbation
	Lithium	Increased lithium toxicity
	Methotrexate	Methotrexate toxicity
Aspirin	Acetazolamide	Increased acetazolamide
	Methotrexate	Methotrexate toxicity
Barbiturates	Alcohol	Enhanced sedation, increased respiratory depression
	Anticoagulants, oral	Decreased anticoagulant effect
	Antidepressants, tricyclics	Decreased antidepressant effect
	Beta-adrenergic blockers	Decreased beta-blocker effect
	Corticosteroids	Decreased steroid effect
	Digitalis glycosides	Decreased digitoxin effect
	Griseofulvin	Decreased griseofulvin effect
	Phenothiazines	Decreased phenothiazine effect
	Quinidine	Decreased quinidine effect
	Rifampin	Decreased barbiturate effect
	Valproic acid	Increased phenobarbital effect

table continues

Table 8.8 continued

Drug	Interacting agents	Resulting effect
Benzodiazepines (chlordiazepoxide, diazepam, lorazepam)	Alcohol	Enhanced sedation
	Barbiturates	Enhanced sedation, increased respiratory depression
Carbamazepine	Anticoagulants (oral)	Decreased anticoagulant effect
	Cyclosporine	Decreased cyclosporine levels
	Diltiazem	Increased carbamazepine effect, possible reduced diltiazem effect
	Doxycycline	Decreased doxycycline effect
	Felodipine	Decreased felodipine effect
	Fluconazole	Increased carbamazepine effect
	Methadone	Decreased methadone level, withdrawal
	Propoxyphene	Increased carbamazepine effect
Clindamycin	Neuromuscular blockers	Enhanced neuromuscular blockade
	Diphenoxylate/atropine	Use caution with use of diphenoxylate (lomotil) for antibiotic associated diarrhea – due to concern for retaining *Clostridium difficile* toxin
Corticosteroids	Barbiturates	Decreased corticosteroid effect
	Insulin	Steroids may increase blood glucose
	Phenytoin	Decreased corticosteroid effect
	Rifampin	Decreased corticosteroid effect
Erythromycin and clarithromycin*	Lovastatin and most statins	Increased risk of myopathy
	Clozapine	Increased clozapine, seizure potential
	Cyclosporin/tacrolimus	Increased immune suppressant toxicity
	Digoxin	Digoxin toxicity

table continues

Table 8.8 continued

Drug	Interacting agents	Resulting effect
	Dofetilide	Increased dofetilide, arrhythmia
	Ergotamine	Ergotism, hypertension and ischemia
	Midazolam, triazolam	Increased benzodiazepine level
	Theophylline	Increased theophylline level
Fluconazole and Ketoconazole	Benzodiazepines	Increased CNS depression
	Cyclosporine, sirolimus, Tacrolimus	Increased immunosuppressant
	Carbamazepine	Increased carbamazepine
	Cisapride	Increased risk arrhythmia
	Phenytoin	Increased level phenytoin
	Rifampin	Decreased antifungal
	Warfarin	Increased anticoagulant effect
Fluoride	Aluminum hydroxide (antacids)	Decreased fluoride absorption
Ketoconazole	Antacids, drugs decreasing GI acid	Decreased ketoconazole absorption
	Pimozide	Increased risk arrhythmia
	Dofetilide	Increased dofetilide, arrhythmia
	Protease inhibitors (HIV)	Increased protease inhibitor level
	Statins (most) (not pravastatin)	Increased risk rhabdomyolysis
	Also see interactions listed above under fluconazole	
	Barbiturates	Increased CNS depression
Meperidine [pethidine]	Curariform drugs	Increased respiratory depression
	Monoamine oxidase inhibitors (phenelzine)	Life-threatening serotonin syndrome, Hypertension
	Selegiline	Serotonin syndrome
	Serotonin antidepressants	Serotonin syndrome
	Sibutramine	Serotonin syndrome

table continues

Table 8.8 continued

Drug	Interacting agents	Resulting effect
Metronidazole	Contraceptives, oral	Reduced contraceptive effect
	Cyclosporine	Increased cyclosporine toxicity
	Warfarin	Increased anticoagulant effect
	Methotrexate	Methotrexate toxicity
Penicillins	Bacteriostatic antibiotics	Reduced penicillin efficacy
	Contraceptives	Reduced contraceptive effect
	Alcohol	Increased CNS depression
	Levodopa	Decreased levodopa effect
	Lithium	Decreased phenothiazine effect
Phenothiazines (promethazine)	Alcohol	Increased respiratory depression
	Carbamazepine	Increased carbamazepine effect
Propoxyphene	Cations, antacids, sucralfate, calcium, didanosine, iron, magnesuim	Decreased absorption
Quinolones	Anticoagulants, oral	Increased bleeding risk
	Hypoglycemics	Increased hypoglycemia
	Probenecid	Increased antibiotic level
	Antidepressants, tricyclics	Hypertension, hypertensive crisis
	Antihypertensive drugs	Decreased antihypertensive effects
Sympathomimetic amines (epinephrine, phenylephrine)	Beta-adrenergic blockers	Hypertension with epinephrine
		Lack of effect when treating anaphylaxis w/ epinephrine
	Halogenated anesthetics	Cardiac arrhythmias
	Digitalis glycosides	Tendency to cardiac arrhythmias
	Indomethacin	Severe hypertension
Tetracyclines	Antacids	Decreased tetracycline absorption
	Bactericidal antibiotics	Reduced antibiotic efficacy

table continues

Table 8.8 continued

Drug	Interacting agents	Resulting effect
	Barbiturates	Decreased doxycycline effect
	Bismuth subsalicylate	Decreased tetracycline effect
	Carbamazepine	Decreased doxycycline effect
	Contraceptives	Reduced contraceptive effect
	Iron, oral	Decreased tetracycline absorption
	Methotrexate	Methotrexate toxicity
	Methoxyflurane [thiopentone]	Increased nephrotoxicity
	Milk and dairy products	Decreased tetracycline effect
	Phenytoin	Decreased doxycycline effect
	Warfarin	Possible increased anticoagulant effect
	Zinc sulfate	Decreased tetracycline absorption

*Azithromycin has little inhibitory effect on CYP3A4 enzymes and so is less likely to be involved in these drug interactions

Table 8.9 Schedules for federally controlled drugs

Category	Interpretation
I	Includes substances for which there is a high abuse potential and no current approved medical use (e.g. heroin, marijuana, LSD, other hallucinogens, certain opiates and opium derivatives).
II	**High potential for abuse.** Use may lead to severe physical or psychological dependence. Prescriptions must be written in ink, or typewritten and signed by the practitioner. Verbal prescriptions must be confirmed in writing within 72 hours, and may be given only in a genuine emergency. No renewals are permitted.
III	**Some potential for abuse.** Use may lead to low-to-moderate physical dependence or high psychological dependence. Prescriptions may be oral or written. Up to 5 renewals are permitted within 6 months.
IV	**Low potential for abuse.** Use may lead to limited physical or psychological dependence. Prescriptions may be oral or written. Up to 5 renewals are permitted within 6 months.
V	**Subject to state and local regulation.** Abuse potential is low; a prescription may not be required.

Table 8.10 Controlled substances

Schedule	Status in Canada
Schedule II	
Narcotic	
Codeine	N
Fentanyl	N
Hydromorphone	N
Levorphanol	N
Meperidine (pethidine)	N
Methadone	N
Morphine (opium)	N
Oxycodone (Percodan, Percocet, Tylox)	N
Oxymorphone	N
Non-narcotic	
Amobarbital	C
Amphetamine	Not available
Methylphenidate	C
Secobarbital	C
Schedule III	
Narcotic	
Paregoric	N
Non-narcotic	
Butabarbital	C
Schedule IV	
Depressants	
Alprazolam	•
Chloral hydrate	•
Chlordiazepoxide	•
Clonazepam	•
Clorazepate	•
Diazepam	•
Fenfluramine	•
Flurazepam	•
Lorazepam	•
Mephobarbital	C
Meprobamate	•
Midazolam	•
Oxazepam	•
Pentazocine	N
Phenobarbital	C
Temazepam	•
Triazolam	•
Narcotics	
Propoxyphene (Darvon)	N
Narcotic commercial preparations	

NB Drugs not covered by Canadian guidelines are indicated with a bullet point

Controlled substances – Canada

In Canada, narcotics are governed by the Narcotics Control regulations and are designated by the letter N. Drugs that are considered subject to abuse and have an approved medical use, and are not narcotics are designated by the letter C.

Table 8.10 lists some of the substances in the United States Schedules II, III and IV. Canadian products are listed in the narcotic and non-narcotic groups for record-keeping purposes.

Controlled drugs – United Kingdom

In the United Kingdom, controlled drugs are regulated by the Misuse of Drugs Act of 1971. These regulations contain five schedules, which are similar to those described above and govern how drugs are stored and prescribed.

Table 8.11 **Risk factors for teratogenicity**

Risk factor	Description
A	Controlled studies in women fail to demonstrate a risk to the fetus in the first trimester, and the possibility of fetal harm appears remote
B	Animal studies do not indicate a risk to the fetus and there are no controlled human studies, or animal studies do not show an adverse effect on the fetus but well controlled studies in pregnant women have failed to demonstrate a risk to the fetus
C	Studies have shown that the drug exerts animal teratogenic or embryocidal effects, but there are no controlled studies in women, or no studies are available in either animals or women
D	Positive evidence of human fetal risk exists, but benefits in certain situations (e.g. life-threatening situations or serious disease for which safer drugs cannot be used or are ineffective) may make use of the drug acceptable despite its risks
X	Studies in animals or humans have demonstrated fetal abnormalities, or there is evidence of fetal risk based on human experience, or both, and the risk clearly outweighs any possible benefit

From Federal Register 1980 44:37434–67. Briggs G C, Freeman R K, Yaffe S J Drugs in Pregnancy and Lactation, Sixth edition. Lippincott Williams & Wilkins, Philadelphia, 2002

DRUGS WITH FETAL EFFECTS FROM MATERNAL EXPOSURE

Risk factors (A, B, C, D, X) have been assigned to all drugs, based on the level of risk for teratogenicity (Table 8.11). Risk factors are designed to help the reader quickly classify a drug for use during pregnancy. They do not refer to breast-feeding risk. The definitions for the factors are those used by the Food and Drug Administration. The definitions in Table 8.11 are from the United States Food and Drug Administration (FDA).

The drugs in Table 8.12 were selected as being of interest to dental practitioners. The risk factor assignments include an 'M' if the risk assignment was from the manufacturer's professional literature. Ratings with an asterisk are drugs over which Briggs et al (2002) differed with the manufacturer.

DRUGS/MEDICATIONS OF CONCERN IN DENTAL PRACTICE (TABLE 8.13)

EMERGENCY ROOM KIT (TABLE 8.14)

FACIAL PAIN – DIAGNOSTIC FEATURES (TABLE 8.15)

FLUORIDE TRAY CONSTRUCTION

Definition

Fluoride trays are used for delivering fluoride gel to dentulous [dentate] patients with xerostomia, such as following head and neck radiotherapy or patients with Sjögren's syndrome.

(See page 351 for continuation of this section)

Table 8.12 Drugs of interest to dentists with fetal effects from maternal exposure (the risk factor assignments include an 'M' if the risk assignment was from the manufacturer's professional literature. Ratings with an asterisk are drugs over which Briggs et al (2002) differed with the manufacturer)

Drug type		Description
Analgesic		
NSAIDs		A combined 2001 population-based observational cohort study and a case-control study estimated the risk of adverse pregnancy outcome from the use of NSAIDs. A positive association was discovered with spontaneous abortions (miscarriages). Use of first-generation NSAIDs during the latter half of pregnancy has been associated with oligohydramnios and premature closure of the ductus arteriosus. Persistent pulmonary hypertension of the newborn may occur if NSAIDs are used in the third trimester.
Acetaminophen	B	In therapeutic doses, apparently safe for short-term use. Continuous, high daily dosage in one mother probably caused severe anemia (possibly hemolytic) in her, and fatal kidney disease in her newborn.
Aspirin	C*	The use of aspirin during pregnancy, especially of chronic or intermittent high doses, should be avoided. The drug may affect maternal and newborn hemostasis mechanisms, leading to an increased risk of hemorrhage. High doses may be related to increased perinatal mortality, intrauterine growth retardation, and teratogenic effects. Low doses, such as 80 mg/day, appear to have beneficial effects in pregnancies complicated by systemic lupus erythematosus with antiphospholipid antibodies. (*Risk factor D if full-dose aspirin used in third trimester.)
Celecoxib	C_M*	Second-generation NSAIDs that should not be used in women attempting to conceive.
Rofecoxib	C_M*	Constriction of the ductus arteriosus in utero is a pharmacologic consequence arising from the use of prostaglandin synthesis inhibitors during pregnancy. (*Risk factor D if used in third trimester or near delivery.)

Table 8.12 continued

Drug type		Description
Diclofenac	B$_M$*	A positive association has been discovered with spontaneous abortions (miscarriages).
Diflunisal	C$_M$*	Constriction of theductus arteriosus in utero is a pharmacologic consequence of these
Etodolac	C$_M$*	agents. Should not beused in women attempting to conceive. (*Risk factor D if used in
Ibuprofen	B$_M$*	third trimester or near delivery.)
Ketoprofen	B$_M$*	
Naproxen	B$_M$*	
Indomethacin	B*	Use of this agent with antihypertensives, particularly the beta-blockers, has been associated with severe maternal hypertension and resulting fetal distress. Should not be used in women attempting to conceive. (*Risk factor D if used for longer than 48 h or after 34 weeks' gestation or close to delivery.)
Phenacetin	B	Possible associations with fetal craniosynostosis, adrenal syndromes and anomalies, anal atresia, accessory spleen, musculoskeletal defects and hydronephrosis.
Anesthetics		
Lidocaine	B$_M$	Possible association with anomalies of the respiratory tract, tumors and inguinal hernias. For anytime use during pregnancy, no evidence of association with large categories of major or minor malformations or defects could be found.
Anticonvulsants		
Carbamazepine	D$_M$	Use in pregnancy is associated with an increased incidence of major and minor malformations, including spina bifida. A fetal carbamazepine syndrome has been proposed consisting of minor craniofacial defects, fingernail hypoplasia, and developmental delay. If the drug is *required* during pregnancy, it should not be withheld because the benefits of preventing seizures outweigh the potential fetal harm.

table continues

Table 8.12 continued

Drug type		Description
Clonazepam	D_M	Toxicity in the newborn, apparently related to this drug are apnea, cyanosis, lethargy, and hypotonia, but no evidence of congenital defects when used alone.
Gabapentin	C_M	Limited human data do not allow an assessment of safety in pregnancy. If *required*, the benefits of therapy appear to outweigh potential risks to the fetus.
Lamotrigine	C_M	First trimester monotherapy exposure possible associations include esophageal malformation, cleft soft palate, and right club foot. Congenital malformations increase when used with other anticonvulsants.
Antidepressant		
Amitriptyline	C_M	Occasional reports have associated amitriptyline with congenital malformations, but the bulk of evidence indicates relative safety during pregnancy, and preferred over other antidepressants.
Dothiepin	D	No fetal risk data available. See Imipramine.
Imipramine	D	Possible association with cardiovascular defects, defective abdominal muscles, diaphragmatic hernia, exencephaly, cleft palate, adrenal hypoplasia, and renal cystic degeneration. Neonatal withdrawal symptoms have been reported.
Fluoxetine	C_M	Available data indicate no relation to major congenital malformations. However, increased risk of spontaneous abortion (miscarriage) and fetal brain development are mildly associated. In one study, infants exposed to the drug late in pregnancy experienced a significant increase in perinatal complications (e.g. prematurity, poor neonatal adaptation, pulmonary hypertension).
Nortriptyline	D	Limb reduction anomalies and neonatal urinary retention have been reported.

table continues

Table 8.12 continued

Drug type		Description
Antihistamines		
Chlorpheniramine	B	Most exposures involve decongestant combinations including adrenergics.
Diphenhydramine	B_M	Possible association with cleft palate (one case-control study).
Promethazine	C	Possible cardiovascular defects. During labor, impaired platelet aggregation, more so in newborn than in mother.
Anti-infectives		
Amebicides		
Metronidazole	B_M	Conflicting safety conclusions; majority of published evidence suggests no significant risk to fetus.
Aminoglycosides		
Amikacin and tobramycin	C*	Eight cranial nerve toxicity is well known. Ototoxicity occurs in humans, has not been reported as an effect of in utero exposure. (*Risk factor D according to manufacturers.)
Gentamicin and neomycin	C	Ototoxicity occurs in humans, has not been reported as an effect of in utero exposure.
Streptomycin	D_M	Small risk of deafness.

table continues

Table 8.12 continued

Drug type		Description
Antibiotics/anti-infectives		
Azithromycin	B$_M$	No association with malformations found.
Bacitracin	C	Although apparently non-toxic to fetus, use with caution at term; possible cardiovascular collapse in newborns.
Chloramphenicol	C	
Chlorhexidine	B	
Clarithromycin	C$_M$	Further study warranted regarding spontaneous abortions (miscarriages).
Clavulanate potassium	B$_M$	Small possibility of spina bifida; other factors and chance may be involved.
Clindamycin and erythromycin	B$_M$	
Polymyxin B	B	
Trimethoprim	C$_M$	Suggestion of structural effects when used during first trimester. (Supplemental folic acid may reduce risk.)
Vancomycin	B$_M$	
Antifungals		
Amphotericin B	B$_M$	
Clotrimazole	B	
Fluconazole	C$_M$	Use during first trimester appears teratogenic (anatomic defects) with continuous daily doses of 400 mg/day or more.
Griseofulvin	C	Possible association with birth of conjoined twins.
Itraconazole	C$_M$	Because of possible dose-related defects, it is considered safer to avoid this drug, if possible, during organogenesis.
		Limb anomalies reported.
Ketoconazole	C$_M$	Possible association with birth defects (unspecified) and spontaneous abortions (miscarriages).
Miconazole	C$_M$	Possible association with congenital malformations (unspecified).
Nystatin	C$_M$	

table continues

Table 8.12 continued

Drug type		Description
Antimalarials		
Dapsone	C_M	If used in combination with pyrimethamine (folic acid antagonist) for malaria prophylaxis, folic acid supplements should be given.
Hydroxychloroquine	C	Malarial prophylactic doses not harmful to fetus. Higher doses for prolonged periods probably represents increased fetal risk.
Antimigraine		
Ergotamine	X_M	Produces a prolonged and marked increase in uterine tone that may lead to fetal hypoxia. Small, infrequent doses do not appear fetotoxic or teratogenic, but idiosyncratic responses may occur that endanger the fetus.
Sumatriptan	C_M	Does not appear to present a major teratogenic risk in humans. The number and follow-up of exposed pregnancies are too limited to assess, with confidence, the safety of this agent.
Antivirals		
Acyclovir	B_M	Drug of choice when indicated.
Famciclovir	B_M	
Foscarnet	C_M	Because of the frequent occurrence of renal toxicity in adults, it is recommended to observe for fetal renal toxicity.
Ganciclovir	C_M	Should only be used during pregnancy for life-threatening disease or in immunocompromised patients with major CMV infections
Valacyclovir	B_M	
Cephalosporins		
Cefazolin	B_M	

table continues

Table 8.12 continued

Drug type		Description
Cholinergics		
Pilocarpine	C_M	A single report of topical use of pilocarpine for glaucoma throughout gestation revealed an infant presenting with hyperbilirubinemia, hypocalcemia, hypomagnesemia, and metabolic acidosis.
Cevimeline		The very limited animal data for Cevimeline, which did not include exposure during organogenesis, and the lack of any reported human pregnancy experience, prevents an assessment of its risk during pregnancy.
Corticosteroids		
Hydrocortisone	C^*	Decrease in birth weight and small increase in the incidence of cleft lip with or without cleft
Cortisone		palate. Should not be withheld if mother's condition requires use of these agents.
Prednisone		(*Risk factor D if used in first trimester.)
Triamcinolone		
Hemostatic		
Aminocaproic acid	C_M	No fetal toxicity observed. No reports describing placental passage have been located.
Tranexamic acid	B_M	No adverse effects during pregnancy have been reported.
Immunosuppresant		
Azathioprine	D_M	Intrauterine growth retardation may be related to the use of this drug.
Mycophenolate	C_M	No reports of use during pregnancy have been located. Because of potential for congenital
Mofetil		defects, manufacturer recommends that women of childbearing potential use effective contraception before and during therapy and for 6 weeks post-therapy.

table continues

Table 8.12 continued

Drug type		Description
Tacrolimus	C_M	Has demonstrated abortifacient properties in three animal species and dose-related teratogenicity in one, but use of this agent during human pregnancy has not been associated with either of these outcomes, although number of exposed fetuses is small.
Thalidomide	X_M	Limb, spinal, jaw, craniofacial and CNS defects along with major organ defects have been reported. Contraindicated during pregnancy and in women of childbearing age who are not receiving two reliable methods of contraception for 1 month prior to starting therapy, during therapy, and for 1 month post-therapy.
Muscle relaxant		
Baclofen	C	Because of its specialized indication to control spasticity secondary to multiple sclerosis and other spinal cord diseases and injuries, its use in pregnancy is anticipated to be limited. Only two reports of use in human pregnancy have been reported, both of which revealed delivery of normal infants.
Carisoprodol	C	No reproductive studies in animals. Two cases of oral clefts in humans in one study reveal the suggestion of a possible association.
Chlorzoxazone	C	Combined data in one human study do not support an association between the drug and congenital defects.
Cyclobenzaprine	B_M	Closely related to the tricyclic antidepressants. No published reports of use in human pregnancy.
Narcotic agonist analgesic		
Codeine	C^*	Significant association with respiratory malformation; milder associations with genitourinary defects, Down syndrome, tumors, umbilical and inguinal hernias. Possible associations have been reported with hydrocephaly and pyloric stenosis. (*Risk factor D if used for prolonged periods or in high doses at term.)

table continues

Table 8.12 continued

Drug type		Description
Fentanyl	C_M*	No reports linking the use of fentanyl with congenital defects have been located. One case report of respiratory muscle rigidity in a newborn. (*Risk factor D if used for prolonged periods or in high doses at term.)
Hydrocodone	C*	Related to codeine. Suggestion of possible association exists between this agent and congenital malformations. (*Risk Factor D if used for prolonged periods or in high doses at term.)
Hydromorphone	B*	Use during pregnancy primarily confined to labor. Respiratory depression in the neonate similar to that produced by meperidine [pethidine] or morphine should be expected. (*Risk factor D if used for prolonged periods or in high doses at term.)
Meperidine [pethidine]	B*	Fetal problems have not been reported from the therapeutic use of this agent in pregnancy except when given during labor. (*Risk factor D if used for prolonged periods or in high doses at term.)
Morphine	C_M*	No reports linking the therapeutic use of morphine with major congenital defects have been located. A possible association with inguinal hernia after anytime use was observed. (*Risk factor D if used for prolonged periods or in high doses at term.)
Propoxyphene	C*	Possible associations after anytime use are: microcephaly, ductus arteriosus persistens, cataract, benign tumors and clubfoot.
Sedative/hypnotic		
Chloral hydrate	C_M	No reports of congenital defects have been located.
Chlordiazepoxide	D	When exposed during the first 42 days of gestation, the following defects have been observed: mental deficiency, spastic diplegia and deafness, microcephaly and retardation, duodenal atresia, and Meckel's diverticulum.

table continues

Table 8.12 continued

Drug type		Description
Diazepam	D	Fetal effects are controversial. Alcohol and smoking may be confounding factors. Continuous use during pregnancy has resulted in neonatal withdrawal. If the maternal condition requires the use of diazepam, the lowest possible dose should be taken. Abrupt discontinuance of this drug should be avoided.
Lorazepam	D_M	High IV doses or continuous oral use may produce 'floppy infant' syndrome. Some association with anal atresia.
Midazolam	D_M	Has a depressant effect on newborns when used for anesthetic induction prior to cesarean sections.
Temazepam	X_M	Possible association with oral cleft. Potential interaction between this agent and diphenydramine, resulting in stillbirth.
Triazolam	X_M	Although no congenital anomalies have been attributed to this agent, other benzodiazepines (e.g. diazepam) have been suspected of producing fetal malformations after first trimester exposure.
Zolpidem	B_M	Data too limited to assess embryonic or fetal safety.

From: Briggs G C, Freeman R K, Yaffe S J 2002 A reference guide to fetal and neonatal risk: drugs in pregnancy and lactation. Lippincott Williams & Wilkins, with permisson.

Table 8.13   Drugs and medications of concern in dental practice

Drug	Concern
Aminophylline	Avoid erythromycin, clarithromycin
Antibiotics	Some antibiotics may cause reduced contraceptive effect (unproven)
Antifungals	Reduced contraceptive effect with itraconazole, fluconazole
Antiplatelet agents (e.g. clopidogrel, dipyridamole/ASA, ticlopidine)	Bleeding
Aspirin*	Potential for bleeding, especially gastric. Potentiation for oral bleeding not established.
Calcium channel blockers (e.g. nifedipine, diltiazem)	Gingival overgrowth, hyperplasia
Coumadin	Bleeding; may be enhanced with aspirin and some NSAIDS, erythromycin, fluconazole, metronidazole, sulfamethoxazole, trimethoprim, gingko. Reduced anticoagulant effect with carbamazepine, nafcillin and vitamin K.
Isoproterenol	Avoid epinephrine
Lithium	Xerostomia, infection, neutropenia, renal failure, stomatitis
MAO inhibitors	Xerostomia, hypotension, tachycardia, arrhythmias
Neuroleptics	Xerostomia, hypotension, tachycardia, arrhythmias, bleeding, thrombocytopenia, infection, neutropenia
Phenytoin	Gingival overgrowth, hyperplasia
Prednisone	Consider supplementation for stressful procedures
Theophylline	Avoid erythromycin, clarithromycin

Arachadonic acid
Endoperoxides
$\downarrow$ cyclo-oxygenase
$\downarrow$ thromboxane $A_2 \rightarrow$ platelet aggregation and vasoconstriction

*Antiplatelet effect due to acetylation of cyclo-oxygenase and suppression of thromboxane A_2 production. At least 95% of thromboxane is required for effective platelet function. A single dose of 100 mg is required to achieve this level, which occurs 15–30 min after ingestion of standard (not controlled release) aspirin. After the last dose there is little or no recovery of thromboxane for 2–3 days. Aspirin has some effect in suppressing platelets released from megakaryocytes over the next several days. Thus, platelet suppression continues for over 48 h. A total turnover of the platelet pool takes about 8 days.

Table 8.14 **Emergency room kit**

Instruments (color-coded)

1. Mirror
2. Locking cotton pliers
3. Dental syringe – aspirating
4. Forceps – Upper/lower universal, ash, anterior, cowhorn
5. Elevators – Woodson, periosteal, number 34, 301, 302, 303
6. Needles 25, 27 or 30 g. short and long
7. Curettes, scalers
8. Scalpel handle (disposable) and blades
9. Needle holder
10. Hemostat (Kelly)
11. Scissors (suture)
12. Tissue pick-ups
13. Explorer
14. Perio probe
15. Calcium hydroxide applicator
16. Spatula
17. Plastic instrument
18. Rubber dam frame, punch, forceps
19. Dappen dish
20. Flashlight – if operating light not available
21. Composite Instrument
22. X-ray holder (XCP, snap-a-ray, styrofoam stabes)

Paper or disposable products

1. Cotton pellets and cotton rolls
2. Gauze – 2 × 2s and 4 × 4s
3. Cotton-tipped applicators
4. Alcohol wipes
5. Calcium hydroxide mixing pads
6. Etching pellets or brush
7. Rubber dam
8. Appropriate suture material
9. Floss
10. Irrigating syringe
11. Number 11 and 15 blades
12. Wooden bite stick
13. Rubber gloves
14. Endodontic irrigating syringes/tips
15. Iodoform gauze (for dry socket)

Materials

1. Calcium hydroxide/barium sulfate paste with needles
2. Composite resin – self-curing or light activated. Etching liquid. Bonding agent
3. Topical anesthetic
4. Calcium hydroxide liner
5. Anesthetic:
   lidocaine 2%, 1:100 000 [1:80 000] mepivacaine bupivacaine
6. Wire or 'nylon' line for splinting
7. Unreinforced ZOE
8. Absorbable gelatin sponge/surgicel/Avitene
9. Vaseline
10. Temporary cement
11. Reinforced ZOE
12. 0.030 wire
13. Erich arch bar
14. No. 0, 2 intraoral films
15. Dry socket paste
16. Topical thrombin (5000 μ/cc, 10 000 μ/cc)
17. Sav-a-tooth solution/Hank's balanced salt solution
18. Cavit, paper points, barbed broches (pulp exturpation)

Miscellaneous

1. Surgical tray
2. Additional forceps and elevators
3. Wire cutters
4. 'Orthodontic' pliers
5. Curing light for composite
6. Endodontic files, solutions and medicaments

Table 8.15 Facial pain – diagnostic features

Disorder	Etiology	Signs and symptoms	Tests	Therapy considerations
Myofascial pain dysfunction (MPD)	Bruxism, clenching, nail biting, gum chewing, lip or cheek biting, pipe smoking, etc. Aberrant occlusion, history of trauma, displaced disc or unknown. Rare in < 18 yo. Secondary to 'stress', anxiety and sometimes depression	Unilateral pain, joint noise, limited function, tenderness to palpation of muscles of mastication, deviation of mandible on opening, emotionally stressed individual, parafunctional habits		Emergency: rest joints and eliminate habits, moist heat, muscle relaxants. Long term splint, refrigerant spray, anesthetic intramuscular injection, counseling. Occlusal adjustment only if clearly contributes to the problem and only when no longer in muscle spasm
Temporomandibular dysfunction (TMD)	Most commonly osteodegenerative arthritis (although rheumatoid arthritis, infection and trauma also possible). Rare in < 18 yo	Pain in joint, crepitus, deviation to affected side, limitation in function	CT or MRI scan to show disc position, if refractory to conservative treatment. TMJ radiograph may show flattening of articular surfaces, spurring of condyles, narrowing of joint, space(s) and ankylosis	Moist heat, anti-inflammatory drugs, cortisone injection, elimination of oral habits, eliminate gross occlusal prematurities

Table 8.15 continued

Disorder	Etiology	Signs and symptoms	Tests	Therapy considerations
Maxillary sinusitis	Viral or bacterial infection of sinus mucosa	Headache, increased temperature, malaise, edema and redness beneath eyes, worst in morning, improves with sitting up, tenderness on sinus palpation	Waters and/or panorex film may suggest sinusitis, but not diagnostic	Antibiotics, decongestants, consider referral to physician/ otolaryngologist
Ear pain	External otitis, foreign body, furunculosis, impacted cerumen, otitis media, mastoiditis, blocked eustachian tube, nasopharyngeal carcinoma	Ear pain must be differentiated from 'otomandibular' syndrome associated with myofascial pain dysfunction	Examine ear canal and TM	Refer to otolaryngologist if otalgic in origin
Iatrogenic pain	Misdirected mandibular injection. Prolonged wide opening during dental procedure	Trismus and pain in area of medial pterygoid muscle 3–4 days postinjection or procedure, and lasting up to several weeks		Analgesics, moist heat, soft diet, jaw-opening exercises
	Altered occlusion from high restoration	Pain in one or more teeth and/or face prosthesis	Check for occlusion prematurities	Adjust occlusion

table continues

Table 8.15 continued

Disorder	Etiology	Signs and symptoms	Tests	Therapy considerations
Parotid gland disease	Infection, tumor	Fever, enlarged gland, purulent exudate from duct	Biopsy, sialogram or CT/MRI	Aggressive antibiotic treatment for infection. May be prolonged treatment in the case of childhood parotitis
Temporal arteritis	Granulomatous lesion of temporal artery	Pain in front of ear, pain on mastication, visual impairment. Similar to MPD	C reaction protein, temporal artery biopsy (lymphocytic infiltration)	Referral to medical specialist immediately for corticosteroid treatment
Eagle's syndrome	Elongation of styloid process	Pain on swallowing, turning of head, extreme pain on palpation of tonsillar fauces	Panoramic, radiograph	Surgical
Trigeminal neuralgia	Disorder of branches of trigeminal nerve	Unilateral lancinating pain of short duration stimulated by specific trigger areas	Anesthetic to trigger zone results in total relief	Referral to specialist

table continues

Table 8.15 continued

Disorder	Etiology	Signs and symptoms	Tests	Therapy considerations
Migraine	Pain may be associated with headache	Unilateral temporal pain, with spasm of temporal muscle, stimulated by vasodilation	No tests. Often have prodromal sensory visceral effects	Refer to specialist
Neoplasms	Tumors involving parotid, trigeminal nerve, nasopharynx, sphenoid sinus	Pain may be associated with numbness or loss of motor function	Direct visualization of all mucosal surfaces and radiographic examination	Referral to appropriate surgical service (e.g. otolaryngologist)
Post-traumatic	Trauma	Set-off by deep pressure at the injury site. Dysesthesias and neurotropic effects noted	Nerve block results in partial relief	Analgesics are effective
Systemic disease	Variable hereditary and emotional factors	Pain is spontaneous, usually in appendages, extraocular muscles. Dysesthesias noted and neurotropic effects in hands	Nerve block results in partial relief	Analgesics are effective

Fluoride Tray Construction (*continued from p. 334*)

Method

- Obtain full arch alginate impressions of both upper and lower teeth.
- Pour a stone or plaster model.
- Trim the model and create a hole through the midpalate and/or midfloor of mouth space.
- Mark the periphery of the tray, on the gingiva of the model, 1–2 mm beyond the gingival margin.
- Heat a sheet of mouth guard plastic on the vacuum former.
- Heat the plastic until it sags at least one inch. Turn the vacuum on and lower the plastic onto the model; allow it to cool.
- Transcribe a line on the plastic with an ink pen over the existing line on the model while it is still on the plaster model. The tray is then removed and trimmed to the marked line.
- Replace the tray on the model and sear all margins carefully until smooth using a Hanau torch with an air stream.
- Allow the tray to cool.
- Deliver the tray to the patient with a prescription for neutral sodium or stannous fluoride, 10–15 drops per tray, to be used every night for 5 min after brushing and flossing. Neutral sodium fluoride may be necessary for patients with mucositis.

HEAD INJURY SHEET

Figure 8.3 shows an example of an instruction sheet for patients with head injuries.

INFECTIOUS DISEASE AND UNIVERSAL PRECAUTIONS

With the current epidemic status of human immunodeficiency virus (HIV), along with hepatitis B and hepatitis C, the proper management of all patients is of paramount importance. Most patients are asymptomatic but points to consider include:

- Approximately 10% of patients with a history of hepatitis B are chronic carriers.
- There is a higher incidence of hepatitis B virus antigen in intravenous drug abusers, alcoholics, institutionalized [residential

Fig. 8.3 **Instruction sheet for patients with head injuries**

_____ (Hospital)   _____ (Doctor's Name)

_____ (Address)   _____ (Phone)

HEAD INJURY SHEET

Dr. _____ has examined you for evidence of brain injury
Signs of trouble could develop later at home, and we ask you to be on
the lookout for them.

SIGNS OF TROUBLE

1. Increasing drowsiness, hard to arouse (If the patient is alert and easily
   awakened, (s)he is probably safe).

2. Other signs:
   Unequal pupil size   Problems with vision or "seeing double"
   Vomiting   Headache
   "Convulsions" (fits)   Bleeding or clear fluid from the ears or nose
   Numbness   Stumbling or other problems with arms or legs
   Confusion

INSTRUCTIONS

Return to this clinic/emergency department if you are concerned or if you
experience any of the signs of trouble listed above.

1. Patient should rest at home for the next 24 hours with someone who
   can check on them at least every four hours.

2. During this period, no alcoholic beverages should be taken.

3. Arousal periodically for children if sleeping

4. Follow-up appointment, if needed. Specify where and when.

care] individuals, renal dialysis patients, recent immigrants and
individuals who work with blood products.

- Hepatitis B antigen/antibody tests determine hepatitis B carrier
  status but are not liver function test markers.
- By the end of 1994, approximately 440 000 cases of AIDS have
  been reported to the Centers for Disease Control (CDC). Of HIV-
  infected individuals, 20–50% develop AIDS in 5–10 years.
- The HIV antibody test is useful to determine whether a person has
  been exposed to the HIV virus. For an individual to be considered

HIV seropositive, two ELISA and one Western blot assays must be positive for HIV antibodies. There is a 'window' period of up to 6 months from infection to seroconversion. A positive HIV antibody test necessitates a physician consult for more specific immune system profile testing (CD4 lymphocyte marker panel) and management. It must be remembered that HIV testing carries with it a social, psychologic and financial (e.g. insurance, loans) stigma and should be used with discretion and reassurance to the patient.

- HIV testing is protected under strict confidentiality laws, which vary by state. It requires pre- and post-test counseling. HIV patients are protected from discrimination under section 504 of the Federal Rehabilitation Act of 1973, as well as by the Americans with Disabilities Act, which came into effect in January 1992. In the United Kingdom, the Disability Discrimination Act of 1995 makes it unlawful to treat people with disabilities differently.

- An increased incidence of concomitant infectious diseases (e.g. TB, hepatitis B and C, venereal diseases) has been seen in HIV patients and should be considered when treating.

Treatment

Treatment decisions should take into account the hematologic and immunologic status of the patient (i.e. need for platelet or antibiotic support) and advisability of elective procedures, etc.

Universal precautions

- Due to the latency of onset of disease and inability to identify all infected individuals, all patients should be treated as if they carry an infectious disease.

- Protective attire should include clothing that covers the arms. Masks, gloves and protective eyewear must be used in situations where there is risk of splashing of bodily fluids. Consideration should be given to scrub suits and OR [theatre] gowns when using high-speed handpieces and with ultrasonic cleaning instruments.

- Operatories [surgeries] where high speed drills are used should be as utilitarian as possible to ensure cleansability.

- To minimize the risk for cross-contamination, protective plastic or aluminum equipment sleeves (e.g. on light handles, X-ray heads) or drapes should be used where possible.

- To avoid cross-contamination, equipment and materials needs should be anticipated. This minimizes the need to enter central supply areas. Preset tub/tray systems should be considered.
- All impressions and equipment should be disinfected/sterilized according to the manufacturer's directions and OSHA/CDC guidelines.
- All intraoral film packets should be disinfected.
- Rubber dam usage with high-speed suction will minimize aerosol spray contamination of the treatment environment.
- Clean-up:
  - All organic debris should be removed from instruments using ultrasonic cleaners where possible and according to the manufacturer's directions. All instruments should be sterilized according to manufacturer's/CDC/OSHA guidelines.
  - All handpieces should be scrubbed clean of any debris, run with water spray for 3 to 5 min, rewiped and sterilized according to manufacturer's directions.
  - All sharps and blood- or saliva-soaked material should be disposed of in biohazard containers.
- It is strongly suggested that the reader become familiar with hospital, national and federal regulations regarding infectious disease issues; they carry with them some significant medicolegal implications.

OPERATING ROOM [THEATRE]: DRESS CODE

The appearance and dress of operating room [theatre] staff must adhere to the principles of safety, infection control and professional standards. Adherence to these standards will lessen the opportunity for workers to serve as potential sources of infection.

The human body is a major source of microbial contamination within the OR [theatre] environment. As it is not possible to sterilize skin, hair and mucous membranes, other measures must be taken to reduce this source of potential pathogens.

Scrubs and gowns

All personnel entering restricted areas of the surgical suite should be attired in operating room apparel. At no time should street clothes be worn within the restricted areas of the surgical suite.

Hair covers

All head and facial hair, including sideburns and neckline, should be covered in semirestricted and restricted areas of the surgical suite:

- The surgical scrub cap or surgical hood should be clean and free of lint. Nets are not acceptable.
- Surgical caps or hoods must be changed upon returning to the surgical suite.

Shoe covers

All personnel entering the restricted areas of the surgical suite should wear shoe covers:

- Shoe covers are removed upon leaving restricted areas of the suite.
- Clean shoe covers are put on upon returning to the restricted area.

Masks

All personnel should wear high-filtration masks in specified restricted areas of the surgical suite:

- Masks should be worn at all times in the OR [theatre] and other designated areas (the room in which the patient's surgical procedure is performed).
- The mask should cover both the nose and mouth and be secured to prevent venting at the sides.
- Masks are worn either on or off. They are not to be saved by hanging around the neck or tucked into a pocket for future use.
- When removing the mask, only the strings should be touched; this reduces contamination of the hands from the nasopharyngeal and oral organisms.

Personal effects

- Nail polish should not be worn by OR [theatre] personnel. Fingernails should be kept clean and short. Artificial nails should not be worn.
- Earrings, if worn at all, must be small and unobtrusive, and worn under a scrub hat.

- Chains and necklaces must be contained inside the scrub shirt. Rings, watches and bracelets should be removed.

OPERATING ROOM [THEATRE]: SCRUB TECHNIQUE

Many hospitals have changed the time-honored hand and arm scrub method with a brush and soap to a brushless scrub with scrub solution alone. One method is as follows:

- Use a nail pick to clean under fingernails to remove dirt and debris. Turn water on and wet hands and arms.
- Hold an open palm under solution dispenser port then depress the foot pump, dispensing approximately a 2-cm blob of solution into palm.
- Begin by cupping palm with solution, then insert opposite hands' fingertips into solution. Then twist fingertips around for a few seconds. Repeat with other hand.
- Rub hands together, beginning with both hands then moving up to forearm region, extending slightly past the elbows.
- Scrub for 90 seconds.
- Rinse thoroughly, then repeat steps 2–4, stopping before the elbow on the second application. Total scrub time is 3 min.

PATIENT TRANSFER

Rationale

The sophisticated rehabilitative and restorative surgical procedures of which dentistry is capable depend on operator visualization and access. These, in turn, depend on appropriate patient positioning and orientation of the light source. Wherever possible, patients should receive restorative dental treatment in a fully adjustable dental chair with articulating headrest, both for the success of the outcome and out of consideration for operator fatigue and stress. In the hospital environment, this ideal can be compromised if patients present to the dental clinic in a wheelchair. However, the wheelchair should not be viewed as an inalterable appendage – it is often merely a transport mechanism necessitated by reason of medico-legal consideration or patient frailty or confusion. For this reason, dentists working in the hospital environment must be comfortable in transferring a patient from wheelchair to dental chair, and vice versa, if the opportunity is not available to incorporate the patient's wheelchair into a custom-made dental unit.

Pretransfer assessment

- Can the patient transfer independently, or with what level of assistance (ask patient; check nursing notes)? Stroke patients tend to overestimate their abilities. Always be prepared to assist the patient when getting up from wheelchair or dental chair.
- If capability is uncertain, can the patient follow directions?
- If the patient has a stronger side, which is it? Always transfer patient to the stronger side!
- If the patient is sitting on a canvas sling, this is evidence that a mechanical/hydraulic lift (a 'Hoyer or C-lift') is necessary for transfer. Such a device can be obtained from the ward or the OR [theatre] but should not be employed without instruction and supervision.
- After dental treatment, a patient with orthostatic hypotension might need to be raised from the prone position in increments and allowed to sit for a few minutes before transfer from the dental chair.
- Whenever possible, utilize the hospital staff to complete the transfer. They may be familiar with the patient and aware of the patient's transfer requirements.
- Ask the transport personnel how the patient was transferred to the wheelchair.
- Back injuries are a common hospital occupational injury, do not attempt a transfer without proper training and assistance.

Minimize physical barriers

- Check the patient for IV lines, drains and cannulas to make sure these are not removed during transfer. Wear gloves during transfer if there is a chance of contact with body fluids.
- Remove waist restraints, vest restraints and leg or arm restraints (such items are only for patient safety or to minimize contractures, and should not be viewed as a sign of a combative or dangerous patient).

- Locate catheter hoses and collecting bags, IV poles, infusion pumps, oxygen lines or other therapeutic attachments in such a way as to pose no impediment to an efficient transfer.
- Remove everything possible from the wheelchair on the side to which transfer will be effected: arm rest, brake arm, leg support, foot support.
- Raise, retract or remove the patient's arm from dental chair to allow unimpeded transfer.

Preparation for the transfer

- For a slideboard assist: position wheelchair parallel to the dental chair. The chair should be at the same height or 3–6 inches lower than the wheelchair.
- For a minimal assist transfer: position wheelchair in the optimal position as described by the patient, but modified to allow the operator clear access to the patient in the event of unsteadiness.
- For a one-person transfer: position the chair parallel to the dental chair, with the patient's stronger side adjacent to the dental chair. The chair should be 3–6 inches lower than the wheelchair.
- For a two-person transfer: position the chair parallel to the dental chair and facing the same direction as the dental chair, with the dental chair 3–6 inches lower than the wheelchair.
- Set the brakes on the wheelchair.
- Explain clearly and slowly the procedure that will be followed in the transfer. Make sure the patient understands his or her role.

The transfer

- Slideboard transfer: the patient will effect the transfer. When complete, release the brakes and move the chair.
- Minimal assist: prior to patient transfer, place a hand on patient's belt or waistband, or beneath patient's arm, to steady patient if necessary. When complete, release the brakes and move the chair.
- One-person transfer: ask hemiplegic patients to hold the dependent arm with the intact arm. For all one-person assists, have patients:
  - bend forward at the waist until nearly doubled over
  - place their weight on the good leg (the one nearer the dental chair)

- ○ rise slowly into the operator's grasp, as the operator gently pulls forward and up
- ○ allow the operator to swivel the patient 90°.
- ○ allow the operator to ease the patient down into dental chair.
- Two-person transfer:
  - ○ make sure the patient's arms are crossed
  - ○ one operator stands, with knees slightly bent, behind patient and grips patient's elbows
  - ○ the other operator stands, with knees slightly bent, at the patient's knees, and grasps the patient's legs behind the knees and the calves
  - ○ the operator behind the patient counts 'one-two-three'; on three, both operators straighten their knees and lift patient out of wheelchair and into dental chair.
- Transferring the patient back to the wheelchair: the return transfer is the reverse of the preceding procedure. Some particular reminders:
  - ○ If the patient had a 'strong side', the wheelchair will need to face the opposite direction that it did before. In addition, any removable portions of the wheelchair will need to be replaced and the hardware on the opposite side removed.
  - ○ As before, position all catheter hoses and collecting bags, IV poles, infusion pumps, oxygen lines or other therapeutic attachments so that they will not interfere with the transfer.
  - ○ When the wheelchair is positioned, lock the brakes.
  - ○ Raise the dental chair so that it is 3–6 inches higher than the wheelchair.
  - ○ When transfer is complete, replace all restraints, hoses, lines, IV poles, etc.

RENAL FUNCTION – ADJUSTMENT OF DOSAGE

Table 8.16 presents general guidelines for use of various doses in renal failure with modification in dose interval according to degree of failure.

Antibiotic and antifungal dosing in renal dysfunction

The initial dose of the antifungal or antibiotic drug should be the same as for a patient with normal renal function to achieve a therapeutic blood level. The maintenance dose should then be reduced. Doses are based on a 70-kg adult (Table 8.17).

Table 8.16 Renal function – adjustment of dosage

Drug	Excretion	Normal	Mild renal failure Creatinine clearance 50–75 cc/min	Moderate renal failure Creatinine clearance 10–50 cc/min	Severe renal failure Creatinine clearance <10 cc/min	Significant dialysis of drug
Narcotic and non-narcotic analgesics						
Codeine	Hepatic >> renal	Every 6 h	Every 6 h	Every 6 h	Every 6 h	Unknown
Meperidine [pethidine]	Hepatic >> renal (10%)	Every 4 h	Every 4 h	Every 4 h	Every 4 h	No (HP)
Acetaminophen [paracetamol]	Hepatic >> renal	Every 4 h	Every 4 h	Every 4 h	Avoid	Yes (H)
Aspirin	Renal	Every 4 h	Every 4 h	Every 4–6 h	Every 8–12 h	Yes (HP)
Barbiturates and benzodiazepines						
Amobarbital Secobarbital	Hepatic	Every 6–12 h	Every 6–12 h	Every 6–12 h	Every 6–12 h	No (HP)
Phenobarbital	Hepatic > renal (30%)	Every 8 h	Every 8 h	Every 8 h	Every 8–16 h	Yes (HP)
Chlordiazepoxide	Hepatic	Every 8 h	Every 8 h	Every 8 h	Every 8 h	No (HP)
Diazepam	Hepatic	Every 8 h	Every 8 h	Every 8 h	Every 8 h	No (HP)
Meprobamate	Hepatic > renal (10%)	Every 6 h	Every 6 h	Every 9–12 h	Every 9–18 h	Yes (HP)
Lidocaine (cardiac)	Hepatic	Intravenous drip or bolus	No change	No change		No (H)

(H) = Hemodialysis
(P) = Peritoneal dialysis

Table 8.17 Dose adjustment after initial dose

Drug	Creatinine clearance normal	> 50 cc/min	30–50 cc/min	10–29 cc/min	< 10 cc/min
Antifungal					
Fluconazole (Difflucan)	200–400 mg q24h	200–400 mg q24h	Decrease dose by 50%		Decrease dose by 50%. Administer dose after hemodialysis
Erythromycin	0.5–1 G q6h	No changes necessary			0.5–1 G q12h
Amoxicillin	250–500 mg q8h or 500–875 mg q12h	No change needed		250–500 q12h	250–500 q24h
Amoxicillin/clavulanate	250–500 mg q8h or 875 mg q12h	No change needed		250–500 q12h	250–500 q24h
Ampicillin IV	1–2 G q4–6h	1–2 G q6h	1–2 G q8h	1–2 G q12h	1–2 G q12–24h Give after HD
Ampicillin/sulbactam (Unasyn)	1.5–3 G q6h	1.5–3 G q6h	1.5–3 G q6–8h	1.5–3 G q12h	1.5–3 G q24h Give after hemodialysis
Dicloxacillin	250–500 mg q6h	No changes necessary			
Penicillin G IV	0.5–4 million units q4h	No change needed		75% of dose	20–50% of dose Give after HD
Penicillin VK	250–500 mg q6h	No change needed			250 mg q6h PO
Ticarcillin/clavulanate (Timentin)	3.1 G q4–6h	3.1 G q6h	2 G q6h	2 G q8h	2 G q12h

table continues

Table 8.17 continued

Drug	Creatinine clearance normal	> 50 cc/min	30–50 cc/min	10–29 cc/min	< 10 cc/min
Ciproflozacin [Ciprofloxacin] PO IV	500–750 mg q12h 400 mg q8–12h	500–750 mg q12h 400 mg q8–12h	500–750 mg q12h 400 mg q8–12h	500–750 mg q24h 400 mg q24h	500–750 mg q24h 400 mg q24h
Cliindamycin	PO: 150–450 mg q6h IV: 600–1200 mg q8h	No changes necessary			
Doxycycline	100 mg q12h IV or PO	No changes necessary. Tetracycline of choice for decreased RF.			Not antianabolic.
Metronidazole (Flagyl)	500 mg IV/PO q8h for *C. difficile*: 250 mg PO QID [200 TDS in the UK]	No changes necessary			

This chart is intended as a guide only. Doses of medications should be verified with a standard reference.

SPLINT CONSTRUCTION – ANESTHESIA

Definition

A carefully molded splint from a vacuum former is used to stabilize periodontally or prosthetically (e.g. crowns, bridges) involved teeth by distributing any forces delivered during intubation over as many additional teeth as possible. Used primarily for maxillary anterior teeth during intubation, it might also be desirable for electro-convulsive therapy.

Method

- Obtain an alginate impression of the maxillary teeth.
- Pour a stone or plaster model.
- A sheet of mouthguard soft plastic and 0.020 thickness hard plastic are placed on the vacuum former, with the 0.020 on top (closest to the heat).
- The sheets are heated until they sag below the vacuum former frame.
- The vacuum is turned on and softened sheets are lowered onto the model.
- When cool, the model is removed and plastic material is trimmed to the gingival area.
- All margins are smoothed lightly with an acrylic bur and a heated Hanau torch flame.
- Disinfection or sterilization as needed.
- Attach to the patient's chart or give to the anesthesiologist.

STEROIDS: TOPICAL AGENTS AND STEROID MILLIGRAM EQUIVALENTS (TABLES 8.18 AND 8.19)

Table 8.18 **Corticosteroids – systemic equivalents**

Agent	Equivalent anti-inflammatory dose (mg)
Cortisone (Cortone)	25
Hydrocortisone (A-hydroCort®, Solu-Cortef®)	20
Prednisolone (AK-Pred®, Prelone)	5
Prednisone (Deltasone®, Orasone)	5
Methylprednisolone (Medrol®, Depo-Medrol®, A-methaPred®, Solu-Medrol®)	4
Triamcinolone (Aristocort®, Aristospan®, Kenacort®)	4
Dexamethasone (Decadron®, Hexadrol®, Dexasone®)	0.75
Betamethasone (Celestone®)	0.6

Table 8.19 **Topical steroids**

Steroid	Generic	Brand	Vehicle
Low potency			
1.0%	Hydrocortisone	Cort-Dome Cortef [Efcortelan]	Cream, lotion, Ointment
2.5%	Hydrocortisone	Synacort	Cream, ointment
Medium potency			
0.1%	Betamethasone valerate	Valisone [Betnovate]	Cream, lotion
0.1%	Triamcinolone acetonide	Aristocort, Kenalog [Adcortyl]	Cream, ointment, lotion
0.025%	Triamcinolone acetonide	Aristocort, Kenalog [Adcortyl]	Cream
High potency			
0.05%	Fluocinonide	Lidex [Metosyn]	Cream, ointment, solution, gel
0.5%	Triamcinolone acetonide	Aristocort A, Kenalog [Adcortyl]	Cream, ointment
Very high potency			
0.05%	Clobetasol propionate	Temovate [Dermovate]	Cream, ointment, gel
0.05%	Halobetasol propionate	Ultravate	Cream, ointment

SUTURE MATERIALS (TABLE 8.20)

VENIPUNCTURE AND BLOOD SPECIMEN TUBES

Definition

Venipuncture is used to insert a needle for administration of fluids, electrolytes, anesthetics, sedation agents and medications, as well as for drawing blood.

Method

- The arm is positioned on the table, bed or arm of chair, and stabilized with other free hand.
- Organize equipment. Wash hands thoroughly and dry.
- Screw needle into blood collection device and place towel under extremity.
- Vein selection is based on which vein is the largest, most easily observable and palpable. This is usually the median cubital vein or cephalic vein in the antecubital fossa, or the metacarpal veins in the dorsum of the hand, the cephalic or basilic veins.
- Tourniquet (either a rubber tubing held with a slip knot or a blood pressure cuff pumped just below diastolic pressure) is applied to upper arm, if selected vein is in antecubital fossa, or forearm, if a vein on dorsum of hand is used.
- Put gloves on.
- Skin site is prepared by rubbing with gauze sponges soaked in 70% alcohol or comparable disinfectant, starting at the vein and circling outward to a 2-inch diameter.
- Remove the cap from the needle. With thumb of same hand, the skin is pulled taut just distal to the planned venipuncture site to prevent the vein from rolling away from the needle tip.
- Cannula needle is placed in line with the vein with bevel up. Needle is inserted, through skin at 15–30° angle.
- When lumen of vein is located, a decrease in resistance to penetration is felt and there is usually a back-flow of blood into the adapter of the infusion tube.

Table 8.20 Suture materials

Material	Composition	Absorption/strength	Reactivity	Use	Advantages	Disadvantages/ contraindications
Absorbable						
Plain gut	Sheep or beef intestine, collagen fibers	Absorption in 70 days. Tensile strength for 7–10 days	Moderate	Ligating vessels, SC closure	Can be used in presence of infection	Reactive. Avoid with sensitivity to collagen or chromium
Chromic gut	Plain gut with chromium salt	50% strength at 12 days	Moderate	SC, fascia, peritoneum closure	Can be used in presence of infection	Reactive. Avoid with sensitivity to collagen or chromium
Polyglactin (Vicryl)	Lactide and glycolide polymer	75% strength at 14 days, gone at 70 days	Minimal	SC, fascia, peritoneal closure	Less reactive, braided	May tattoo if dyed
Non-absorbable						
Silk	Organic (fibroin)	Progressive degranulation of fiber over time	Acute	Most tissues	Easily handled	Not for use with sensitivity to silk
Nylon (Ethilon) (Nurolon)	Long-chain aliphatic polymers	Gradual loss of tensile strength over time	Minimal	Most tissues ophthalmic	Easily adjustable tension	Has memory, may slip
Polyester fiber (Mersilene)	Ethylene terephthalate	No absorption	Minimal	Most tissues	Less reactive, dependable, lasting strength, good tie down	Braided, may tattoo if dyed
Polypropylene (Prolene)	Isotactic crystalline Stereoisomer of polypropylene	No absorption	Minimal	Most tissues	Monofilament, permanent strength, non-reactive, no-slip	
Steel	316L stainless steel	Indefinite strength Non-absorbable	Minimal	Abdominal surgery, orthopedic	Non-reactive, no-slip	Difficult to work with, special cutter, allergic potential

From: Ethicon, Inc. 1999 Wound closure manual.

- The angle of the needle is decreased until it is flush with the skin and the plastic catheter moved cautiously up the vessel lumen. The cannula needle is removed and discarded in the sharps container.
- The tourniquet is relaxed.
- The IV tubing (line) is connected to the catheter hub and adequate fluid flow is assured.

  Note: if the site is also to be used for blood drawing, a plastic syringe should be connected to the catheter hub and blood withdrawn from the vein prior to connection of the IV line. A needle is then placed on the plastic syringe and the blood is injected into the specific blood drawing tube for the desired lab test.
- Anchoring the catheter and securing the arm board:
  - the catheter is taped flush with the skin
  - a 5-inch strip of tape is placed under the hub of the needle and each end is wrapped tightly and diagonally, criss-crossing over the junction of the catheter and the hub. Additional tape can be used to secure the IV tubing against the arm

Table 8.21 **Commonly used evacuated blood specimen tubes**

Stopper color	Additive	Action, notes
Red	None	
Gold	Inert silicon gel	Acts as a separator between red blood cells and serum after centrifuging
Purple	Ethylenediamine tetraacetic acid (EDTA)	Chelates calcium from the blood, thus preventing clotting; the potassium salt of EDTA is usually used
Blue	Sodium citrate	Same action as for EDTA; the anticoagulant of choice for coagulation studies
Gray	Potassium oxalate	Same action as for EDTA; is also a glycolytic inhibitor for glucose determinations
Green	Heparin	Prevents clotting by deactivating thrombin and thromboplastin; both sodium and lithium salts are used

- Method of blood drawing with Vacutainer system.
  - The glass collection tube can be connected to the system and allowed to fill $^2/_3$–$^3/_4$ with blood while the system is held in place. When stabilizing the system, the first glass collection tube can be removed and replaced by additional tubes as needed (Table 8.21).
  - When enough blood has been collected, the tourniquet is relaxed and the needle (with system and last collection tube in place) is withdrawn while applying pressure at the site with a gauze sponge. Hold pressure for 2–3 min, longer if the patient is on anticoagulant therapy.
  - Attach proper labels to each tube of blood and fill out appropriate forms.
  - Dispose of equipment properly.
  - Remove gloves and wash hands.

References

Briggs G C, Freeman R K, Yaffe S J 2002 Drugs in pregnancy and lactation, sixth edn. Lippincott Williams & Wilkins, Philadelphia

British Medical Association 2002 British National Formulary, vol. 41. British Medical Association, London.

Dajani A S et al 1997 Prevention of bacterial endocarditis – recommendations by the American Heart Association. Journal of the American Medical Association 227:1794–1801.

Ethicon, Inc. 1999 Wound closure manual. Ethicon, Inc., Somerville, NJ

Federal Register Department of Health, Education and Welfare. Food and Drug Administration. 21 CFR Parts 201 and 202. 1980 44:37434–67

Gahart B L Intravenous medications. A Handbook for Nurses and Allied Health Professionals. In: Gahart B L, Nazareno A R, eds, 2003: Edition 19. WB Saunders & Co.

Trissel L A Handbook on injectable drugs. 2003: Edition 12 American Soc Health-System Pharmacists.

Chapter 9

Laboratory tests
(from Lehmann and Henry 2001)

HEMATOLOGY

Collected in a tube containing EDTA (violet top)

Complete blood count (CBC) [FBC] and differential

Test	Normal conventional units [SI units]		Significance if high	Significance if low	Oral findings
Red blood cell (RBC) count	Adult male:	$4.5–9 \times 10^6/\mu L$ [$4.5–9 \times 10^{12}/L$]	Polycythemia	Anemia	Pale, atrophic oral mucosa possible large trabecular pattern on radiograph in chronic anemia
	Adult female:	$4.5–5.1 \times 10^6/\mu L$ [$4.1–5.1 \times 10^{12}/L$]			
RBC indices					
Mean corpuscular volume (MCV)	Adult:	$80–96 \ \mu m^3$ [80–96 fL]	Macrocytosis	Microcytosis	Note: High or low MCV not equal to high or low hematocrit
Mean corpuscular hemoglobin (MCH)	27.5–33.2 pg		Hyperchromia	Hypochromic anemia	
Mean corpuscular hemoglobin concentration (MCHC)	33.4–35.5% [concentration fraction: 0.334–0.355]		Hyperchromia	Hypochromic anemia	
Hemoglobin	Adult male:	14.0–17.5 gm/dL [140–175 g/L]	Polycythemia	Anemia	
	Adult female:	12.3–15.3 gm/dL [123–153 g/L]			

table continues

Hematocrit	Adult male: 41.5–50.4% [volume fraction: 0.415–0.504] Adult female: 35.9–44.6% [0.359–0.446]	Polycythemia	Anemia
Reticulocyte count	0.5–1.5% [number fraction: 0.005–0.015]	Increased number of RBC put into circulation. Nucleated RBC may be present. Hemolytic anemia or iron deficiency anemia responding to treatment	
Sedimentation rate	Men < 50 yrs: < 15 mm/hour Men 50–85 yrs: < 20 mm/hour Men > 85 yrs: < 30 mm/hour Women < 50 yrs: < 20 mm/hour Women 50–85 yrs: < 30 mm/hour Women > 85 yrs: < 42 mm/hour	Infection, infarction, trauma or tumor may be present, pregnancy	Sickle-cell anemia
White blood cell (WBC) count	4400–11 000/μL [4.4–11.3 × 10⁹/L]	Evaluation for infection or malignancy	Hematologic neoplastic, disease (early leukemia), drug-induced neutropenia, cyclic neutropenia, agranulocytosis, viral infection, overwhelming bacterial infection
Segmented neutrophils (polys)	41–78% [number fraction: 0.41–78]	Infection, inflammation toxic states, tissue destruction, certain drugs (adrenal acute hemorrhage), stress	Agranulocytosis, drug-induced neutropenia, viral infection, infectious diseases, chemical-induced, hypersplenism, collagen–vascular disorder	Enlarged gingiva, oral ulcers or other infection secondary to immunosuppression from disease and/or therapy

table continues

Complete blood count (CBC) [FBC] and differential *continued*

Test	Normal conventional units [SI units]	Significance if high	Significance if low	Oral findings
Band neutrophils (bands)	0–6% [0.0–0.06]	Immature neutrophils, indicates rapid production of cell line, often seen in infection		
Lymphocytes	23–44% [0.23–0.44]	Usually accompanies a normal or elevated WBC. Viral infections, mononucleosis, infectious lymphocytosis, hypoadrenalism hypothyroidism	Immunodeficiencies, adrenal–corticosteroid exposure, severe debilitating illness, defects of lymphatic circulation	
Monocytes	0–7% [0.0–0.07]	Chronic infectious (e.g. tuberculosis), bacterial endocarditis, granulomatous disease		
Eosinophils	0–4% [0.0–0.04]	Parasitic diseases, certain allergic diseases, chronic skin diseases, various miscellaneous diseases (sarcoidosis, Hodgkin's disease, metastatic carcinoma)		
Basophils	0–2% [0.0–0.02]	Chronic hypersensitivity states, no specific allergen, myeloproliferative disorders		
Glycosylated hemoglobin	5.5–9% of total hemoglobin	Diabetes mellitus		

Coagulation tests

Test	Normal conventional units [SI units]	Significance if high	Significance if low	Oral findings
Bleeding time	Normal range is usually 2–8 minutes	Depends on device used von Willebrand's disease or other coagulation defects in which one or more factors are missing, such as vitamin K deficiency, hemophilia, liver disease, or the presence of circulating anticoagulants		
Clot retraction	Complete by 4 hours at 37°C.	Platelet disorders: thrombocytopenia, thrombasthenia		
Clotting time (capillary tube coagulation)	3–6 minutes	Hemophilias, fibrinogen deficiency, heparin administration, vitamin K deficiency, liver disease		
Fibrinogen level[a]	200–400 mg/dL [2.0–4.0 g/L]	Pregnancy	Afibrinogenemia, hypofibrinogenemia, dysfibrinogenemia	
Activated partial thromboplastin[a] time (APTT)	25–35 seconds A control test is run at the time of each test	Will detect many coagulation defects but will not detect platelet defects nor deficiency of factor VII; may be normal in vitamin K deficiency (or administration of warfarin)		

table continues

Coagulation tests *continued*

Test	Normal conventonal units [SI units]	Significance if high	Significance if low	Oral findings
Platelet count	150 000–450 000/µL [150–450 × 10⁹/L]	Thrombocytosis, inflammatory reactions, (rheumatic fever, rheumatoid arthritis, septicemia), or resulting from blood disorders (hemorrhage, iron deficiency anemia, hemolytic anemia), malignancy, post-operative, postsplenectomy	Thrombocytopenia; immunologic or idiopathic thrombocytopenia purpura, cancers, drugs, infectious mononucleosis, systemic lupus erythematosus, viral diseases (chickenpox, smallpox, rubella, measles); secondary to splenomegaly and hypersplenism, Gaucher's, lymphoma, miliary tuberculosis, sarcoidosis, myeloproliferative disorders, nonsplenic sequestration (cavernous hemangioma, disseminated intravascular coagulation, thrombocytopenic purpura), mechanical destruction (cardiac valve prosthesis), miscellaneous (hemorrhage, multiple blood transfusions, chronic alcoholism), deficient production (bone marrow suppressive drugs), physical agents (ionizing radiation), bone marrow replacement metastatic tumor	

table continues

Prothrombin time (PT)	A control is run with the test. Normal range is usually 10–13 sec or within 2 sec of control	Will detect deficiencies of factors II, V, VII and X, fibrinogen and vitamin K, will also detect warfarin administration
International normalized ratio (INR)	Therapeutic range usually 2–4	See PT
Thrombin time (TT)	Usually 17–25 seconds	Heparin, qualitative abnormalities of fibrinogen or hypofibrinogenemia
Tourniquet test for capillary fragility after 5 minutes	< 10 petechiae in a 2.5 cm circle	Quantitative and qualitative platelet disorders, small vessel disease, coagulation defects
Factor VIII assay	50–150% of normal (control sample) activity	Hemophilia A, von Willebrand's disease
Factor IX assay	50–150% of normal (control sample) activity	Hemophilia B, Christmas disease
Bethesda inhibitor assay	< 0.4 Bethesda units	Antibodies to specific coagulation factors. Each Bethesda unit decreases factor concentration by 50%

[a]Note: Collect in vacutainer containing 3.8% sodium citrate.

Other tests

Sickle-cell tests

Sickle screen	No sickled RBCs	Sickled RBCs represent sickle cell anemia or heterozygous state
Hemoglobin electrophoresis		Gives a complete characterization of hemoglobins present in the RBCs (e.g. nomal fetal, sickle, thalassemia hemoglobins). Can differentiate homozygous individual from heterozygous carrier state

HIV tests

CD4	300–1300/μL [0.3–1.3 × 10^9/L]	AIDS, inherited lymphocytopenia, chemotherapy, radiotherapy, glucocorticoids, autoimmune disease	
HIV RNA (viral load)	0 copies in 1 cc of plasma	HIV	
Anti-HIV (HIV antibody)	Negative	HIV	

table continues

Viral hepatitis tests

HBs Ag	Negative	Acute or chronic hepatitis B
HBs Ab (antibody to HBV surface antigen)	Absence or presence	Hepatitis B or prior immunization
Anti-HCV (antibody to HCV)	Negative	Hepatitis C
HCV RNA	Negative	Hepatitis C

Tuberculosis tests

Purified protein derivative (PPD)	< 10 mm induration	Previous TB exposures

Syphilis tests

Rapid plasmin reagin (RPR) test	Negative, non-reactive	Presence of syphilis antibody, antiphospholipid syndrome

BLOOD CHEMISTRY

Test	Normal conventional units [SI units]	Significance if high	Significance if low	Oral findings
Total protein	6.0–7.8 g/dL [60–78 g/L]	Albumin: pregnancy, malnutrition, chronic hepatic disease, nephrotic syndrome, major infection, surgical and accidental trauma, eclampsia, uremia		
Albumin	3.5–4.5 g/dL [32–45 g/L]			
Globulins	2.3–3.5 g/ml [23–35 g/L]			
Albumins/globulins ratio	2:1			
Protein electrophoresis				
Albumin	52–65% [fraction 0.52–0.65]	Globulin: pregnancy, obstructive jaundice, uncontrolled diabetes mellitus, nephrotic syndrome, infectious disease, sarcoidosis, amyloidosis, subacute and chronic liver disease, rheumatoid erythematosis, Hodgkin's disease	Globulins: acute hepatocellular necrosis, intravascular hemolytic anemia, severe infections, some neoplastic, diseases, viral hepatitis, cirrhosis, lymphomas, lymphatic leukemia, nephrotic syndrome, scleroderma	
Alpha globulins	9.5–18% [0.095–0.18]			
Beta globulins	8–14% [0.08–14]			
Gamma globulins	12–22% [0.12–0.22]			
IgG	800–1801 mg/dL [8.0–18.0 g/L]	Cirrhosis of liver, infection	Antibody deficiency	
IgA	113–563 mg/dL [1.1–5.6 g/L]			
IgM	54–222 mg/dL [0.5–2.2 g/L]			

table continues

Test	Normal conventional units [SI units]	Significance if high	Significance if low	Oral findings
Calcium	Adults: 9.2–11.0 mg/dL [2.30–2.74 mmol/L]	Vitamin K intoxication, metastatic or lytic tumors of bone, milk alkali syndrome, hypoparathyroidism, hyperparathyroidism	Hypoparathyroidism, vitamin D deficiency states (rickets, osteomalacia), renal failure, acute pancreatitis	Hyperparathyroidism: pattern of alveolar bone trabeculation, loss of lamina dura, presence of large multiloculated radiolucencies Hypoparathyroidism; increased bone density, enamel hypoplasia, candidiasis
Phosphorus, inorganic	2.3–4.7 mg/dL [0.74–1.52 mmol/L]	Renal disease, hypoparathyroidism	Hyperparathyroidism, adult rickets, may indicate increased carbohydrate metabolism or use of drugs that elevate carbohydrate metabolism (epinephrine, insulin)	
Cholesterol	150–250 mg/dL [3.88–6.47 mmol/L]	Primary disorders of lipid metabolism, uncontrolled diabetes mellitus, obstructive jaundice, hypothyroidism, nephrosis, pancreatitis, acute alcoholism	Hyperparathyroidism, acute hepatitis, malnutrition	

table continues

Test	Normal conventional units [SI units]	Significance if high	Significance if low	Oral findings
Glucose	70–110 mg/dL [3.9–6.1 mmol/L]	Diabetes mellitus, surgical removal of the pancreas, corticosteroid therapy	Hepatic disease, Addison's disease, excess insulin	Diabetes mellitus: acetone breath, dryness of oral mucosa with burning and diffuse erythema, severe chronic peridontal disease, lowered resistance to infection may lead to impairment of normal healing process
Uric acid (nitrogenous waste-product of nucleoprotein breakdown)	Male: 4.0–8.5 mg/dL [0.24–0.51 mmol/L] Female: 2.7–7.3 mg/dL [0.16–0.43 mmol/L]	Gout, any pathologic process leading to increased nuclear catabolism (leukemia, lymphomas, toxemia of pregnancy, polycythemia vera, lead poisoning and pneumonia), renal disease secondary to decreased renal tubular secretion		
Creatinine	0.6–1.2 mg/dL [53–106 µmol/L] Clearance: Male: 107–139 cc/min. [1.78–2.32 cc/s] Female: 87–107 cc/min. [1.45–1.78 cc/s]	Renal impairment, severe muscle disease, hyperparathyroidism, amphotericin B, ascorbic acid, MI, trauma With advancing age, BUN and Creat. values are less useful as indices of renal function, for the following reason: the		Renal failure: Bad taste from urea in saliva, parotitis, oral mucosal breakdown with non-specific ulcerations, chronic periodontal disease, acute necrotizing ulcerative

table continues

Test	Normal conventional units [SI units]	Significance if high	Significance if low	Oral findings
	Clearance is more sensitive in detection of renal disease since creatinine may not be elevated until 50% of the tissue is destroyed	age-related decline in lean body mass results in reduction of protein degradation and thus less BUN to be cleared. Decline in muscle mass with age results in less creatinine. Yet overall BUN and Creat. levels remain unchanged due to diminished clearance capacity		gingivitis, gingival hemorrhage, ecchymoses of the oral mucosa due to abnormal thrombocyte function, neuropathy with tingling or numbness of the tongue, osteodystrophy seen as fibrocystic lesions of the thinning of the lamina dura and cortical bone of the alveolus
Phosphatases Acid phosphatase (greatest activity at pH of 5)	Total: 0.13–0.63 U/L [2.2–10.5 U/L]	Cancer of prostate that has metastasized or broken through the capsule; rectal exams with prostatic massage may cause a transient rise (up to 24 hours)		
Alkaline phosphatase (greatest activity at pH of 9)	20–130 IU/L [20–130 U/L]	Bone diseases with osteoblastic activity (hyperparathyroidism, Pagets disease, adult rickets, metastatic malignancy, hypervitaminosis D), biliary tract disease, liver disease,		

table continues

Test	Normal conventional units [SI units]	Significance if high	Significance if low	Oral findings
		growing children, second and third trimesters of pregnancy, phenothiazines, erythromycin, oxacillin, some oral contraceptives, alcoholic liver disease, viral or chronic hepatitis		
Transaminases				
Total serum glutamine oxaloacetic transaminase (SGOT, AST)	8–33 U/L at 37°C	Disease with destruction of the tissue in which it is found (e.g. myocardial infarction, liver disease, skeletal muscle disease); drugs (e.g. ampicillin, cephalothin, cloxacillin, erythromycin, indomethalcin. methotrexate, opiates); infectious mononucleosis, Reye's syndrome		
Serum glutamic pyruvic transaminase (SGPT, ALT)	4–36 U/L at 37°C	Liver disease, many drugs/ diseases that elevate SGOT also elevate SGPT		
GGT (gamma glutamyl transpeptidase)	5–40 IU/L at 37°C [5–40 U/L]	Liver disease, particularly sensitive to alcohol ingestion		
LDH (lactic dehydrogenase)	80–120 units at 30°C [38–62 U/L at 30°C] (lactate → pyruvate)	Damage to any tissues in which it is found (e.g. myocardial infarction, muscular dystrophy, megaloblastic anemia)		

OTHER BLOOD DETERMINANTS

Test	Normal conventional units [SI units]	Significance if high	Significance if low	Oral findings
Blood urea nitrogen (BUN)	8–23 mg/dL [2.9–8.2 mmol/L]	Renal azotemia, prerenal azotemia, decreased glomerular filtration rate With advancing age, BUN and Creat. values are less useful as indices of renal function, for the following reason: the age-related decline in lean body mass results in reduction of protein degradation and thus less BUN to be cleared. Decline in muscle mass with age resulting in less creatinine. Yet overall BUN and Creat. levels remain unchanged due to diminished clearance capacity	Severe liver disease, rapid overhydration, low protein diets	
Bilirubin				
Conjugated (direct)	< 0.3 mg/dL [< 5 μmol/L]	Liver disease, intrahepatic disruption, bile duct disease, extrahepatic bile duct obstruction		
Unconjugated (indirect)	< 0.1–1.0 mg/dL [2–17 μmol/L]	Retention-type jaundice (hepatocellular), hemolysis, RBC degradation, defective hepatocellular uptake/conjugation		

table continues

Test	Normal conventional units [SI units]	Significance if high	Significance if low	Oral findings
Creatine phosphokinase (CPK)	Males: 55–170 U/L at 37°C Females: 30–135 U/L	Muscle disease; acute myocardial, pulmonary or cerebral infarction		
Iron (serum iron)	60–150 µg/dL [10.7–26.9 µmol/L] (males slightly higher than females)	Hemolytic anemias, hemochromatosis, pernicious anemia	Iron deficiency anemia, anemias secondary to chronic infection	In anemic patients, oral mucosa may have a pale appearance
Total iriron binding capacity (TIBC)	250–400 µg/dL [44.8–71.6 µmol/L]	Iron deficiency anemia, anemia secondary to blood loss	Liver disease, anemias secondary to chronic infection, malnutrition	
Serum osmolality	280–295 mOsm/kg [280–295 mmol/kg]	Water loss, chronic renal disease with a rising blood urea nitrogen, increased serum glucose	Inappropriate antidiuretic hormone secretiion, Addison's disease	
Oral glucose tolerance test (GTT)	Pretest: 70–110 mg/dL [3.9–6.1 mmol/L] 60 min: 20–50 mg/dL above fasting [1.1–2.8 mmol/L above fasting] 120 min: 5–15 mg/dL above fasting [0.3–0.8 mmol/L above fasting]	Diabetes mellitus, hyperthyroidism, Cushing's disease	Severe liver damage	

table continues

Test	Normal conventional units [SI units]	Significance if high	Significance if low	Oral findings
Triglycerides	10–190 mg/dL [0.11–2.15 mmol/L]	Prolonged consumption of high caloric foods; alcohol	Low caloric intake, vegetarians	
Electrolytes Sodium (Na)	136–142 mEq/L [136–142 mmol/L]	Hypernatremia: excessive water loss (vomiting, diarrhea, severe sweating)	Hyponatremia: cirrhosis, congestive heart failure, adrenal insufficiency, nephrosis, excessive use of diuretics, inappropriate secretion of antidiuretic hormone, water intoxication	
Potassium (K)	3.8–5.0 meq/L [3.8–5.0 mmol/L]	Hyperkalemia: release of cellular potassium as in crush injuries, after surgery, hemolysis of red blood cells, renal failure, and acidosis	Hypokalemia: insufficient intake, vomiting, diarrhea, nasogastric suction, use of diuretic medications	
Chloride (Cl)	95–103 mEq/L [95–103 mmol/L]	Generally will follow serum sodium	Vomiting	
Magnesium (Mg)	1.3–2.1 mEq/L [0.65–1.05 mmol/L]	Renal failure. large doses of antacids that contain Mg	Alcoholism, diabetic acidosis, malabsorption hypocalcemia, hypokalemia, neuromuscular irritability	
Adrenocorticotropic hormone (ACTH)	08:00 hours, peak: 25–100 pg/cc [25–100 ng/L] 18:00 hours, trough: 0–50 pg/cc [0–50 mg/L]	Addison's disease, ectopic ACTH syndrome, pituitary adenoma, Cushing's syndrome, primary adrenal insufficiency, stress	Primary adrenocortical hyperfunction, secondary hypoadrenalism	

URINALYSIS

Test	Normal conventional units [SI units]	Significance if high	Significance if low	Oral findings
Color	Clear to straw	Red to red-brown: hemoglobin, beets; greenish-orange: bilirubin; orange-brown; urobilin; brown-black: homogentistic acid; yellow-brown: rhubarb	Cloudy: precipitated phosphates, urates, mucus, bacteria, erythrocytes, leukocytes; milky: pyuria, fat	
Odor	Faintly aromatic	Bacteria, asparagus, fecal contamination		
Specific Gravity	1.016–1.022	Glucose, protein, dehydration, uncontrolled diabetes mellitus	Overhydration, diabetes insipidus, chronic nephritis	
Chemical Examination				
pH	4.6–8.0	Dietary, febrile illness in children	Ketosis, systemic acidosis	
Protein	40–150 mg in 24 hours; dipstick negative trace	Exercise, emotional stress, pregnancy, fever, prolonged exposure to cold, nephritis, destructive lesions of the kidney, nephrotic syndrome, congestive heart failure, ascites, chemical poisoning		

table continues

Test	Normal conventonal units [SI units]	Significance if high	Significance if low	Oral findings
Glucose	Negative dipstick	Hyperglycemia: diabetes mellitus, dextrose administration, Cushing's disease, pheochromocytoma, ingestion of large dose of glucose, stress, pancreatic disease, pregnancy, renal tubular/CNS dysfunction		
Ketones	0	Incomplete fat metabolism, starvation, malnutrition, fever, severe vomiting or diarrhea, pregnancy, diabetic or alcoholic ketoacidosis		
Hemoglobin	0	Renal pathology, malignant hypertension, hemolytic anemia, malaria, scurvy, incompatible blood transfusions		
Bilirubin	0	Obstructive jaundice, hepatitis		
Bence–Jones protein	0	Multiple myeloma		
Amylase	35–260 Somogyi units/h [6.5–48.1 U/h]	Pancreatitis, mumps, salivary gland inflammation, occasionally perforated peptic ulcer		

table continues

Test	Normal conventonal units [SI units]	Significance if high	Significance if low	Oral findings
Microscopic examination				
White blood cells	0–2	Urinary tract infection, renal disease with casts, pyelonephritis		
Red blood cells	1–3	Renal disease, trauma, anticoagulant therapy, excessive physical exertion		
Epithelial cells	Several	Renal cells: renal disease; transitional cells: bladder, ureter or kidney pelvis disease; squamous cells: urethral or vaginal disease		
Casts	Described by constituent	Hyaline CHF, mild kidney disease or damage, dehydration; Epithelial cell: moderate kidney disease; CMV waxy cast: renal disease, transplant rejection		
Crystals		May indicate nephrolithiasis or gout		

THYROID

Test	Normal conventional units [SI units]	Significance if high	Significance if low	Oral findings
Hormones Thyroid-stimulating hormones (TSH)	0.5–5 μIU/cc	Hypothyroidism	Hyperthyroidism, secondary Hypothyroidism	
Total triiodothyronine (T_3)	80–200 mg/dL [1.23–3 nmol/L]	Hyperthyroidism	Hypothyroidism	
Total thyroxine (T_4)	5.5–12.5 μg/dL [71–161 nmol/L]	Hyperthyroidism	Hypothyroidism	
T_3 Resin uptake	25–38 relative % uptake [0.25–0.38 relative uptake fraction]			
Radioactive iodine (RAI) uptake test	5–30% in 24 hours	Hyperthyroidism	Hypothyroidism	

CEREBROSPINAL FLUID

Test	Normal conventional units [SI units]	Significance if high	Significance if low	Oral findings
Glucose	40–80 m/dL [2.8–4.4 mmol/L]		Purulent meningitis, CNS leukemia	
Protein	12–60 mg/dL [120–600 mg/L]	Meningitis, brain tumor.		
White blood cells	0–5 lymphocytes/µL (adult) with up to 20 in children	MS, Guillain–Barré syndrome		
Red blood cells	0	Local trauma, subarachnoid hemorrhage		

ARTERIAL BLOOD GASES

Test	Normal conventional units [SI units]	Significance if high	Significance if low	Oral findings
pH	7.38–7.42			
PCO_2	35–45 min Hg [4.7–5.3 kPa]			
PO_2	95–100 mm Hg [12.7–13.3 kPa]			
O_2 Saturation	94–100% [0.94–1.00 fraction saturates]			

References

Lehmann H P, Henry J B 2001 Appendix 5: SI Units. In: Henry J B (ed) Clinical diagnosis and management by laboratory methods, 20th edn. W B Saunders, Philadelphia, p 1426–1441

Examples of hospital charts

BRIEF HISTORY AND PHYSICAL EXAMINATION RECORD

Date: 26 September 2003

Informant: Patient, patient's old chart

Present illness: Patient is a 33 yo white male admitted for multiple extractions (×12) and restorative dental treatment. This is one of many admissions for this patient who has chronic kidney disease s/p cadaveric kidney transplant, which has subsequently failed and has been removed. He is on dialysis, with a shunt, on M, W, F, at the Dialysis Unit from 1800 to 2300. Pt. also has chronic hepatitis B and a heart murmur of mitral valve prolapse.

Past medical history:
Heart murmur.
HBV positive, chronic active carrier with some cirrhosis.
Renal failure, M, W, F via left/right arm shunt.

Past operations/admissions: <u>Hospital admissions</u>: Multiple, including cadaveric kidney transplant (June 2001). Removal of transplanted kidney, exploratory laparotomy (September 2001).
<u>Operations</u>: See above. Also, T & A as a child.
<u>Current medication</u>: Benadryl [Piriton], amphogel [Maalox], cimetidine, multivitamins, folic acid, Lomotil.
<u>Allergies</u>: None known.

Social history: (+) EtOH, cigarettes. Single, unemployed, lives with sister.

System review:
<u>Cardiorespiratory</u>: History of heart murmur of mitral valve prolapse with regurgitation.

Neg. history for rheumatic fever, angina, MI.

<u>Gastrointestinal</u>: History of chronic GI hypermotility. Chronic hepatitis B.

<u>Genito-Urinary</u>: Cadaveric kidney transplant and subsequent failure. On dialysis.

<u>Physical examination</u>: B/P 100/70 mmHg, Temp 98.6°F (37°C), Pulse 72, R 20.

<u>General</u>: 33 yo male, slightly obese in NAD.

<u>HEENT</u>: NC/AT, PERRLA, EOMs full without nystagmus. Neck supple. Pharynx clear.

Multiple decayed teeth; advanced periodontal disease; 4 impacted 3rd molars.

<u>Lungs</u>: Clear to A/P.

<u>Heart</u>: RRR nl, S1, S2, II/VI SEM.

<u>Abdomen</u>: BS+, soft, non-tender, 3^+ hepatomegaly, without organomegaly.

<u>Rectal</u>: Deferred.

<u>Musculoskeletal</u>: Extremities slightly wasted. Full range of motion and reflexes.

<u>Neurological</u>: Alert and oriented × 3. Cranial Nerves II-VI grossly intact.

Diagnosis:
1. Impacted 3rd molar teeth ×4, gross caries ×8, and advanced periodontal disease
2. Mitral valve prolapse
3. Chronic hepatitis B
4. Chronic renal failure

Plan: Extractions ×12 and restorative dental treatment (17 September 2003) under general anesthesia with pre-operative antibiotic prophylaxis. Routine meds and penicillin G (dose) IV q4h.

D.A. Jones, DDS

PROGRESS NOTES

Patient's identification stamp

Date: 27 September 2003

Anesthesia Note: Pt. is a 33 yo white male with a history of chronic renal disease. He had cadaveric kidney transplant which has subsequently been removed. He has GI hypermobility, a heart murmur and chronic hepatitis B. Patient has a shunt in R arm and is dialyzed M.W.F.

Past Operations: Multiple under general anesthesia without complications. ·

Exam: 33 yo white male NAD, BP 160/90 mmHg, Pulse 72, R 20, Temp 98.6°F (37°C)

Labs:

13	95	Creat 9.2	BUN 36
5.8	28	WBC: 5.0	Hct: 16.5
PT 12.6/12.2		INR 1.2	PT T 30.2

Mouth: Good opening, hyperextention of neck. Gross caries. Ant. teeth stable, crowns.

Lungs: Clear to A/P

Cardiac: S1, S2, RR, II/VI SEM

Procedure: Multiple extractions, restorative dentistry, scaling.

Anesthesia plan: General anesthesia, naso-tracheal intubation pending transfusion. Avoid R arm.

L. V. Vandam, MD

REQUEST FOR CONSULTATION

Date: 27 September 2003

To Doctor: Renal service

Probable diagnosis: Caries/periodontal disease

Information desired: Pt. is a 33 yo white male followed in Renal Clinic with multiple decayed and impacted teeth. He will go to the OR (27 September 2003) for extractions, restorative dentistry, and scaling. Request any management precautions or suggestions re: renal disease.

D.A. Jones, DDS

PROGRESS NOTES – THE PREOPERATIVE NOTE

Date: 27 September 2003

Preoperative diagnosis: Caries, periodontal disease, and impacted teeth
Chronic renal disease
Chronic hepatitis B
Mitral valve prolapse with regurgitation.

Plan: Extractions ×12, and restorative dentistry under general anesthesia
with penicillin coverage

Surgeon: Dr Jones

EKG: Within normal limits

CXR: Slight infiltrate, RLL; slight cardiac enlargement

U/A: Within normal limits

Allergies: None known

Labs:

131	95
5.8	28

Creat 9.2   BUN 36
Hct 16.5   PT 12.6/12.2   INR 1.2   PTT 30.2
WBC 5.0

Patient to receive 2 units washed, irradiated prbc (packed red blood cells).
Type [group] and hold 2 units washed, irradiated packed red blood cells.

Consent signed.

D.A. Jones, DDS

PROGRESS NOTES – BRIEF OPERATIVE NOTE

Date: 27 September 2003

Preoperative diagnosis: Caries, impacted teeth and periodontal disease. Chronic renal disease. Chronic hepatitis B.

Postoperative diagnosis: Same.

Surgeon: Dr Jones

Procedure: Extractions ×12, restorative treatment, and scaling under penicillin prophylaxis.

Anesthesia: General (nasotracheal).

EBL: 200 cc

Fluids: 200 cc 0.9% NaCl

Complications: None.

Plan: Hct on floor. If < 25, 1 unit washed, irradiated prbc. Hematocrit in am. Discharge to home tomorrow.

D.A. Jones, DDS

PROGRESS NOTES – POSTOPERATIVE NOTE

Date: 27 September 2003

Vital signs: Stable T 98.9° BP 100/70 P 72 R 16

Lungs: Clear to A/P (auscultation and percussion)

Extraction sites: Without bleeding

Patient awake, alert, comfortable
Hct 29   IV TKO (to keep open)

D.A. Jones, DDS

DISCHARGE NOTE

Date: 28 September 2003

Discharge patient to home

Rx: Oxycodone/Acetaminophen [paracetamol] po q4h PRN. Disp. 10

Routine meds

Return to dental clinic 30 September 2003 at 09:00 h.

D.A. Jones, DDS

DISCHARGE SUMMARY

Patient name: John Doe

Hospital number: R 7699 30571

Date of admission: 26 September 2003

Date of discharge: 28 September 2003

Staff physician: David A. Jones, DDS

Family physician: James Smith, MD

History of present illness: Mr Doe was admitted 26 September 2003 for removal of eight grossly decayed molars, and four impacted third molars, restorative dentistry and scaling under general anesthesia and penicillin prophylaxis. Patient has not received routine dental care since childhood.

Past medical history: Significant for chronic renal disease. The patient received a cadaveric renal transplant that failed and was later removed. The patient is on dialysis Mondays, Wednesdays and Fridays at the Kidney Center. He has a shunt in place. He has chronic hepatitis B and a heart murmur. He has had multiple hospital admissions for procedures including kidney transplant, removal of the transplant, and exploratory lap.
Medications on admission: Benadryl 25 mg po PRN itch, Maalox 600 mg po tid, Cimetidine 300 mg po bid, Multivitamin with iron 1 tab po qd, Folic Acid 50 ug po qd, Darvon po q4h PRN pain, Lomotil.

Physical exam: Patient is a 33 yo white male, slightly obese, in no acute distress. Pupils are equal, round and reactive to light and accommodation. Extraocular movements are full and without nystagmus. Neck is supple and without nodes. Lungs are clear to auscultation and percussion. Cardiac exam shows S1, S2 with a II over IV systolic ejection murmur, regular rhythm. The abdomen is soft, non-tender, with hepatomegaly and normal bowel sounds. Neurologic status was intact to gross exam.

Laboratory data: sodium 131, chloride 95, potassium 5.8, carbon dioxide 25, creat. 9.2, BUN 36. WBC 5.0, Hct 16.5, PT 12.6/12.2, PTT 30.5.

Hospital course: The patient was admitted 26 September 2003 and dialyzed that evening. He was transfused 27 September 2003 preoperatively and intraoperatively with two units of irradiated, washed packed red blood cells. He was taken to the operating room in the afternoon of 27 September 2003 where, under general anesthesia, 12 teeth were removed and routine restorative treatment was done on the remaining teeth. His postoperative course was benign and he was discharged the morning of 28 September 2003 with a hematocrit of 28. He is to be followed by Dr David Jones.

Discharge diagnosis: Chronic renal failure. Chronic hepatitis B. Multiple extractions, dental restorations and scaling while in the hospital.

Operations and procedures: Extractions (×12), restorative dentistry, dental scaling. Estimated disability: None.

David A. Jones, DDS
cc: Dr Sigmon

PHYSICIAN'S ORDERS [REQUESTS]

		Patient's identification stamp
		Drug allergies: None known

Date	Time	Physician's orders
27 Sept 03	11:00	Admit to Dental, Dr Jones
		<u>Diagnosis</u>: Gross caries × 8, periodontal disease, impacted 3rd molars × 4. Chronic renal failure and chronic hepatitis. Mitral valve prolapse.
		<u>Condition</u>: Good
		<u>Allergies</u>: None known
		<u>Vital signs</u>: Per routine
		<u>Activity</u>: Ad lib
		<u>Diet</u>: Ad lib/NPO after midnight
		<u>Meds</u>: Benadryl 25 mg [Piriton 4 mg] PO PRN itch
		Maalox 600 PO tid
		Cimetidine 300mg PO bid
		Multivitamin with iron 1 tab PO qd
		Folic Acid 50 PO qd
		Renal consult
		Dialysis this pm.
		DA Jones, DDS
27 Sept 03		Transfuse 2 units packed rbc washed and irradiated; IV 0.9% NaCl TKO
27 Sept 03		Penicillin G (dose) IV on call to OR [theatre]
		DA Jones, DDS

PHYSICIAN'S ORDERS [REQUESTS]

		Patient's identification stamp
Drug allergies: None known		

Date	Time	Physician's orders

27 Sept 03	15:00	Post-Op Orders:
		Admit to floor via recovery room
		Diagnosis: Extractions ×12, restorative treatment, dental scaling. Chronic renal failure. Chronic hepatitis B. Mitral valve prolapse.
		Condition: Stable
		Allergies: None known
		Vital signs: Per routine
		Activity: Bed rest tonight; Ad lib tomorrow
		Diet: Clear liquids advance to soft diet as tolerated
		IV: 0.9% NaCl 75 cc/h until adequate POs then TKO
		O_2: 40% humidified O_2 via mask × 8 hour to prevent hypoxia
		Meds: Benadryl [Piriton] 25 mg PO PRN itch
		          Maalox 600 mg PO tid
		          Multivitamin with iron 1 tab PO qd
		          Folic Acid 50 mg PO qd
		          Oxycodone/Acetaminophen (co-codanol) PO q4h PRN pain
		Labs: Hct this evening - if less than 25, transfuse 1 unit irradiated, washed rbc. Hct in am
		Nursing: HOB 30°
		Ice to side of face 20 min/hour ×12 hours
		No rinsing or spitting ×24 hours
		                                        D.A. Jones DDS

DISCHARGE NOTE

Patient's identification stamp

Date	Time	Physician's orders
28 Sept 03	20:00	Discharge to home

Return to dental clinic 30 September 2003 at 09:00.

D.A. Jones DDS

OPERATIVE NOTE

Patient's identification stamp

Preoperative diagnosis: Impacted third molars. Grossly decayed molars. Multiple other carious teeth. Periodontal disease. Chronic renal failure. Hepatitis B. Mitral valve prolapse.

Postoperative diagnosis: Same

Operations: Extraction of molars (×12), Routine restorative treatment, scaling.

Surgeon: David A. Jones, DDS

Assistant: G. V. Black, III, DDS

Anesthesia: General nasotracheal

Indications for operation: Patient is 33 yo white male with grossly decayed first and second molars (×8), deep horizontally impacted mandibular third molars and deep vertically impacted maxillary third molars. The patient has chronic renal disease for which he is now dialyzed through a shunt in his right arm. He has chronic hepatitis B and mitral valve prolapse.

Procedure: The patient was brought to the operating room [theatre] with an intravenous line in place through which he was receiving his second unit of washed, irradiated packed red blood cells. He had received penicillin prophylaxis on call to the OR [theatre]. Once under adequate general anesthesia via nasotracheal intubation, the patient was prepped and draped in the usual manner. A rubber dam was placed to isolate all teeth from second premolar to second premolar, in the maxilla and mandible. The maxillary lateral and central incisors were prepared on the gingival third of the buccal surface. The teeth were cleaned with pumice. The teeth were acid etched and then filled with Silux – universal shade – and polished. All four maxillary premolars required MOD amalgams with a deep excavation on the distal of #13, requiring vitrebond base. Matrix bands and wedges were placed. The amalgam was packed and carved. The lower right premolars required excavations and the placement of amalgam on the gingival third of the buccal surface. All teeth except the molars were gross scaled using curettes. The field was irrigated and suctioned dry. The rubber dam was removed. The first and second molars were removed starting in the upper left quadrant with the second molar, first molar and then third molar. The teeth were extracted using elevators and forceps. An incision was made over the maxillary third molar region. The tissue was reflected. An air drill was utilized to remove overlying bone. The tooth was identified, and removed with elevators. The area was curetted with normal saline and closed with 3-0 chromic gut suture. The lower left, upper right and lower right molars were extracted in a similar manner. The mouth was irrigated with normal saline and the throat pack was removed. The patient was brought to the Recovery Room awake and responsive.

D.A. Jones DDS

Examples of emergency room admissions

EMERGENCY ROOM ADMISSION

Date: 2 October 2003
Time: 04:30
Patient name: Darryl Johnson
Chief complaint: 'My face hurts and I can't get my teeth together'
History of present illness: This 27 yo male was involved in an alleged act of interpersonal violence outside of a nightclub approximately 2.5 hours ago. He reports that he had been consuming alcohol since early last evening. He says that three men beat and kicked him as he was leaving the club. He apparently lost consciousness for a brief period and when he became responsive was lying in a pool of blood. Passers-by summoned an ambulance, which brought the patient to the hospital.
Past medical history:
Hospitalization: Gun shot wound right abdomen in 1998, went to County Hospital
Operations: As above
Medications: None
Allergies: Penicillin
Social history:
EtOH: Patient reports approximately 40 drinks per week
Tobacco: 24 pack-years (or give the number of cigarettes per day)
Other recreational drug use: None
Review of systems:
Skin: Multiple scars from previous trauma
Head: No previous history of head injury
Eyes: No history of visual disturbances
Ears: No hearing disturbances, tinnitus, vertigo, infections
Nose and sinuses: No history of trauma or sinusitis
Mouth and throat: Multiple teeth previously extracted, occasional sore throat
Neck: No lumps, goiter, or pain
Respiratory: No cough, wheezing, pneumonia, TB

<u>Cardiac</u>: No known cardiac disease or HTN; no dyspnea, orthopnea, chest pain, or palpitations

<u>GI</u>: Good appetite; no nausea, vomiting, indigestion, diarrhea, bleeding, constipation, pain, jaundice, gallbladder, or liver problems

<u>Urinary</u>: No dysuria, frequency, hematuria, or nocturia

<u>Genito-reproductive</u>: No abnormalities or dysfunction

<u>Musculoskeletal</u>: No joint pain, muscular pain, or functional disturbances

<u>Neurologic</u>: No fainting, seizures, motor or sensory loss, no memory disturbances

<u>Psychiatric</u>: No known psychiatric illness

<u>Endocrine</u>: No thyroid dysfunction, temperature intolerance, diaphoresis, or diabetes

<u>Hematologic</u>: No history of excessive bleeding, no anemia

Physical examination:

Pulse 84 regular, R 20, BP 140/86 mmHg, Temp 98.5°F (37°C) (axillary)

<u>Skin</u>: R abdominal scar secondary to old GSW, multiple scars on upper extremities from previous lacerations

<u>Head</u>: Contusions and abrasions over R occipital scalp and R forehead, moderate edema over L face

<u>Eyes</u>: Visual acuity grossly normal, subconjunctival hemorrhage O.S., pupils react to light, mild anisocoria, EOMI, normal retinal exam, anterior chamber clear.

<u>Ears</u>: Impacted wax obscures R TM, L TM intact, L EAC narrowed secondary to edema, pain to palpation over L tragus and preauricular region, auditory acuity grossly normal, no hemorrhage or drainage

<u>Nose</u>: Nasal bridge mobile and tender to palpation, intranasal exam reveals blood clots and areas of active bleeding, septal deviation and edema obstructing nasal airway

<u>Mouth</u>: R posterior open bite, only occlusal contact on L posterior molars: mucosal color normal, no oropharyngeal lesions, missing teeth numbers (give the teeth numbers)

<u>Neck</u>: Tender to palpation, trachea midline, edema in L submandibular region

<u>Nodes</u>: None palpable

<u>Thorax and lungs</u>: Thorax symmetrical, no tenderness to palpation, clear to auscultation and percussion

<u>Heart</u>: RRR without S3, S4, or murmur, no bruits, JVP normal

<u>Abdomen</u>: Old RUQ abd scar; no masses or tenderness; liver, spleen, kidneys not palpable, liver of normal size

<u>Genitalia</u>: Normal, without lesions

<u>Rectal</u>: Negative, brown stool, negative for occult blood

<u>Peripheral vascular</u>: Pulses all 4+, no pedal edema or ulcers

<u>Musculoskeletal</u>: No deformities, normal ROM

<u>Neurologic</u>: CN II–XII grossly normal with exception of left V2 and V3 (describe the deficit), motor and sensory function otherwise intact, DTR 2$^+$ bilat and equal, mental status apparently normal

Radiographs: Left mandibular ramus fracture, naso-ethmoidal and orbital fracture extending through left infraorbital foramen and medial aspect of left infraorbital rim

Assessment: This patient is an otherwise healthy 27 yo male who was allegedly assaulted this morning. Although he reports a brief episode of unconsciousness, he is alert and oriented ×3. He is presently wearing a cervical collar and is on a spine board. Left mandibular ramus and naso-ethmoidal and orbital fracture. Facial contusions and abrasions

Plan: Admit to oral and maxillofacial surgery, Dr V. H. Kasanjian. IV antibiotics, to OR [theatre] for ORIF of facial fractures

W. Guy, DMD

PHYSICIAN'S ORDERS [NOTES]

		Patient's identification stamp
Date	**Time**	**Physician's orders**
2 Oct 03	05:00	Admit to oral and maxillofacial surgery – Dr Kasanjian
		<u>Diagnosis</u>: Left mandibular ramus fracture, naso-ethmoidal and orbital fractures
		<u>Condition</u>: Good
		<u>Allergies</u>: PCN
		<u>Vitals</u>: q 4 h
		<u>Activity</u>: Bed rest
		<u>Diet</u>: NPO. Void on call to OR [theatre]
		<u>Meds</u>: Ancef 1g (cefuroxime 750 mg) IV stat, then 500 mg q 6 h, Demerol (pethidine) 50 mg/ Phenergan 25 mg IM q 4 hrs PRN pain IV at 150 mL/h
		Please page resident at 2568 when patient called to OR [theatre] or if any problems or questions
		W. Guy, DMD

CONSULTATION

Date: 2 October 2003

Time: 05:15

To: Neurosurgery

From: Oral and maxillofacial surgery

Request: 27 yo male with left mandibular ramus and naso-ethmoidal and orbital fractures. Allegedly assaulted early this morning. Please evaluate C-spine preoperatively for ORIF of facial fractures.

W. Guy, DMD

PREOPERATIVE NOTE

Date: 2 October 2003

Time: 05:00

Preoperative diagnosis: Left mandibular ramus and naso-ethmoidal and orbital fractures

Operation planned: ORIF facial fractures

Anesthesia: General/Nasal ET tube

Surgeons: V H Kazanjian DMD, MD

Resident: W Guy, DMD

ECG: NSR

CXR: NAD

Allergies: Penicillin

UA: Yellow/clear, sp gr 1.014, pH 6.9, micro: neg

Labs:

135	93	11	Hgb 13.5	PT 11.5	INR 1.0
5.0	29	0.9	Hct 40.5	PTT 22	

Consent: Signed

Neurosurgery consult: Pt seen, C-spine cleared

W. Guy, DMD

OPERATIVE NOTE

Patient's identification stamp

Date: 2 October 2003

Time: 11:00

Preoperative diagnosis: Left mandibular ramus, and naso-ethmoidal and orbital fractures

Postoperative diagnosis: Same

Surgeons: V H Kazanjian DMD, MD and W Guy, DMD

Anesthesia: General/nasal ET tube

EBL: 100 cc

Fluids: 1500 cc IV crystalloids

Specimens: None

Cultures: None

Complications: None

W. Guy, DMD

POSTOPERATIVE NOTE

Patient's identification stamp

Date: 2 October 2003

Time: 17:00

Patient without complaint, mild/mod discomfort from edema, AVSS, B.P. 125/85, P 80, R 18

Oral intake: 200 cc Urine output: 700 cc

Lungs: clear. Out of bed to bathroom, occlusion stable, dressings intact, surgical wounds closed primarily

Diagnosis: Patient following normal post-op course
Plan: Encourage PO intake and ambulation, IV TKO (to keep open), anticipate discharge in morning

W. Guy, DMD

DISCHARGE NOTE

Patient's identification stamp

Date: 3 October 2003

Time: 08:00

Patient without complaint. Mild discomfort controlled with Ibuprophen (Ibuprofen). Vitals stable. Oral intake: 2000 cc; Urine output: 1700 cc

<u>Lungs</u>: clear, occlusion stable, dressings intact, surgical wounds closed primarily

<u>Diagnosis</u>: Good post-op course, ready for discharge

<u>Plan</u>: Discharge to home and return to OMFS clinic in 1 week for F/U

W. Guy, DMD

POSTOPERATIVE NOTES AND ORDERS (REQUESTS)

Patient's identification stamp

Date: 2 October 2003

Time: 11:00

<u>Operation</u>: ORIF left mandibular ramus, and naso-ethmoidal and orbital fracture

<u>Condition</u>: Stable. Vitals q 15 min until stable, then q 1 hr, then q 4 hrs

<u>Allergies</u>: Penicillin

<u>Activity</u>: Out of bed with assistance this PM

<u>Diet</u>: Soft

IV D5$^1/_2$ NS at 125 cc/hr

Ancef 500 mg (cefuroxime 750 mg) IV q 6 h

Morphine sulfate 2 mg IV × 4 max in PARR only

Demerol (pethidine) 50 mg/Phenergan 25 mg IM q 4 h PRN moderate to severe pain

Ibuprophen (Ibuprofen) 600 mg PO q 6 h PRN mild to moderate pain

Compazine 10 mg (Stemetil 125 mg) IM q 4 h PRN nausea or vomiting

Ephedrine nasal spray 2 squirts each nostril PRN congestion

Humidified 40% oxygen via face mask

Record intake and output

Elevate HOB 30 degrees

Light oral suction at bedside

Coughing and deep breathing q 2 hrs while awake

Please page (pager #) for any questions or if:

BP systolic	> 180 or < 100 mmHg
BP diastolic	> 100 or < 50 mmHg
Pulse	> 100 or < 50
Temp	> 101.5°F (38.5°C)

Severe nausea or vomiting

No void by 8 h post-op

W. Guy, DMD

FURTHER POSTOPERATIVE NOTE

Patient's identification stamp

Date: 2 October 2003

Time: 17:00

1. IV to TKO
2. Discontinue oxygen
3. Encourage PO intake and ambulation

W. Guy, DMD

DISCHARGE INSTRUCTIONS

Patient's identification stamp

Date: 3 October 2003

Time: 08:00

1. Discharge to home
2. Keflex (cefalexin) 500 mg PO QID × 7 days
3. Ibuprophen (Ibuprofen) 600 mg PO q 4-6 hrs PRN pain
4. Return to OMFS clinic 10 October 2003 at 0900

W. Guy, DMD

OPERATIVE NOTE (DICTATED)

Name: Darryl Johnson

Unit Number: 07 3359 113

Hospital location:

Date of operation: 2 October 2003

Date: 2 October 2003

Surgeons: V H Kazanjian and W Guy

Preoperative diagnosis: Left mandibular ramus fracture and left naso-orbito-ethmoid fracture

Postoperative diagnosis: Same

Operation: ORIF left mandibular ramus fracture ORIF left naso-orbito-ethmoid fracture

Anesthesia: General via nasal endotracheal tube

Specimens: None

Blood loss: 100 cc

Fluid replacement: 1500 cc

Indications and consent: This 27 yo male sustained facial injuries including a L mandibular ramus fracture, a naso-ethmoidal and orbital fractures, as well as contusions and lacerations. He has a malocclusion consisting of a right posterior open bite and left posterior occlusal prematurity. The patient also has pain over the left mandibular ramus and midface. He is unable to respire nasally due to septal deviation. The nature of the injuries and prognosis with and without treatment have been explained to the patient. He has given his consent for necessary treatment.

Procedure: The patient was taken to OR [theatre] #7 and placed on the operating table in a supine position. An IV was already in place in the right forearm. General anesthesia was induced and the patient was nasally intubated. The patient was then positioned, prepped and draped in the usual fashion. A moistened throat pack was placed in the oropharynx. Maxillomandibular fixation, using 25-gauge stainless steel wire, was applied to establish proper occlusion. A skin marker was used to draw a line between the inferior aspect of the left tragus and the antegonial notch. A curvilinear line was drawn just beneath the middle third of this line. 6 cc 0.5% lidocaine with 1:200 000 epinephrine was infiltrated subcutaneously in this region. A 15 blade was used to incise through skin and subcutaneous tissue. Bleeding along the skin edges was coagulated using electrocautery. Lack of paralysis was confirmed by the anesthesiologist. Dissection was carried down to the lateral aspect of the mandibular ramus in a layered fashion. A nerve stimulator was used to test each layer prior to incising. The buccal and marginal mandibular branches of the facial nerve were located and protected with retractors. The fracture was identified, reduced and rigidly fixed with a double-Y Wurzburg miniplate and six 2.0 mm diameter, 7 mm length screws. IMF was released and occlusion was verified. The wound was irrigated and muscle was closed with 3-0 chromic gut in an interrupted fashion. Subcutaneous interrupted 4-0 chromic gut sutures were then placed, followed by skin closure with continuous 5-0 nylon sutures. 6 cc 2% lidocaine with 1:100 000 [1:80 000] epinephrine was used to infiltrate submucosally over the nasal septum. The deviated nasal septum was then straightened with an Ashe forceps and scalpel handle. A further 6 cc 2% lidocaine with 1:100 000 [1:80 000] epinephrine was then infiltrated in the maxillary vestibule. An incision was made at the depth of the left maxillary vestibule with a 15 blade. A periosteal elevator was used to expose the left anterior maxillary wall and the fracture site. The fractured segment involving the anterior maxilla and nasal bone was reduced and stabilized using a 6 hole straight Luhr microplate with six 4 mm screws. The wound was irrigated with normal saline and closed using 3-0 chromic gut suture to reappose the zygomaticus levator muscles. The mucosa was closed with 4-0 chromic gut suture in running horizontal mattress fashion. Arch bars were removed and the oral cavity was irrigated and suctioned. The throat pack was removed and the oro- and nasopharynx were suctioned. The left facial wound was dressed with bacitracin and Telfa. The nose was dressed externally with Steri-strips and an Aquaplast splint. The patient was allowed to wake and was extubated. He was then taken to the recovery room in stable condition.

W. Guy, DMD

DISCHARGE SUMMARY

Patient: Darryl Johnson

Date of admission: 2 October 2003

Date of discharge: 3 October 2003

Physician: V H Kasanjian DMD MD

History of present illness: This 27 yo male came to hospital after allegedly being assaulted at a local night club. He sustained a left mandibular ramus and naso-ethmoidal and orbital fractures, and facial contusions and abrasions.

Past medical history: The patient is otherwise in good health. His previous history is significant for other traumatic wounds.

Physical exam: Well-developed, well-nourished 27 yo male in mild/moderate distress secondary to facial injury. The patient presented with cervical collar in place but C-spine injury was ruled out shortly after arrival. Significant L facial edema was present with tenderness to palpation over the L mandibular ramus. Contusions and abrasions were present over the R face. Multiple pre-existing edentulous areas were present and there was a R posterior open bite with occlusal prematurity of the L posterior teeth. There was tenderness to palpation over the nasal bridge and gross mobility of the nasal bones. The intranasal exam exhibited hemorrhage and septal deviation. Subconjunctival ecchymosis was present and mild anisoiconia (apparently pre-existing) was present. There was a palpable step at the L infraorbital rim. The patient exhibited sensory deficit of the V2 and V3 distributions. All other findings were within normal limits with the exception of old traumatic scars on the abdomen and extremities. All laboratory data were within normal limits. Radiographic evaluation was consistent with the clinical diagnosis.

Hospital course: The patient was admitted through the ER [A&E], placed on IV antibiotics and scheduled for surgery. The patient was taken to the OR [theatre] where ORIF of facial fractures was performed. The patient tolerated the procedure well, was extubated in the OR [theatre] and taken to the recovery room in stable condition. The remainder of the patient's postoperative course was uneventful and he was deemed ready for discharge the following morning. Upon discharge the patient was consuming PO fluid and solids, ambulating and urinating without difficulty.

Discharge diagnosis: Facial fractures

Operations and procedures:
ORIF left mandibular ramus fracture
ORIF left naso-ethmoidal and orbital fractures

Disability: Patient will be able to return to normal activities over the next 2 weeks

Discharge medications:

Cefalexin 500 mg PO QID × 7 days

Ibuprophen (ibuprofen) 600 mg q 6 hrs PRN pain

Follow-up care: Return to OMFS clinic on 10 October 2003 at 11:40

W. Guy, DMD

Antifungal treatment regimes

Topical agents

- Clotrimazole troches (10 mg 5×/day for 10 days).
- Miconazole cream (dab on corners of mouth QID).
- Miconazole and 1% hydrocortisone cream (Daktacort) (dab on corners of mouth QID).
- Nystatin–triamcinolone acetonide (Mycolog II) ointment (dab on corners of mouth QID).
- Nystatin ointment (thin layer inner of denture tid).
- Chlorhexidine rinse (10 cc swish and spit bid).

Note: Nystatin liquid is cariogenic.

Systemic agents

- Diflucan (fluconazole) (200 mg leading dose followed by 100 mg/day for 1 week).

Steroidal treatment regimes

Topical steroid agents

Mildly-potent corticosteroids
- Triamcinolone.
- 0.05% betamethasone.

Potent corticosteroids (limit use to 2 weeks)
- 0.05% fluocinonide gel (Lidex).
- 0.05% clobetasol gel (Temovate).
- Dexamethasone (Decadron) elixir (0.5 mg/5 cc 10 cc rinse and spit, QID for 2 weeks).

Systemic steroids (in collaboration with patient's physician)

- Prednisone (10 mg tablets, 4 in morning for 5 days, then decrease by one tablet each successive day).

Alternative/corticosteroid-sparing agents

- Azathioprine, thalidomide, pentoxifylline.
- Dapsone (titrate up to 75 mg bid).

Antiviral treatment regimes

- Acyclovir (800 mg QID for 1 week).
- Valacyclovir (500 mg bid for 1 week).

Psychotropics/chronic pain

Tricyclic antidepressants

- Dothiepin (25 to 75 mg daily).
- Amitriptyline (10 or 25 mg tablets: start 1 tablet before bedtime for 1 week, then titrate dose as needed up to 75 mg before bedtime).
- Clonazepam (Klonopin) [Rivotril] (0.25 mg at bedtime for 1 week followed by weekly dose escalation to 0.75 mg/d).
- Venlafaxine (Effexor) (up to 37.5 mg bid).

Appendix 7

The salivary gland

Salivary stimulants

- Pilocarpine (5 mg qid).
- Cevimeline (30 mg tid).

Salivary substitutes

- Carboxymethyl cellulose (0.5% aqueous solution or OTC saliva substitute; use as frequently as needed).

Appendix 8

Topical fluoride concentrates

- Fluoride gel: neutral NaFl 1.1% (Prevident or Gel-Kam 0.4% stannous fluoride) (brush on for 2 min expectorate qd).

Antibiotic treatment regime

- Tetracycline mouthwash (250 mg/15 cc H_2O; swish 1 min and expectorate 3×/day for 4 days).

Emergency kit

Injectable drugs

Epinephrine 1:1000 dilution – preloaded syringe (1 cc/mL) for subcutaneous administration

Antihistamine – diphenhydramine (Benadryl) [chlorpheniramine maleate (Piriton)]10 cc/mL ampules

Hydrocortisone 300 mg ampule [100 mg vials of powder for reconstitution] for IV injection

D50W 50 cc ampule for IV injection, 0.5.g/cc

Epinephrine 1:10 000 dilution for IV injection (0.1 mg/cc)

Lidocaine 2% for IV injection, 100 mg/5 cc, 5 cc vial

Atropine for IV injection, 0.1 mg/cc, 10 cc vial

Diazepam for IV injection, 5 mg/cc, 2 cc vial

Narcan for IV injection, 0.4 mg/cc, 1 cc vial

Morphine for IV injection, 10 mg/cc, 19 cc vial

Other drugs

Oxygen

Albuterol [salbutamol] – metered dose inhaler

Nitroglycerin tablets 0.4 mg [or metered dose (0.4 mg per release) spray] (sublingual tablets must be < 1 year old stock)

Aspirin 160–350 mg

Equipment

Tourniquets

Magill intubation forceps

Syringes l0 cc volume

Wall suction device, suction tubing, Yankauer suction tip

Oxygen nasal cannula or face mask

Nasopharyngeal airway, oropharyngeal airway sizes 7 and 8

Laryngoscope and endotracheal tubes

14-gauge intravenous catheter for needle cricothyroidotomy

Normal saline 0.9%, 1000 cc bags

18- and 20-gauge angiocatheters for IV fluid administration

Bag valve mask

Emergency medications

Medication	Use	Adult dose	Method of action
Atropine	To cause vagal blockade in cases of bradycardia or excess salivation. Avoidance with history of glaucoma and iris–lens adhesions	0.4–0.6 mg IM or IV	Muscarinic acetylcholine blockade
Aromatic ammonia	Syncope	1 cap to nose	Noxious stimuli
Aspirin	Acute myocardial infarction	160–350 mg PO	Platelet inhibition
Diazepam	Status epilepticus, severe recurrent convulsive seizures. Avoid with hypersensitivity	2–5 mg IV	Sedative, muscle relaxant
Diphenhydramine [chlorphenamine maleate]	Dermatologic allergic reaction. Avoid with infants, lactating mothers, those on monoamine oxidase inhibitors or with hypersensitivity	10–20 mg IV/IM for adult. 0.5 mg/kg dose for child	Antihistamine with anticholinergic and sedative effects
Phenytoin*	Control of grand mal status epilepticus. Avoid with hypersensitivity, sinus bradycardia, sinoatrial block, arteriovenous block	50 mg/minute IV in normal saline for maximum 15 mg/kg	Anticonvulsant at the motor cortex
Epinephrine	Anaphylaxis, asthma	0.3 cc of 1:1000 SC adults. 0.01 cc/kg for children	Sympathetic receptor stimulant receptor action
Hydrocortisone	Acute adrenal insufficiency, severe allergic reaction	300 mg IV	Anti-inflammatory adrenal cortical steroid
Albuterol [salbutamol] metaproterenol	Bronchospasm associated with acute and chronic bronchial asthma, or pulmonary emphysema. Avoid with cardiac arrhythmias, tachycardia and with use of epinephrine	Inhalation of metered dose inhaler 2 puffs/dose	Bronchodilation
Morphine	Pain due to myocardial infarction	4–10 mg IM, 2–4 mg IV.	Narcotic analgesic

Medication	Use	Adult dose	Method of action
Naloxone	Complete or partial reversal of opioid depression	2.0 mg IV, IM or SC for adult; 0.01 mg/kg IV, IM, SC for child	Pure narcotic antagonist
Sodium bicarbonate*	Metabolic acidosis	1 mEq/kg IV	Maintenance of pH
Succinylcholine*	To cause skeletal muscle paralysis for intubation	1.5 mEq/kg IV	Short-acting muscle relaxant and depolarizing agent
Nitroglycerin	Prophylaxis treatment and management of angina	1–2 tablets (or metered spray) sublingual or in buccal pouch every 5 min or prophylactically 5–10 min prior to strenuous activity	Relaxes smooth muscle, vasodilation

* These drugs should be used only by clinicians fully trained in their use

Index